Artificial Intelligence

A tool for effective diagnostics

Online at: https://doi.org/10.1088/978-0-7503-5964-1

IOP Series in Artificial Intelligence in the Biomedical Sciences

Series Editor

Ge Wang, Clark and Crossan Endowed Chair Professor,
Rensselaer Polytechnic Institute, Troy New York, USA

About the Series

The *IOP Series in Artificial Intelligence in the Biomedical Sciences* aims to develop a library of key texts and reference works encompassing the broad range of artificial intelligence, machine learning, deep learning and neural networks within all applicable fields of biomedicine. There is now significant focus in using advancements in the field of AI to improve diagnosis, management, and better therapeutic options of various diseases. Some examples and applications incorporated would be AI in cancer diagnosis/prognosis, implementing artificial intelligence, data mining of electronic health records data, ambient intelligence in hospitals, AI in virus detection, AI in infectious diseases, biomarkers and genomics utilizing machine learning and clinical decision support with AR. These are just a few of the many applications that AI and related technologies can bring to the biomedical sciences. The series contains two broad types of approach. Those addressing a particular field of application and reviewing the numerous relevant artificial intelligence methods applicable to the field, and those that focus on a specific AI method which will permit a greater in-depth review of the theory and appropriate technology.

A full list of titles published in this series can be found here:
https://iopscience.iop.org/bookListInfo/iop-series-in-artificial-intelligence-in-the-biomedical-sciences#series.

Artificial Intelligence

A tool for effective diagnostics

Edited by
Smith K Khare
Applied AI and Data Science Unit, The Faculty of Engineering, The Maersk Mc-Kinney Møller Institute, University of Southern Denmark, Odense, Denmark

and

Centre for Clinical Artificial Intelligence, Odense University Hospital, Odense, Denmark

Sachin Taran
Department of Electronics and Communication Engineering, Delhi Technological University (DTU), Delhi, Shahbad Daulatpur, New Delhi 110042, India

Ankush D Jamthikar
Rutgers Robert Wood Johnson Medical School, Rutgers University, Newark, NJ, USA

IOP Publishing, Bristol, UK

ISBN 978-0-7503-5964-1 (ebook)
ISBN 978-0-7503-5962-7 (print)
ISBN 978-0-7503-5965-8 (myPrint)
ISBN 978-0-7503-5963-4 (mobi)

DOI 10.1088/978-0-7503-5964-1

Version: 20241101

IOP ebooks

British Library Cataloguing-in-Publication Data: A catalogue record for this book is available from the British Library.

Published by IOP Publishing, wholly owned by The Institute of Physics, London

IOP Publishing, No.2 The Distillery, Glassfields, Avon Street, Bristol, BS2 0GR, UK

US Office: IOP Publishing, Inc., 190 North Independence Mall West, Suite 601, Philadelphia, PA 19106, USA

Dedicated to my father, Shri. Kashiram Narayanrao Khare, my mother, Mrs Madhuri Khare, my wife Amrita, and my handsome son Adyant.

—Dr Smith K Khare

Dedicated to my mother, Smt. Sushma Diwakar Jamthikar.

—Dr Ankush D Jamthikar

Contents

Preface

Artificial intelligence (AI) has the potential to facilitate the integration of intelligent healthcare systems and human–machine interfaces in a variety of ways. Advancements in AI are changing the landscape of the healthcare system, enabling automated and accurate disease diagnosis and patient tracking, which are improving patient outcomes. AI algorithms are data driven and require a large and diverse type of real-world patient data set. This book attempts to describe the use of AI in various human–machine interface systems and effective diagnostics, focusing on the detection of Alzheimer's disease (AD), focal and non-focal seizures, abnormal heartbeats, leukemia, electrocardiogram rhythms, human attention, and human emotions.

This book is a comprehensive guide that provides the medical research community with all the information it needs to analyze and study physiological and physical signals and blood smear images. Physiological signal analysis includes the analysis of electronic healthcare records (EHRs), electrocardiograms (ECGs), and electroencephalograms (EEGs), while physical signal analysis includes the analysis of human speech. To explore the effective analysis of complex physiological variables, this book describes the analysis of time-series data in the time, frequency, time–frequency, and nonlinear domains. It presents methods for exploring such complex signals that use optimal signal processing techniques and adaptive AI techniques which can be applied in different use cases.

Chapter 1 introduces the techniques used for effective diagnostics and the human–machine interface of AI. It covers the role of explainable AI, uncertainty quantification, and the privacy of AI models in healthcare applications.

Chapter 2 discusses recent advancements in emerging technology in healthcare management systems (HMSs). It examines recent research and thus talks about the use of new technologies in healthcare, along with important enabling aspects and significant applications. This chapter emphasizes the greatest challenges that blockchain technology (BT), AI, and the Internet of Things (IoT) typically face and discusses the most pressing difficulties that need to be addressed so that these new technologies can be better used in HMSs.

Chapter 3 covers the integration of EHRs and IoT devices in healthcare. It highlights proactive emerging trends aimed at ensuring that patients continue to receive high-quality care in an increasingly digital age.

Chapter 4 discusses how EEG signals can be used for the detection of attention deficit hyperactivity disorder (ADHD) using machine learning (ML) and/or deep learning techniques, as well as state-of-the-art approaches. It provides a review of EEG signals used for the detection of ADHD.

Chapter 5 provides a comparative analysis of different classification algorithms used to achieve practical application accuracy. It also highlights the importance of using artifact removal techniques to maintain the integrity of EEG data for reliable analysis.

Chapter 6 explores the use of a simpler wavelet filter bank to decompose EEG signals. This approach uses orthogonal filters with rational coefficients to reduce the complexity of AD detection. The model uses two open-source AD data sets and different classifiers; its highest performances are an AD detection accuracy of 97.60% for two-class classification and an accuracy of 96.95% for three-class classification.

Chapter 7 presents a novel automated system called EEG-focal that classifies EEGs into focal and non-focal groups using an empirical wavelet transform (EWT). The results show that the EEG-focal system achieves a classification accuracy of 93%, making it a robust and reliable tool for physicians in operating rooms.

Chapter 8 uncovers the potential for the linear and nonlinear features of EEG signal rhythms to be used in the development of an efficient automatic computer-based system called EEG-seizure, which is used to recognize epileptic attacks. The system achieves 100% accuracy using cascade forward neural networks combined with the best feature selection (FS) technique.

Chapter 9 offers an overview of various stages of ECG analysis, beginning with an understanding of the conduction system and the interpretation and processing of ECG data. The chapter then explores the concept of time–frequency representation (TFR) for ECG analysis. In addition, it presents a preliminary analysis method that employs the TFR to convert ECG signals into images, which are then used to predict cardiac rhythm abnormalities, such as atrial fibrillation.

Chapter 10 presents a real-time implementation of ECG beat identification using the R-peaks of the ECG signal, employing both fractional-order differential (FOD) and Hilbert transformation (HT) techniques. The model has obtained an accuracy and a sensitivity of 97.24% and 70.47%, respectively, using an artificial neural network (ANN) classifier.

Chapter 11 explores the integration of advanced ML techniques into the detection and classification of leukemia using blood smear images. It highlights the limitations of traditional diagnostic methods in accurately distinguishing between different leukemia subtypes, emphasizing the need for more sophisticated computational approaches.

Chapter 12 presents emotion recognition using EEGs and galvanic skin response (GSR). These biomarkers are important for affective computing and human–machine interfacing. EEG and GSR signals contain useful information for emotion classification.

Chapter 13 explores how the human voice is an essential tool for conveying emotions and proposes a novel speech emotion recognition (SER) framework which is based on the combination of EWT and a cubic support vector machine (CSVM). The system is designed for multiclass SER and uses a combination of the auditory spectrogram, cepstral coefficients, spectral descriptors, periodicity, and harmonicity for feature extraction.

Chapter 14 demonstrates the applicability of EEG signals for imagined speech applications using Hjorth parameters and entropy features. It discusses the importance of studying the inherent characteristics of imagined speech signals to enhance the performance of imagined speech recognition systems and, potentially, advance toward ‘mind reading’ capabilities in the future.

Chapter 15 explores brain–computer interface (BCI) technology that can assist impaired persons in communicating with the outside world. The effective categorization of various motor imagery activities can improve the dependability of BCI systems. This chapter describes the classification of focused and drowsy states by a suitable ML algorithm using singular spectrum-analysis-based features.

Acknowledgments

Dr Smith expresses his heartfelt debt to his father, mother, wife Amrita, adorable son Adyant, and his in-laws for their unending inspiration throughout the completion of this novel book titled 'Artificial Intelligence: A Tool for Effective Diagnostics and Human–Machine Interface'. Dr Smith sincerely thanks the unit leader and colleagues at the Applied Artificial Intelligence and Data Science Unit, University of Southern Denmark, Denmark. He also expresses his gratitude to the director and head of department, The Maersk Mc-Kinney Møller Institute, University of Southern Denmark, Denmark. Dr Smith is deeply grateful to his mentor and advisers for their unwavering support, insightful guidance, and constant encouragement throughout his research journey.

Dr Taran expresses his heartfelt indebtedness to his parents, wife, and lovely daughters Vedika and Manogyaa for their unending inspiration throughout the completion of this novel book titled 'Artificial Intelligence: A Tool for Effective Diagnostics and Human–Machine Interface'. Dr Taran thanks his university vice-chancellor, head of department, and colleagues at the Department of Electronics and Communication Engineering (ECE) at Delhi Technological University (DTU).

Dr Ankush expresses his heartfelt gratitude to his mother, who has been a constant source of support and motivation throughout his journey toward success. He is deeply thankful for her enduring love and unwavering belief in him. Additionally, he wishes to extend his sincere thanks to his mentors and advisers, who have consistently guided and mentored him throughout his research career. Their invaluable advice and direction have been pivotal in shaping his professional path. Dr Ankush would also like to express his profound appreciation to all the authors who have contributed to this book. Their research work and support have significantly enriched the comprehension of knowledge within the research community.

We want to thank all our friends, well-wishers, and all those who keep us motivated to do more and more, better and better. We sincerely thank all the contributors for their writing about the relevant theoretical background and real-time applications described in Artificial Intelligence: A Tool for Effective Diagnostics and Human–Machine Interface. We are also deeply grateful to many whose names are not mentioned here. We appreciate and wish to acknowledge their help during this work.

We humbly thank T Michael Slaughter, Senior Commissioning Manager, and all the editorial staff (IPEM–IOP) of IOP Publishing for their great support, necessary help, appreciation, and quick responses. We also thank IOP Publishing for allowing us to contribute to a relevant topic with a reputed publisher. We are grateful to all those with whom we have enjoyed working during this project.

This book is dedicated to all researchers and innovators pursuing their research journey for continuous advancement. Finally, we would also like to thank God for showering us with his blessings and strength to perform this type of novel and quality work.

Editor biographies

Smith K Khare

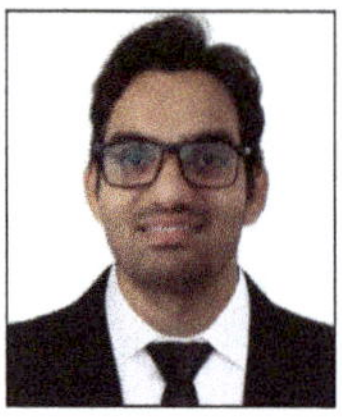

Dr Smith K Khare is an assistant professor at the Faculty of Engineering, The Maersk Mc-Kinney Møller Institute, University of Southern Denmark, Denmark. He also works as a researcher in the Center for Clinical Artificial Intelligence (CAI-X) at Odense University Hospital, Denmark. He works together with clinical professionals to aid clinicians in automated decision-making using advanced engineering and AI techniques. Prior to this, he was a postdoctoral fellow at the Department of Electrical and Computer Engineering at Aarhus University. Smith Khare is an engineer and holds a PhD in electronics and communications from the Indian Institute of Information Technology, Design and Manufacturing, Jabalpur, India.

He has published more than 50 articles in peer-reviewed journals, book chapters, and international conferences. He also serves as a guest editor and academic editor for reputed journals. He is a technical reviewer for leading international journals published by the IEEE, Elsevier, Springer, and Wiley. Smith was among the top 2% most-cited scientists within his subfield of engineering and technology twice in 2023 and 2024, according to Elsevier. He has also received various national and international awards. According to Google Scholar, his publications have around 1740 citations, his h index is 25, and his i-10 index is 33 (as of May 2024). His primary research interests include AI, ML algorithms, biomedical signal processing, and deep learning.

Sachin Taran

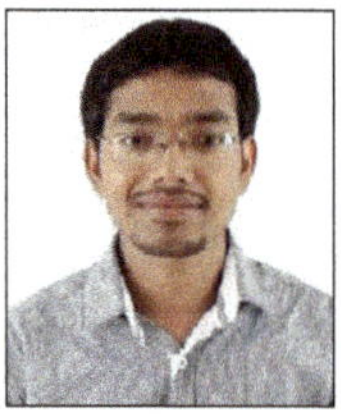

Dr Sachin Taran is a motivated teaching professional with approximately 12 years of teaching and research experience in electronics and communication engineering. Dr Taran is currently working as an assistant professor at the Department of Electronics and Communication Engineering, Delhi Technological University (DTU), Delhi. He received a PhD degree from the Indian Institute of Information Technology, Design and Manufacturing, Jabalpur, India, and a postdoctoral degree from Nanyang Technological University (NTU), Singapore. Dr Taran served as an assistant professor at the Department of Electronics and Communication, Shangvi Innovative Academy, Indore, India, from 2009 to 2010. He served as an assistant professor at the Department of Electronics and Communication at Medicaps University, Indore, India, from 2010 to 2015. His research interests include AI, signal processing, time–frequency analysis, and ML. He received the Commendable Research Award from Delhi Technological University (DTU), Delhi, India, in 2020, 2021, 2022, and 2023. He has authored or co-authored more than 50 research articles in various reputed international publishers' journals, such as those of the IEEE, Elsevier, Springer, the Internet Engineering Taskforce (IET), and the IOP. His work has been cited 1468 times in the last five years; his h index is 20, and his i-10 index is 28. Dr Taran has also served as a technical reviewer for leading international journals published by the IEEE, Elsevier, Springer, the IET, etc.

Ankush D Jamthikar

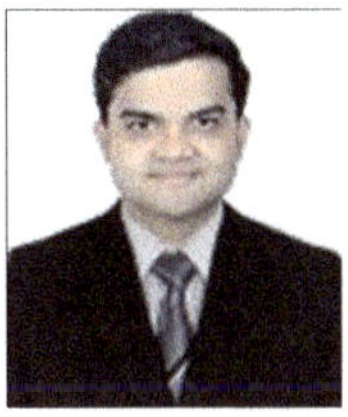

Dr Ankush D Jamthikar is an accomplished postdoctoral fellow at the Division of Cardiovascular Disease and Hypertension, Rutgers Robert Wood Johnson Medical School, Rutgers University, NJ, USA. He earned his BTech in Electronics and Communications Engineering from the Government College of Engineering, Amravati, India, followed by MTech and PhD degrees from Visvesvaraya National Institute of Technology, Nagpur, India, focusing on cardiovascular disease risk assessment. A prolific contributor to the field, Dr Jamthikar has authored approximately 50+ international journal articles, conference papers, and book chapters, predominantly in cardiovascular/stroke risk stratification and AI; he boasts an h index of 22 and an i index of 32. His research primarily centers on leveraging AI in medical imaging, particularly ultrasound, to advance stroke and cardiovascular risk stratification methodologies. Dr Ankush D Jamthikar is not only a distinguished researcher but also contributes significantly to the academic community as an editorial board member of the journal Artificial Intelligence in Health. He holds roles as a guest editor or academic editor for several scholarly journals. His expertise is further recognized through his service as a technical reviewer for prominent international journals published by the IEEE, Elsevier, Springer, and Wiley, ensuring rigorous scholarly standards across the fields of medical imaging and AI.

List of contributors

Hesam Akbari
Department of Information Science, University of North Texas, Texas, USA

Sunil Athawale
Department of Electronics and Communication Engineering, Motilal Nehru National Institute of Technology, Allahabad, India

Ankit Baisoya
Department of Electronics and Communication Engineering, Delhi Technological University (DTU), New Delhi, India

Ayan Banerjee
Institute of Technical Education and Research (ITER), Siksha 'O' Anusandhan (SOA), Bhubaneswar, Odisha, India

Amit Kumar Dwivedi
Department of Electronics and Communication Engineering, Delhi Technological University (DTU), New Delhi, India

Pranjali Gajbhiye
Woxsen University, Hyderabad, Telangana, India

Pradnya Ghare
Department of Electronics and Communication Engineering, Visvesvaraya National Instiute of Technology, Nagpur, MH, India

Asmar Hafeez
Department of Electronics and Communication Engineering, Delhi Technological University (DTU), New Delhi, India

Mehrab Hosain
Department of Electronics and Communication Engineering, Delhi Technological University (DTU), New Delhi, India

Ankush D Jamthikar
Rutgers Robert Wood Johnson Medical School, Rutgers University, NJ, USA

Shyam Joshi
Woxsen University, Hyderabad, Telangana, India

Pramod H Kachare
Ramrao Adik Institute of Technology, DY Patil University, Nerul, Mumbai, India

Ashwin Kamble
Acuradyne Medical Systems, SINE, IIT Bombay, Mumbai, India

Vikram Singh Kardam
Department of Electronics and Communication Engineering, Delhi Technological University (DTU), New Delhi, India

Smith K Khare
The Faculty of Engineering, The Maersk Mc-Kinney Møller Institute, University of Southern Denmark, Denmark

Joseph Nixon Kiro
Department of Computer Applications, National Institute of Technology (NIT), Raipur, Chhattisgarh, India

Wael Korani
Department of Information Science, University of North Texas, Texas, USA

Madhu Kumari
Department of Electronics and Computer Engineering, National Institute of Advanced Manufacturing Technology (NIAMT), Ranchi, India

Shalini Mahato
Department of Electronics and Computer Engineering, National Institute of Advanced Manufacturing Technology (NIAMT), Ranchi, India

Sanjay L Nalbalwar
Dr Babasaheb Ambedkar Technological University, Lonere, Maharashtra, India

Nikhil
Department of Electronics and Communication Engineering, Delhi Technological University (DTU), New Delhi, India

Jeebananda Panda
Department of Electronics and Communication Engineering, Delhi Technological University (DTU), New Delhi, India

Anukul Pandey
Department of Electronics and Communication Engineering, Delhi Technological University (DTU), New Delhi, India

Govind Prasad
Department of Electrical and Electronics Engineering, Birla Institute of Technology & Science (BITS) Pilani, Pilani Campus, Rajasthan, India

Digambar V Puri
Ramrao Adik Institute of Technology, DY Patil University, Nerul, Mumbai, India; Dr Babasaheb Ambedkar Technological University, Lonere, India

Khushboo Rani
ITER, Siksha 'O' Anusandhan (SOA), Bhubaneswar, Odisha, India

Ravi
Department of Electronics and Communication Engineering, Delhi Technological University (DTU), New Delhi, India

Bhawna Sachdeva
Department of Electronics and Communication Engineering, Delhi Technological University (DTU), New Delhi, India

Sandeep Saharan
Woxsen University, Hyderabad, Telangana, India

Sandeep B Sangle
Ramrao Adik Institute of Technology, DY Patil University, Nerul, Mumbai, India

Anirvina Sharma
Nazareth Hospital, Prayagraj, Uttar Pradesh, India

Sandeep Kumar Singh
Department of Electronics and Communication Engineering, Motilal Nehru National Institute of Technology, Allahabad, India

Vansh Singh
Department of Electronics and Communication Engineering, Delhi Technological University (DTU), New Delhi, India

Vineet Singh
Woxsen University, Hyderabad, Telangana, India

Bam Bahadur Sinha
Department of Computer Science and Engineering, National Institute of Technology (NIT), Sikkim, India

Vikas Kumar Sinha
Department of Electronics and Communication Engineering, National Institute of Technology Rourkela, India

Annapureddy Srija Reddy
Department of Electronics and Communication Engineering, Motilal Nehru National Institute of Technology, Allahabad, India

Sachin Taran
Department of Electronics and Communication Engineering, Delhi Technological University (DTU), New Delhi, India

Tanishqa Tyagi
Department of Electronics and Communication Engineering, Delhi Technological University (DTU), New Delhi, India

Ujjwal Kumar Upadhyay
Department of Electronics and Communication Engineering, Delhi Technological University (DTU), New Delhi, India

Contributor biographies

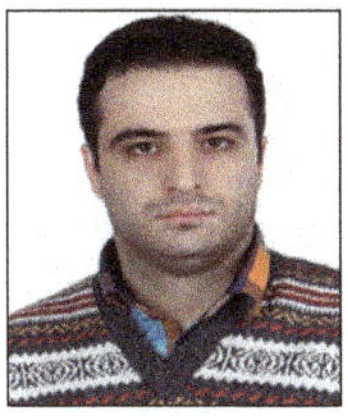

Hesam Akbari is a PhD candidate in data science at the Department of Information Science, University of North Texas, Texas, USA. As a neuroscientist, he conducts research in biomedical signal and image processing and ML. He has had several scientific articles published by high-quality journals and conferences. In his PhD work, he focuses on the detection of mental disorders using EEG signals.

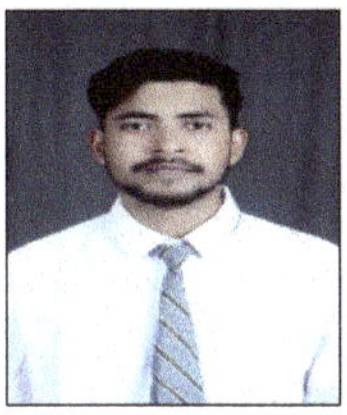

Sunil Athawale completed a bachelor of technology (BTech) degree in electronics and communication engineering at the Motilal Nehru National Institute of Technology, Allahabad, India, in 2024. He has a strong background in web development, having worked on projects such as Zyaka and GoFood. He has a keen interest in programming and excels at solving problems related to data structures. His active areas of research are data science, data analysis, ML, and AI.

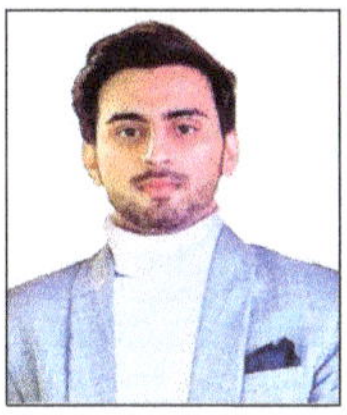

Ankit Baisoya is currently working as a software development engineer. He received his bachelor of technology degree in electronics and communication engineering from Delhi Technological University (DTU), New Delhi, India, in 2022.

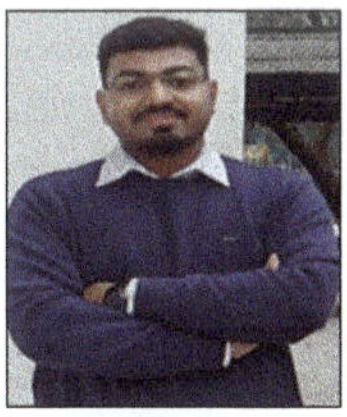

Mr Ayan Banerjee is pursuing an MTech degree in computer science engineering at ITER, Siksha 'O' Anusandhan (SOA), Bhubaneswar, Odisha, India. He has authored a paper presented at an IEEE international conference. His research interests include the IoT, electronic healthcare, and AI–ML.

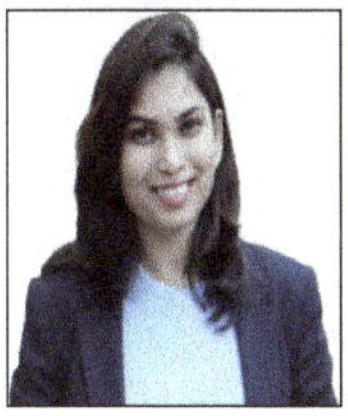

Dr Pranjali Gajbhiye, an expert in the field of neuroscience, has a wealth of experience as an industry expert, educator, researcher, and trainer. Holding positions as both an assistant professor and a neuroscientist specializing in analytics, she boasts a strong educational foundation obtained at the National Institute of Technology and BITS, culminating in her MTech and PhD qualifications. Her research is focused on human–machine interaction, ML, and deep learning techniques. With a focus on biomedical signal processing and neurology, Dr Pranjali possesses a unique ability to decipher human psychology through brain signals. In addition, she spearheads the Human Machine Interaction Lab within the AI Research Centre at Woxsen University, Hyderabad, Telangana, India.

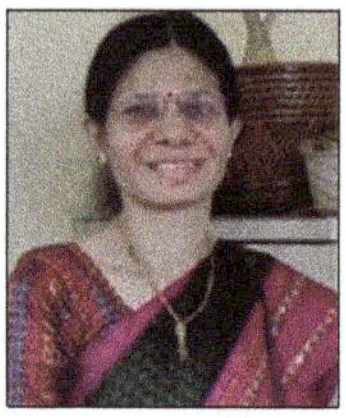

Dr Pradnya H Ghare (Senior Member, IEEE) received MTech and PhD degrees from the Department of Electronics and Communication Engineering, Visvesvaraya National Institute of Technology (VNIT), Nagpur, India, in 2012 and 2017, respectively. She is an assistant professor in the Department of Electronics and Communication Engineering at VNIT, Nagpur, India. She has had several research papers published by reputed journals and conferences. Her research areas include wireless sensor networks (WSNs), body area networks, and the IoT. She has also developed some IoT-based products.

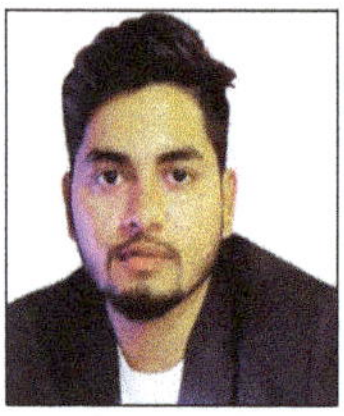

Asmar Hafeez is currently working as an MTech student in the Department of Electronics and Communication Engineering, Delhi Technological University (DTU), New Delhi, India. He received his BTech degree in electronics and communication engineering from the Dr A.P.J. Abdul Kalam Technical University (AKTU), Lucknow, Uttar Pradesh, India, in 2022.

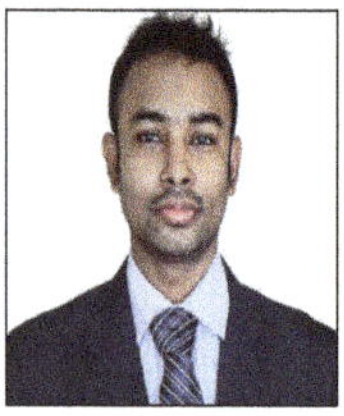

Mehrab Hosain is currently working as an operations and system engineer at Channel i, Impress Telefilm Ltd, Bangladesh. He holds a master of technology degree in signal processing and digital design awarded by Delhi Technological University (DTU), New Delhi, India, in 2023; a master of engineering degree in computer science and engineering awarded by the University of Information Technology and Sciences (UITS), Dhaka, Bangladesh, in 2022; and a bachelor of science degree in electrical and electronic engineering awarded by Bangladesh University of Business and Technology (BUBT), Dhaka, Bangladesh, in 2016. His research interests include digital security, ML, signal processing, forensic science, and combating deepfake technology. In addition, he is an adjunct faculty member at Tagore University of Creative Arts (TUCA), Dhaka, Bangladesh.

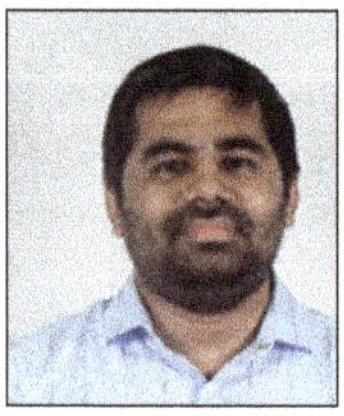

Pramod H Kachare received his Bachelor of Engineering (BE) degree in electronics and telecommunication engineering from the Don Bosco Institute of Technology, University of Mumbai, India, in 2012 and his MTech degree in electronics and telecommunication engineering from the Veermata Jijabai Technological Institute Matunga, University of Mumbai, India, in 2015. He joined the Ramrao Adik Institute of Technology, DY Patil University, Nerul, Mumbai, India, in 2015 as an assistant professor in electronics and telecommunication engineering. His research interests are speech and signal processing, ML, and metaheuristic optimization. He has published articles in several peer-reviewed journals and conferences, and serves as a reviewer for various international journals and conferences.

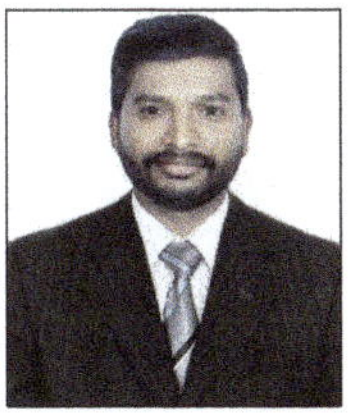

Dr Ashwin Kamble received his BE degree from the MET Institute of Engineering, Bhujbal Knowledge City, Nashik, India, in 2011; his MTech degree from Veermata Jijabai Technological Institute (VJTI), Mumbai, India, in 2015; and his PhD degree from Visvesvaraya National Institute of Technology (VNIT), Nagpur, India, in 2023. He has served as an assistant professor at the Veermata Jijabai Technological Institute Matunga, University of Mumbai, India; the Ramrao Adik Institute of Technology, DY Patil University, Nerul, Mumbai, India; and the Shah & Anchor Kutchhi Engineering College, Mumbai, India. He is currently working as a signal processing engineer at Acuradyne Medical Systems, SINE, IIT Bombay, Mumbai, India. His research interests include biomedical signal processing, ML, and deep neural networks.

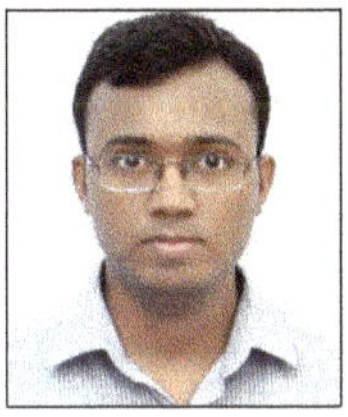

Vikram Singh Kardam is currently working as a research scholar at the Department of Electronics and Communication Engineering, Delhi Technological University (DTU), New Delhi, India. He received his BTech degree in electronics and communication engineering from Chhatrapati Shahuji Maharaj University (CSJM) Kanpur, Uttar Pradesh, India, and his MTech degree from Delhi Technological University (DTU), New Delhi, India.

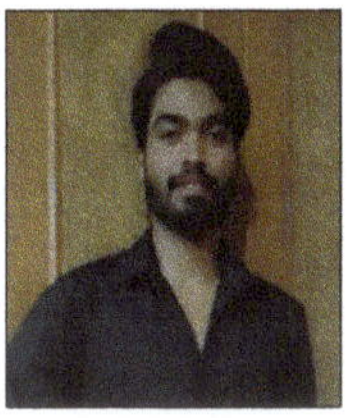

Mr Joseph Nixon Kiro is currently working on a master of computer applications (MCA) degree at the National Institute of Technology (NIT), Raipur, Chhattisgarh, India. His research interests include ML-based disease prediction systems, autonomous driving, computer vision, and image processing techniques. His work has been published ten times in international conference proceedings, journals, and books.

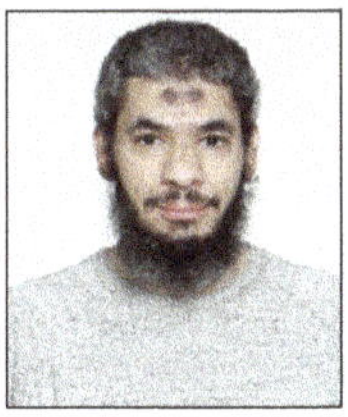

Dr Wael Korani is an assistant professor of data science in the Department of Information Science, University of North Texas, Texas, USA. Since 2003, Dr Korani has been an active researcher in the field of AI, including ML, data mining, and optimization. He has proposed solutions to several AI problems in different research areas, including computer science, engineering, and medical sciences.

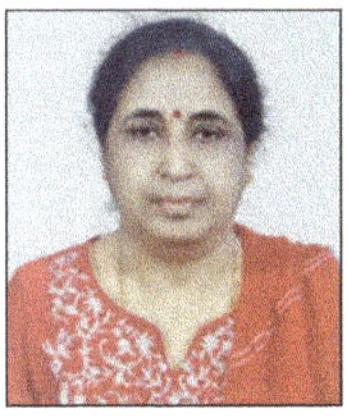

Dr Madhu Kumari holds a BTech (electronics and telecommunication), an MTech (electronics), and a PhD (economic analysis of renewable energy resources). She is currently working as an associate professor and head of the Department of Electronics and Computer Engineering, National Institute of Advanced Manufacturing Technology (NIAMT), Ranchi, India. She has worked in the fields of smart vehicles, smart cities, IoT-based smart agriculture, and water distillation in rural areas for health and hygiene. Since 2000, she has been working in a computer literacy program for the tribal community. Her research areas include digital image processing, semiconductors, chip design for solar photovoltaic cells, smart communication systems, the application of the IoT in power generation, and antenna system design.

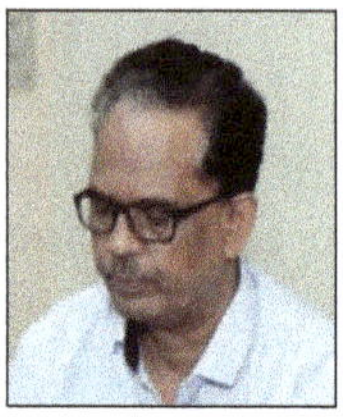

Sanjay L Nalbalwar works as a professor and the head of the Department of Electronics and Telecommunications Engineering at the Dr Babasaheb Ambedkar Technological University, Lonere, Maharashtra, India. He received his BE in 1990 and his Master of Engineering (ME) degree in 1996 from the Shri Guru Gobind Singhji Institute of Engineering and Technology (SGGSIET), Nanded, India, and his PhD from the Indian Institute of Technology Delhi, New Delhi, India, in 2008. He has published more than 270 papers in Scopus- and Science Citation Index (SCI)-indexed peer-reviewed journals and conferences. His areas of interest include signal and image processing. He is a member of the IEEE and the Institution of Electronics and Telecommunication Engineers (IETE). He serves as a reviewer for various journals published by Elsevier and Springer.

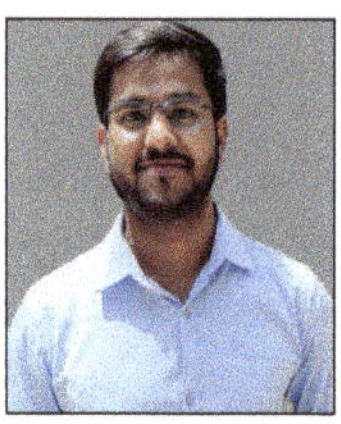

Mr Nikhil is a final-year BTech student in electronics and communication engineering at Delhi Technological University (DTU), New Delhi, India. He has a strong academic background and actively participates in research projects. He has gained practical industry experience through internships in the technical hardware industry during his time at college. Nikhil is dedicated to advancing in his field, particularly in the areas of communication systems and signal processing.

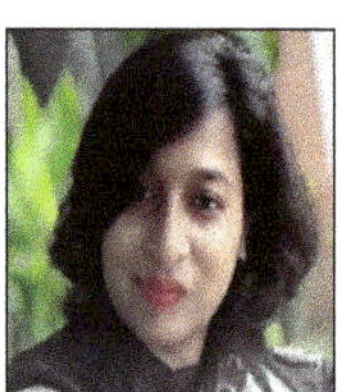

Dr Shalini Mahato is currently working as an assistant professor in the Department of Electronics and Computer Engineering, National Institute of Advanced Manufacturing Technology (NIAMT), Ranchi, India. She has more than seven years of teaching and industrial experience. She completed her PhD in computer science and engineering at the Birla Institute of Technology, Mesra, Jharkhand, India, in 2021. She completed her MTech (computer systems and technology) degree in 2013 and her BTech (computer science and engineering) degree in 2008 at Maulana Abul Kalam Azad University of Technology, West Bengal, India. She has worked as a developer at Tata Consultancy Services (TCS). She has contributed to more than 26 research papers, out of which seven are SCI indexed and ten are Scopus indexed. Her project was selected for the MSME Idea Hackathon 2022 sponsored by the Ministry of Micro, Small, and Medium Enterprises (MSME) Innovative Scheme, Government of India. She was the winner of the MSME Idea Hackathon 2022. She has three Indian patents filed under her name. Her areas of interest include ML, soft computing, and biomedical signal processing.

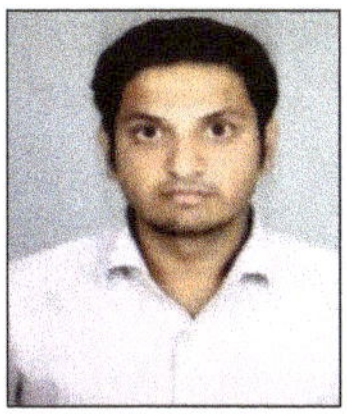

Anukul Pandey was born in Jamui, Bihar, India. He received his MTech and PhD degrees in electronics and communication engineering in 2013 and 2019, respectively. He is currently serving as an assistant professor at Delhi Technological University (DTU), New Delhi, India. His research interests include ML, biomedical signal and image processing, data compression, and steganography.

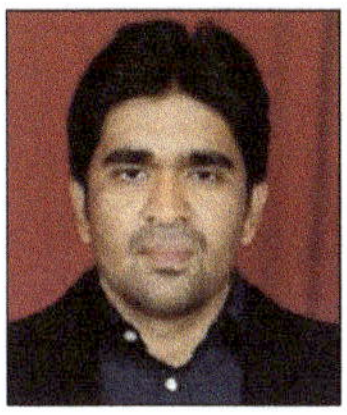

Dr Govind Prasad holds a BTech degree in electronics and communication engineering from MP Christian College of Engineering and Technology, Bhilai, Chattisgarh, India; an MTech degree in very large-scale integration (VLSI) design and embedded systems from the National Institute of Technology Rourkela, India; and a PhD degree from the International Institute of Information Technology, Naya Raipur, Chhattisgarh, India. He joined the Indian Institute of Technology Gandhinagar, Gujarat, India, as a postdoctoral researcher from 2022 to 2023. Since March 2023, he has worked for the Faculty of Engineering at ITER, Siksha 'O' Anusandhan (SOA), Bhubaneswar, Odisha, India, where he is currently an assistant professor. He has authored or co-authored one Indian patent, one book chapter, more than twelve research papers in peer-reviewed international journals, and more than twenty IEEE international conference papers. He has received the Best Citation Award from Wiley and the Best Paper Award from the IEEE. His research interests include radiation-hardened static random-access memory (SRAM) memory design, mixed-signal VLSI design, and the IoT.

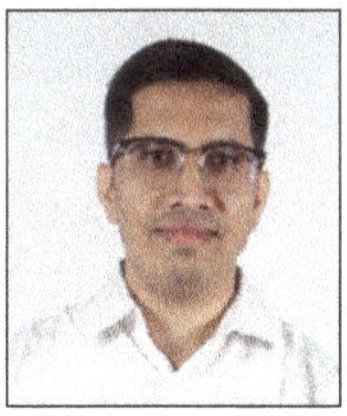

Dr Digambar V Puri completed his BTech and PhD degrees in electronics and telecommunication engineering at the Dr Babasaheb Ambedkar Technological University, Lonere, Maharashtra, India, in 2012 and 2023, respectively, and his MTech at Veermata Jijabai Technological Institute Matunga, University of Mumbai, India, in 2015. He is currently working as an assistant professor in electronics and telecommunication at the Ramrao Adik Institute of Technology, DY Patil University, Nerul, Mumbai, India. His research interests include biomedical signal processing, pattern recognition, ML, data analysis, and image processing. He has published articles in various high-impact-factor peer-reviewed journals and conferences. He has written a book on 'Signals and Systems' for Nirali Publications. He serves as a reviewer for various journals published by Elsevier and Springer.

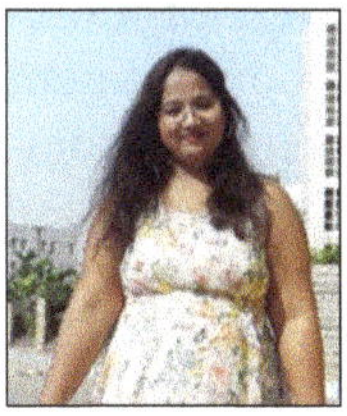

Ms Khushboo Rani is pursuing an MTech degree in computer science engineering at ITER, Siksha 'O' Anusandhan (SOA), Bhubaneswar, Odisha, India. She has authored/co-authored an IEEE international conference. Her research interests include the IoT, electronic health-care, and AI–ML.

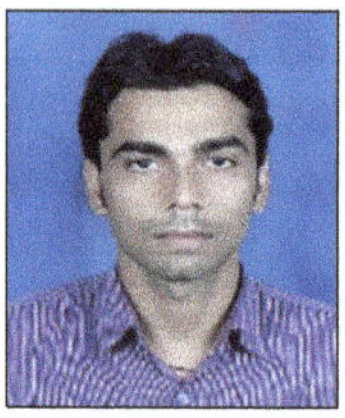

Mr Ravi has worked at the Department of Electronics and Communication Engineering at Galgotias College of Engineering and Technology, Greater Noida, Gautam Budh Nagar, Uttar Pradesh, India, since October 2023. He is a research scholar at Delhi Technological University (DTU), New Delhi, India. He received his BTech degree in electronic and telecommunication engineering from the Visveswaraya Institute of Engineering and Technology, Gautam Budh Nagar, India, in 2009 and his MTech degree in instrumentation and signal processing from the Indian Institute of Technology Roorkee, Roorkee, Uttarakhand, India, in 2015. His research interests include biomedical signal processing, pattern recognition, ML, and deep neural networks.

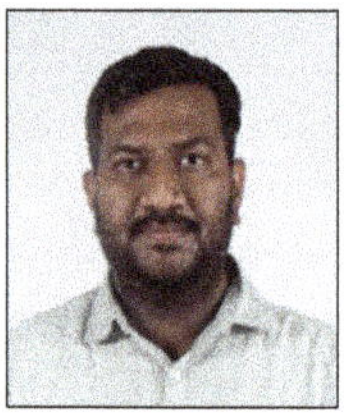

Sandeep B Sangle received his BE degree from the University of Pune, Pune, Maharashtra, India, in 2012 and his ME and PhD degrees from the Ramrao Adik Institute of Technology, DY Patil University, Nerul, Mumbai, India, in 2016 and 2023, respectively. He joined the Department of Electronics and Telecommunication Engineering at the Ramrao Adik Institute of Technology in 2014, where he is currently working as an assistant professor. His research focuses on speech processing, biomedical signal processing, statistical methods, ML, and deep learning. He has published articles in various high-impact, peer-reviewed journals and conferences. He serves as a reviewer for various international conferences.

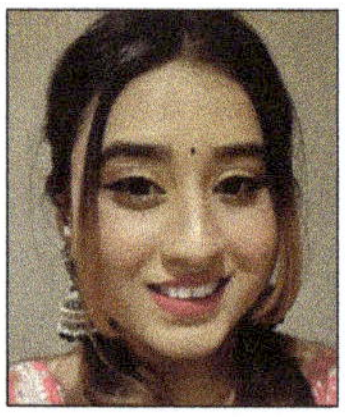

Dr Anirvina Sharma obtained a Bachelor of Medicine and Bachelor of Surgery (MBBS) degree from the D. Y. Patil Education Society, Kolhapur, Maharashtra, India, in 2022. Licensed to practice medicine in Maharashtra, Delhi, and Uttar Pradesh, Dr Anirvina Sharma also holds full registration and a license to practice in the UK. Currently, she works as a resident in the Department of Surgery at Nazareth Hospital, Prayagraj, Uttar Pradesh, India. In this role, she is deeply involved in both clinical practice and day-to-day clinical and non-clinical teaching, as well as in the clinical governance of the hospital. Trained to the European Resuscitation Council standard, she is an Advanced Life Support provider. Having taken additional courses in clinical teaching and clinical governance, Dr Anirvina Sharma is dedicated to continuous professional development. She was awarded third prize for a research proposal presentation at the National 2nd Year MBBS Alliance, showcasing a commitment to medical research and innovation. Her current research interests include cardiovascular health, medical technology and innovation, health disparities, and the management of chronic diseases.

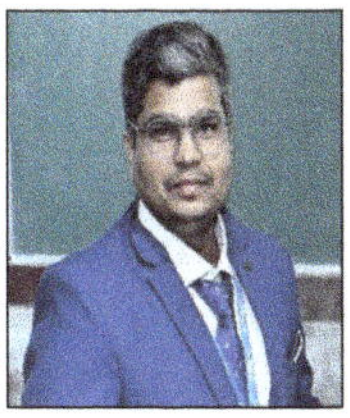

Sandeep Kumar Singh received a BE in Electronics and Communication Engineering from Rajiv Gandhi Proudyogiki Vishwavidyalaya University, Bhopal, Madhya Pradesh, India, in 2010; an MTech degree in microelectronics (ME) and VLSI design from the Motilal Nehru National Institute of Technology, Allahabad, India, in 2013; and a PhD degree in electronics and communication engineering from Visvesvaraya National Institute of Technology (VNIT), Nagpur, India, in 2020. He works for the Department of Electronics and Communication Engineering, Motilal Nehru National Institute of Technology, Allahabad, India, as an assistant professor. Before this, he held the position of research associate at the Institute of Communications Engineering, National Sun Yat-sen University (NSYSU), Taiwan, from 2020 to 2023. He leads research in the areas of AI and ML, unmanned aerial vehicles (UAVs), reconfigurable intelligent surfaces (RISs)/intelligent reflecting surfaces (IRSs), finite blocklength codes, next-generation multiple access schemes such as non-orthogonal multiple access (NOMA) and rate splitting multiple access (RSMA), simultaneous wireless information and power transfer (SWIPT), massive multiple-input multiple-output (**MIMO**), full-duplex radio, and orthogonal frequency-division multiplexing (OFDM).

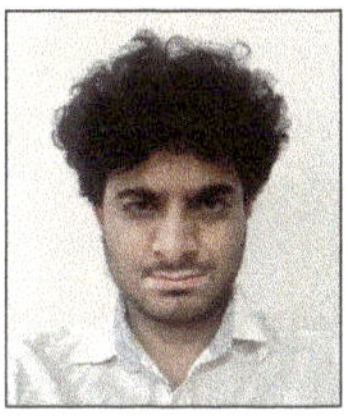

Vansh Singh is currently working as a senior software development engineer. He received his bachelor of technology degree in electronics and communication engineering from Delhi Technological University (DTU), New Delhi, India.

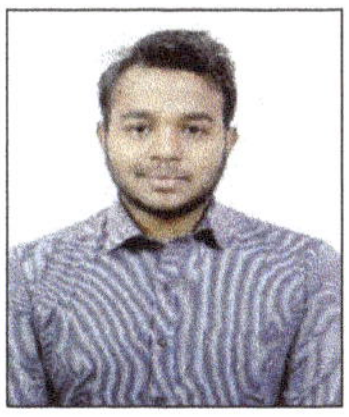

Vineet Singh received a BTech degree in electronics and telecommunications from the International Institute of Information Technology, Pune, India, in 2021 and an ME degree in the field of information and communication technology from the Asian Institute of Technology, Thailand, in 2023. He is currently working as a research associate at the AI Research Centre, Woxsen University, Hyderabad, Telangana, India. His current research mainly focuses on telemedicine and AI in healthcare and sustainable development goals (SDGs). With a passion for research, he is likely to be found delving into cutting-edge technologies, contributing to the academic community, and potentially aiming to address real-world challenges through his work.

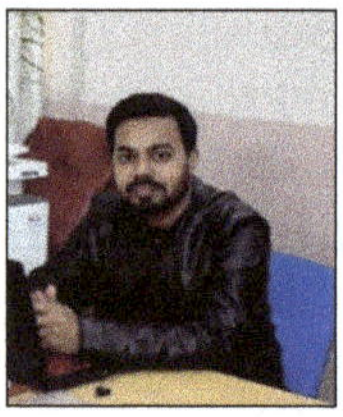

Dr Bam Bahadur Sinha is currently serving as an assistant professor in the Department of Computer Science and Technology at the esteemed National Institute of Technology (NIT), Sikkim, India. Dr Sinha has a wealth of academic experience, having previously held faculty positions at prestigious institutions including the Indian Institute of Information Technology Ranchi, India; the Institute of Information Technology Dharwad, India; and the National Institute of Technology Andhra Pradesh, India. His academic journey boasts remarkable achievements, culminating in the attainment of a PhD in computer science and engineering from the National Institute of Technology Nagaland, India, in 2020, following his earlier success in securing a gold medal during his MTech studies in 2017. Dr Sinha's scholarly contributions are evident through his extensive publication record, comprising 41 research articles, among which 16 are indexed by SCI/SCIE and four by Scopus, alongside 18 international conference presentations and three book chapters.

Notably, Dr Sinha's intellectual property portfolio includes three copyrights and two design patents, underscoring his innovative endeavors within the field. His scholarly pursuits extend beyond traditional publications, as evidenced by his authorship of the book 'Panorama of Deep Learning Based Recommender System: Development and Challenges,' a notable addition to the Massachusetts Institute of Technology bookstore. Dr Sinha's research interests encapsulate the forefront of technological innovation, spanning ML, deep learning, and optimization techniques. His multidisciplinary expertise positions him as a pivotal figure in advancing the frontiers of computational intelligence.

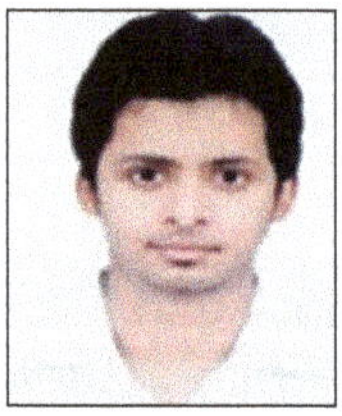

Vikas Kumar Sinha received his MTech degree from the Manipal Institute of Technology, Karnataka, India, in 2015, after acquiring his bachelor of engineering degree in electronics and telecommunication engineering from the Government Engineering College Bilaspur, Chhattisgarh, India, in 2012. During his studies, he interned at the Council of Scientific and Industrial Research—Central Scientific Instruments Organization (CSIR-CSIO), Chandigarh, India, in 2014–15. He is currently pursuing a PhD in the Department of Electronics and Communication Engineering, National Institute of Technology Rourkela, India. He has also worked as an assistant professor at the J K Institute of Engineering, Bilaspur, Chhattisgarh, India. He has reviewed many papers in multiple journals. His research interests are diverse and impactful, focusing on optimization techniques, biomedical signal processing, and embedded systems. He has published multiple papers in different conferences and SCI-indexed journals. His work is geared toward advancing the frontiers of technology and improving practical applications in these critical areas. Through his dedicated and innovative approach, Vikas Kumar Sinha is making significant contributions to both the academic community and the broader field of electronics and communication engineering.

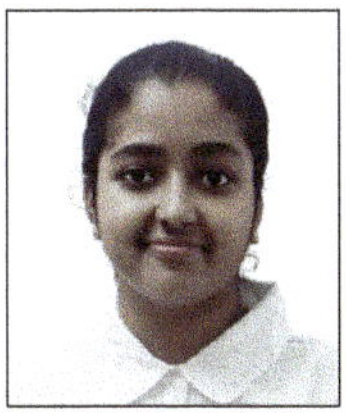

Annapureddy Srija Reddy completed a Bachelor of Technology (BTech) degree in electronics and communication engineering from Motilal Nehru National Institute of Technology, Allahabad, India, in 2024. Her active areas of research are data science, data analysis, ML, and AI for healthcare systems.

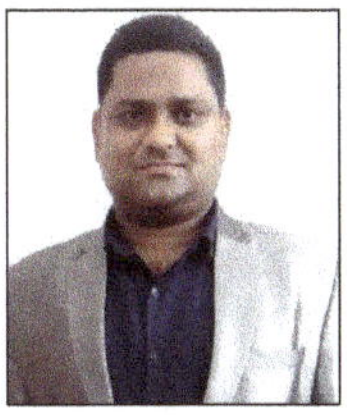

Dr Gopal Singh Tandel has over 20 years of experience, including 16 years in teaching and four years in research. He obtained his doctorate from Visvesvaraya National Institute of Technology (VNIT), Nagpur, India. His academic qualifications include an MTech and a BE in computer science and engineering in 2008 and 2005, respectively, awarded by the Rajiv Gandhi Proudyogiki Vishwavidyalaya University, Bhopal, Madhya Pradesh, India. With 15+ publications in SCI-indexed and peer-reviewed international/national journals/conferences boasting a high impact factor, he holds an h index of 8+ and has been cited more than 720 times. Dr Tandel has successfully passed national-level exams such as the Graduate Aptitude Test in Engineering (GATE) and the University Grants Commission National Eligibility Test (UGC NET) and has been an expert speaker in various faculty development programs. His research interests encompass image processing, healthcare, computer vision, and parallel computing. He specializes in data structures and algorithms, computer networks, operating systems, database management systems (DBMSs), computer architecture, computer graphics, microprocessors, digital circuits, and systems.

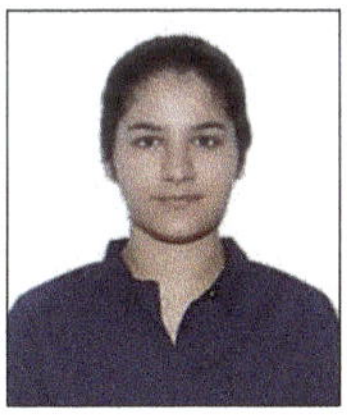

Tanishqa Tyagi is a dedicated Research Scholar at the Department of Electronics and Communication at Delhi Technological University (DTU), New Delhi, India. She received her BTech degree in electronics and communication engineering from Shiv Nadar University, Greater Noida, Uttar Pradesh, India, in 2019 and her MTech degree in signal processing and digital design from Delhi Technological University (DTU) in 2023. Her academic pursuits are focused on advancing knowledge in the field of electronics and communication. With a deep enthusiasm for research, she frequently engages in investigating innovative technologies, making active contributions to academia, and is likely focused on addressing practical challenges through her work.

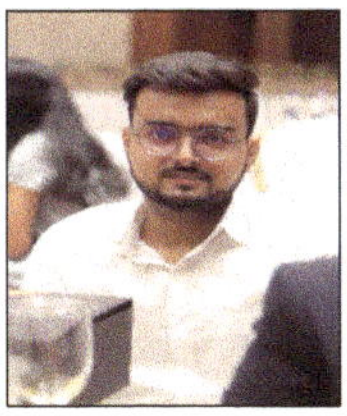

Ujjwal Kumar Upadhyay is currently working as a software development engineer. He holds a bachelor of technology degree in electronics and communication engineering from Delhi Technological University (DTU), New Delhi, India.

Chapter 1

Introduction to AI-driven diagnostics and human–machine interfaces

Smith K Khare, Ankush Jamthikar and Sachin Taran

The use of artificial intelligence (AI) in healthcare has revolutionized diagnostic techniques in recent years, leading to more accurate, efficient, and timely patient care. This chapter investigates the efficacy of AI-driven systems for diagnostics and human–machine interfaces. It provides an overview of the pipeline for automated decision-making systems and introduces the role of existing AI models used for automated diagnosis and the development of the human–machine interface. In the following section, we discuss potential challenges of the current systems, which limit their real-time implementation in clinical settings. These challenges include concerns about data privacy; decision fairness; the requirement for huge, annotated data sets; and the potential for algorithmic bias.

1.1 Introduction

In the last decade, rising technological development has resulted in manifold uses of AI. AI makes use of human-like intelligence for the specific applications it is developed for and tries to behave and think like humans. This property of AI has been widely used in applications such as robotics, transportation, manufacturing, and healthcare. AI accomplishes this using its subfield of machine learning (ML), which performs algorithmic computations to make decisions about new and unseen data without human intervention. Recently, deep learning (DL) algorithms, a type of ML, have performed self-learning tasks by automatically extracting and classifying features from large amounts of structured, semi-structured, and unstructured information, such as physiological signals, medical images, text, facial data, speech, audio, and video [1].

Manual analysis of such data is time-consuming and tedious [2]. Therefore, AI plays a crucial role in analyzing such data and making decisions based on it. Physiological signals, physical signals, and medical imaging have been used in the

doi:10.1088/978-0-7503-5964-1ch1

monitoring of various physiological and pathological conditions [3–5]. Physiological conditions include drowsiness, emotions, sleep, human attention, and motor imagery tasks. Similarly, pathological conditions include schizophrenia, depression, Parkinson's disease (PD), Alzheimer's disease (AD), focal/non-focal seizures, stroke, hypertension, attention deficit hyperactivity disorder (ADHD), myocardial infarction, atrial fibrillation, etc [6, 7]. Early detection and diagnosis of these physiological and pathological conditions can be helpful in effective medication and treatment [8]. Manual monitoring of such physical and physiological conditions can be time-consuming, error-prone, biased, and tedious. In addition, physical signals such as those obtained via the monitoring of facial data and text can lead to false positives and bias and require extensive computation [9, 10]. Similarly, the monitoring of pathological conditions such as seizures, AD, PD, and ADHD can be performed using medical imaging techniques such as magnetic resonance imaging (MRI), computed tomography (CT), and positron emission tomography (PET) [5, 11, 12]. However, these techniques are prone to radiations, computationally expensive, and costly, and they require trained professionals [5, 11, 12]. Therefore, physiological signals are widely preferred and play a crucial role in the timely detection and diagnosis of physiological and pathological conditions. Physiological signals provide a direct measure of neural, physical, and cardiac activities and they are noninvasive, cost-efficient, and nonintrusive [13, 14].

1.2 Pipeline for automated decision-making

The process of automated decision-making for the monitoring of physiological and pathological conditions involves various steps. These steps include acquiring the data, preparing the data for analysis, data analysis, feature extraction, and classification/regression. The steps involved in automated decision-making are shown in figure 1.1. The following subsections briefly explain the role of each step in terms of its contribution to effective data analysis and decision-making for diagnostics and the human–machine interface.

1.2.1 Input source

The first stage in the pipeline of automated decision-making is an input source. The input source may be physical, demographic, physiological, and/or facial or medical

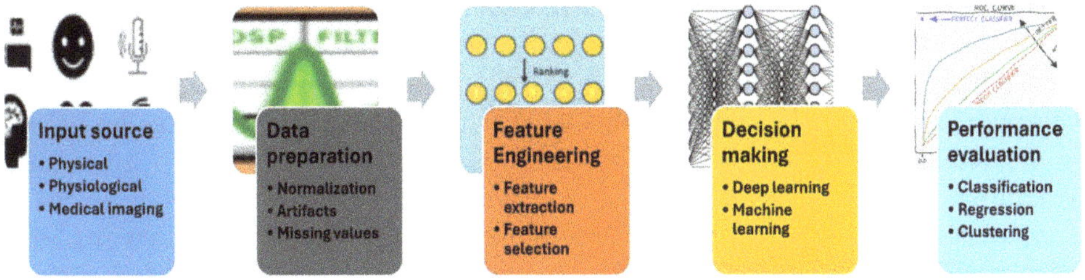

Figure 1.1. Pipeline of the traditional decision-making model.

images. Physical data includes speech, audio, text, and facial data. Demographic data or details include age, gender, race, educational level, habits, smoking history, alcohol history, economic background, marital status, and many more. Physiological signals are direct measurements of physiological, neurological, or cardiological activity in terms of electrical activity; they include electroencephalograms (EEGs), galvanic skin response (GSR), respiration (RSP), electrocardiograms (ECGs), electromyograms (EMGs), electrooculograms (EOGs), photoplethysmograms (PPGs), electrodermal activity, and electronic health records. Similarly, imaging data includes facial images, CT, ultrasound, MRI, functional MRI, mammography, and PET.

1.2.2 Data preparation

Preprocessing is an important stage in data analytics and ML, since it transforms raw data into a clean and useful state. Preprocessing ensures that the data is uniform, proper, and appropriate for analysis or model training. Preprocessing processes differ according to the nature of the data. Preprocessing steps include outlier detection, the management of missing values, and normalization.

1.2.3 Feature engineering and selection

Feature extraction and selection are two fundamental strategies used in ML to lower data complexity and boost model efficacy. Feature extraction transforms the original features into a lower-dimensional space, usually by generating new features that capture significant data more efficiently. This can help to minimize computing complexity and eliminate duplicate or noisy characteristics. Feature selection entails selecting the subset of the original features that is most relevant to the desired variable. This can help boost system interpretation, decrease overfitting, and improve the model's accuracy [15].

1.2.4 Classification strategies

Intelligent healthcare has proven to be highly beneficial. It enhances and accelerates service delivery, enables healthcare institutions to achieve distinction, and increases medical staff productivity by lowering the time and effort required to complete tasks. Furthermore, it assists patients' attempts to protect their money from unnecessary expenditure. Some well-known ML models used for various applications include support vector machines (SVMs), artificial neural networks (ANN), naive Bayes (NB) classifiers, ensemble models (random forest, XGBoost, CatBoost), decision trees, and *k*-nearest neighbors [1]. DL is a branch of ML that focuses on developing and training neural networks with multiple layers to learn from complicated data structures. DL models can automatically learn hierarchical characteristics from raw data, making them ideal for efficient healthcare systems. DL models include convolutional neural networks (CNNs), feedforward neural networks (FNNs), long short-term memory networks (LSTMs), gated recurrent units (GRUs), variational autoencoders (VAEs), recurrent neural networks (RNNs), and generative adversarial networks (GANs) [1].

1.2.5 Performance evaluation

Performance metrics are used to assess the efficacy and quality of ML models. The parameters that are used to evaluate ML performance depend on the type of problem-solving involved, e.g. classification, regression, or clustering, and the goals of the analysis. The evaluation of classification models includes metrics such as recall (sensitivity), accuracy, specificity, area under the curve and receiver operating characteristics, F1 score, and precision. The evaluation metrics for regression models include mean absolute error, mean square error, root mean square error, and the coefficient of determination. Finally, clustering-based models include evaluation metrics such as the silhouette score, adjusted Rand index, homogeneity, and completeness.

1.3 Effective diagnostics and human–machine interfacing using AI techniques

Technological advancements have led to a boom in healthcare applications, particularly in diagnosis and the human–machine interface. The following subsection explores the role of physiological signals and medical imaging in developing effective diagnostics and human–machine interfaces using AI techniques.

1.3.1 Effective diagnostics using physiological signals and medical imaging

The integration of AI-based technologies with physiological signals, coupled with advanced medical imaging, is transforming the landscape of healthcare diagnostics and treatment. Techniques such as electroencephalography and electrocardiography are pivotal; EEGs capture the brain's electrical activity, which can help in diagnosing neurological disorders, and ECGs monitor the heart's electrical impulses to detect cardiovascular conditions. AI's role in enhancing the analysis of ECG signals is particularly transformative; it employs sophisticated machine learning algorithms to analyze these signals for subtle irregularities that might indicate cardiac abnormalities. This capability enables the early detection of potentially life-threatening conditions such as arrhythmias and myocardial infarctions, often before they become clinically apparent. ECGs, as a primary screening method, have consistently attracted the attention of physicians and researchers aiming to extract meaningful insights. Several recent studies have highlighted the role of AI in predicting cardiovascular events using ECG signal analysis [16–19].

Furthermore, the application of AI extends to medical imaging [20–25]. Technologies such as MRI, CT scans, and x-rays are significantly augmented by AI to improve image processing speeds, enhance resolution and clarity, and facilitate automatic and precise interpretation. These advancements enable radiologists to detect and diagnose a range of conditions quickly and with greater accuracy. Beyond mere diagnostics, AI also contributes to predictive healthcare, utilizing vast data sets of imaging and physiological signals to forecast disease progression. This predictive power supports the customization of treatment plans tailored to the individual nuances of each patient's condition, promoting more effective treatments and optimizing outcomes.

In essence, the amalgamation of AI with traditional diagnostic methods such as EEGs, ECGs, and medical imaging is not only enhancing the precision and efficiency of medical diagnostics but is also paving the way for a new era in personalized and predictive medicine, where technology and healthcare converge to deliver unprecedented patient care.

1.3.2 Effective human–machine interfacing using physiological signals

There are various methods by which speech feature extraction can be achieved, which gradually increases the accuracy of a digital system. The major advantage of selecting a feature extraction method is to build a capable and efficient speech processing system. This chapter highlights the various feature extraction methods used in speech recognition systems. Linear predictive coefficient (LPC), mel-frequency cepstral coefficient (MFCC), perceptual linear prediction (PLP), relative spectral perceptual linear prediction (RASTA-PLP), and wavelet transform (WT) are the most used methods of feature extraction [26–29]. The various techniques used to extract features from signals have their own advantages and disadvantages. Studies have supported the popularity of WT by proving that it is good at operating on signals that change over time, i.e. nonstationary signals.

As an emerging communication technique, the brain–computer interface (BCI) aims to build a direct connection between the human brain and a computer [30]. It allows control of an external device using a direct link to the user's brain. In this system, activity patterns detected in EEG signals from the brain are evaluated and presented to the subject in visual or audio form so that he/she can learn to control the signals just by thinking. An example would be to imagine doing a task. This establishes a direct pathway that can assist people with disabilities to communicate. It provides humans with an alternative communication channel by translating neural responses into a computer command [31, 32]. The aim of a brain–computer interface (BCI) is to provide a communication channel for patients who have lost normal communication abilities due to severe motor impairments. Brain–computer interfacing is an emerging technology that performs computer-aided control using brain activity alone. It has found widespread application in areas such as neuro-prosthetics, rehabilitation, and entertainment.

Some of the notable work with EEG-based BCI is as follows. Late positive potential-based features have been used as the input of an SVM to develop a more specialized emotion recognition system [30]. A hierarchical network structure with different subnetwork nodes has been proposed for emotion recognition [31]. Two-stage filtering using EEG signals has been suggested for discrete emotion recognition [33]. A human emotion recognition system has been developed based on EEG signals using nonlinear data-driven decomposition techniques such as adaptive tunable Q WT and adaptive variational mode decomposition [34, 35]. Heart rate variability (HRV) has been recorded by ECG and used to trigger an alarm when a driver feels sleepy or fatigued [36]. Adaptive Hermite decomposition [37] and clustering–variational mode decompositions [38] have been suggested for the detection of drowsiness. Flexible analytic WT [39] and variational nonlinear chirp-mode decomposition [40] have been explored using EEG signals and various ML techniques. Tunable Q-factor wavelet transform (TQWT)-based features have been suggested for drowsiness detection and motor imagery tasks [41, 42]. Signal-dependent orthogonal transform-based feature extraction and ML-based classification strategies have been adopted for motor imagery (MI) classification using EEG signals [43]. Nonstationary decomposition-based algorithms such as empirical mode decomposition combined with Hilbert transform [44], ensemble empirical mode decomposition [45], and rational dilation WT [46] have been suggested for MI task classification using EEG signals and multiple classification algorithms.

1.4 Challenges in today's automated decision-making systems

AI has become an essential component of modern technological advancement, enabling better diagnostics and human–machine interfaces. However, most of the existing systems available for the detection and diagnosis of human–machine interfaces and diagnostics have not been clinically deployed due to uncertainty, a lack of explainability, and concerns about privacy. Figure 1.2 presents an overview of the challenges in today's decision-making models.

1.4.1 Explainable artificial intelligence

Many AI models are 'black boxes,' with decision-making mechanisms that are hidden and difficult for humans to understand. The opaque nature of AI models raises concerns among clinical experts and stakeholders, restricting the clinical applications of these models. Explainable artificial intelligence (XAI) has been developed with the goal of making AI judgments more transparent and intelligible.

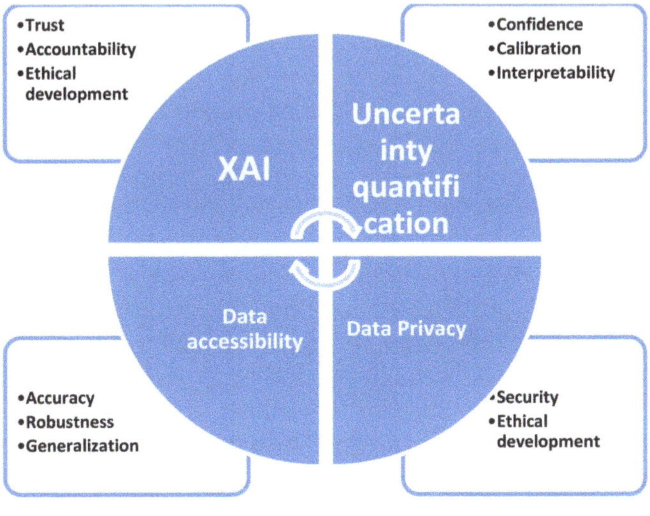

Figure 1.2. Graphical overview of the current challenges encountered by AI models.

XAI plays an important role for several reasons, including trust, accuracy, fairness, responsibility, compliance, and AI system improvement [47–49]. XAI plays a crucial role in achieving the objectives discussed below.

1.4.1.1 Trust and transparency

Traditional AI models, particularly DL models, sometimes function as 'black boxes,' making judgments without revealing information about how those decisions were reached. XAI simplifies these processes, allowing consumers to comprehend the reasoning behind AI judgments. This openness is critical for fostering confidence between AI systems and stakeholders, ensuring that AI is perceived as a trustworthy and accountable tool.

1.4.1.2 Accountability and compliance

Healthcare standards require automated selections to be explainable. As an example, the European Union's General Data Protection Regulation (GDPR) includes the 'right to explanation,' which allows the stakeholders of automated decision-making systems to receive an explanation about how and why a particular AI model has made a decision in a specific instance. XAI increases trust and responsibility by justifying the decisions produced by ML or DL models, thereby helping stakeholders to understand their decisions and also helping to achieve compliance with legislation.

1.4.1.3 Improving AI models

Model explainability provides techniques to identify the biases and faults in an automated AI model. Therefore, XAI helps scientists, researchers, clinicians, and end-users to understand decisions, allowing their biases and errors to be identified. Such transparency and understanding are critical ways of enhancing AI models, improving trust in the model, and ensuring effective and equitable functioning across multiple scenarios and populations.

1.4.1.4 Enhancing user adoption and satisfaction

Ensuring trust and confidence is crucial for AI models to be implemented in a real-time healthcare environment. XAI has the potential to offer transparent, sensible, and intelligent explanations to users, which may improve user satisfaction and acceptance.

1.4.1.5 Facilitating collaboration between humans and AI

The applicability of XAI provides a strong collaborative bridge between users and AI models for verifying, comprehending, and contesting the decisions of AI systems. This hand-in-hand dynamics between AI and the users, especially clinicians, can provide subtle information to clinicians that allows them to verify and validate their own decisions during diagnosis, treatment, medication, and even when monitoring the future risks of the decisions.

1.4.1.6 Ethical AI development
Societal norms and ethical standards are also key factors in the successful implementation of AI in the real world. XAI may help in reducing data abuse, thereby promoting the development of intelligent decision-making models.

1.4.2 Role of uncertainty quantification
Uncertainty quantification (UQ) is the science of studying uncertainty in the decisions produced by ML and DL models. It becomes crucial to evaluate the confidence of the model in decision-making when the model or the data is affected by unknown data and insufficient sources of information. Factors causing uncertainty in the decisions can be due to intrinsic randomness, noise in the input, measurement errors, parameter and model approximations, and unpredictability in the input data [2, 50]. Therefore, uncertainty analysis plays an important role in assessing the fairness and confidence in the predictions made by an AI model. The impact of UQ analysis on the model is discussed below.

1.4.2.1 Model confidence
Assessing the level of confidence in decisions produced by ML and/or DL models is crucial, especially when a model is designed for healthcare applications which can have serious repercussions. The analysis of uncertainty using UQ provides certainty and confidence in decisions and provides insights about the doubtfulness of the models' decisions. Therefore, performing UQ for a model helps users and decision-makers to take preventive and appropriate actions based on their confidence in the AI model.

1.4.2.2 Decision-making in the presence of uncertainties
The science of UQ gives stakeholders an insight into the robustness and dependence of the decisions made by AI models. This helps them to make intelligent and effective decisions, even in the presence of uncertainties. In the medical domain, the science of UQ helps clinicians and physiological experts to determine whether to rely on the decisions of AI–ML models, opt for expert suggestions, or seek extra testing.

1.4.2.3 Model calibration
The science of UQ facilitates precise and accurate calibration of AI–ML models. It also determines the chances of accurately estimating the likelihood of actual outcomes. An uncalibrated or poorly calibrated AI–ML model may make poor decisions due to overconfidence or underconfidence. UQ helps researchers and stakeholders to tune their developed AI models properly and accurately, which results in accurate and reliable decision-making.

1.4.2.4 Risk assessment and risk management
Accessing and evaluating risk is a crucial aspect of healthcare engineering. Integrating UQ evaluation into an AI–ML model results in forecasting the most likely outcomes and estimating the entire spectrum of expected outcomes and their

corresponding likelihood. Therefore, UQ enables risk management and risk assessment of complex AI models.

1.4.2.5 Model interpretability

UQ improves the readability of ML models by providing more context for decisions. Understanding the uncertainty associated with decisions can help consumers to better trust and comprehend the results of ML algorithms.

1.4.3 Need for multimodal data

Multimodal data analytics is crucial for developing a robust, detailed, accurate, and effective model for diagnosis and human–machine interfacing. The availability of diverse and huge data sets provides generalization, dependability, and accuracy during the training, verification, and testing of AI applications in healthcare. Multimodal medical data sets are composed of multiple types of information including electronic healthcare records (EHRs), medical imaging, clinical notes, and physiological data. Analysis of such diverse data may provide crucial insights and reveal the characteristics of pre-medical or medical conditions. The integration of multimodal data with recent AI, ML, DL, or their hybrid combinations may result in improved reliability, accuracy, and precision in clinical use. However, the lack of public data sets and multimodal data impedes multidirectional research.

1.4.4 Data privacy

With the rising usage of AI in multiple domains such as healthcare, medical robotics, and human–machine interfaces, it becomes crucial that patient and user data are protected from different attacks. This reflects an urgent need for a strong privacy-preserving system that safeguards patient data and meets ethical requirements. A strong privacy-preserving system allows data sensitivity, safeguards data from breaches, improves cybersecurity, and maintains regulatory compliance. This can be achieved by using techniques such as data encryption, federated learning, and differential privacy.

1.5 Conclusions

This book thoroughly explores various advanced techniques that utilize physiological signals and healthcare data to enhance diagnostic accuracy. AI and its subsets, ML and DL, are dramatically transforming the analysis and diagnosis of numerous physiological and pathological conditions. By processing vast amounts of diverse data types, such as physiological signals and medical images, AI tools offer more efficient, precise, and unbiased monitoring and diagnosis compared to traditional manual methods. These technological advancements are especially vital for the early detection and management of conditions such as AD, PD, and epilepsy. AI leverages noninvasive and cost-effective techniques, thereby optimizing healthcare outcomes and reducing dependency on more invasive, expensive, and resource-intensive methods. This book also underscores the potential of a series of AI-based techniques that significantly enhance medical diagnostics, proving invaluable for researchers and physicians in the field. The development of AI in healthcare is not only advancing medical research but also significantly improving patient care.

References

[1] Khare S K, Khan A M, Bajaj V and Sinha G R 2023 Introduction to smart healthcare and the role of cognitive sensors *Cognitive Sensors, Volume 2: Applications in Smart Healthcare* (Bristol: IOP Publishing) p 1–1

[2] Pope C, Ziebland S and Mays N 2000 Qualitative research in health care. Analysing qualitative data *BMJ (Clinical Research Ed.)* **320** 114–6

[3] Yaacob H, Hossain F, Shari S, Khare S K, Ooi C P and Acharya U R 2023 Application of artificial intelligence techniques for brain-computer interface in mental fatigue detection: a systematic review (2011–2022) *IEEE Access* **11** 74736–58

[4] Khare S K, Gadre V M and Acharya U R 2023 ECGPsychNet: an optimized hybrid ensemble model for automatic detection of psychiatric disorders using ECG signals *Physiol. Meas.* **44** 115004

[5] Khare S K, Gaikwad N B and Bajaj V 2022 VHERS: a novel variational mode decomposition and Hilbert transform-based EEG rhythm separation for automatic ADHD detection *IEEE Trans. Instrum. Meas.* **71** 1–10

[6] Ferguson S Understanding psychological disorders https://healthline.com/health/psychological-disorders#sleep

[7] Lin W H, Zhang H and Zhang Y T 2013 Investigation on cardiovascular risk prediction using physiological parameters *Comput. Math. Methods Med.* **2013** 272691

[8] Di Luca M, Nutt D, Oertel W, Boyer P, Jaarsma J, Destrebecq F and Quoidbach V 2018 Towards earlier diagnosis and treatment of disorders of the brain *Bull. World Health Organ.* **96** 298

[9] Siuly S, Khare S K, Bajaj V, Wang H and Zhang Y 2020 A computerized method for automatic detection of schizophrenia using EEG signals *IEEE Trans. Neural Syst. Rehabil. Eng.* **28** 2390–400

[10] Khare S K and Bajaj V 2022 A hybrid decision support system for automatic detection of Schizophrenia using EEG signals *Comput. Biol. Med.* **141** 105028

[11] Khare S K, Bajaj V and Acharya U R 2021 PDCNNet: an automatic framework for the detection of Parkinson's disease using EEG signals *IEEE Sens. J.* **21** 17017–24

[12] Khare S K and Acharya U R 2023 Adazd-Net: automated adaptive and explainable Alzheimer's disease detection system using EEG signals *Knowledge-Based Syst.* **278** 110858

[13] El-Dahshan E S A, Bassiouni M M, Khare S K, Tan R S and Acharya U R 2024 ExHyptNet: an explainable diagnosis of hypertension using EfficientNet with PPG signals *Expert Syst. Appl.* **239** 122388

[14] Khare S K and Bajaj V 2021 A CACDSS for automatic detection of Parkinson's disease using EEG signals *2021 Int. Conf. on Control, Automation, Power and Signal Processing (CAPS)* (Piscataway, NJ: IEEE) 1–5

[15] Khare S K, Blanes-Vidal V, Nadimi E S and Acharya U R 2023 Emotion recognition and artificial intelligence: a systematic review (2014–2023) and research recommendations *Inf. Fusion.* **102** 102019

[16] Martínez-Sellés M and Marina-Breysse M 2023 Current and future use of artificial intelligence in electrocardiography *J. Cardiovasc. Dev. Dis.* **10** 175

[17] Han C, Kang K W, Kim T Y, Uhm J S, Park J W, Jung I H, Kim M, Bae S, Lim H S and Yoon D 2022 Artificial intelligence-enabled ECG algorithm for the prediction of coronary artery calcification *Front. Cardiovasc. Med.* **9** 849223
[18] Huang P S *et al* 2022 An artificial intelligence-enabled ECG algorithm for the prediction and localization of angiography-proven coronary artery disease *Biomedicines* **10** 394
[19] Khurshid S *et al* 2022 ECG-based deep learning and clinical risk factors to predict atrial fibrillation *Circulation* **145** 122–33
[20] Gore J C 2020 Artificial intelligence in medical imaging *Magn. Reson. Imaging* **68** A1–4
[21] Chassagnon G, Vakalopoulou M, Paragios N and Revel M P 2020 Artificial intelligence applications for thoracic imaging *Eur. J. Radiol.* **123** 108774
[22] Zhou L Q, Wang J Y, Yu S Y, Wu G G, Wei Q, Deng Y B, Wu X L, Cui X W and Dietrich C F 2019 Artificial intelligence in medical imaging of the liver *World J. Gastroenterol.* **25** 672–82
[23] Sechopoulos I, Teuwen J and Mann R 2021 Artificial intelligence for breast cancer detection in mammography and digital breast tomosynthesis: state of the art *Semin. Cancer Biol.* **72** 214–25
[24] Dack E, Christe A, Fontanellaz M, Brigato L, Heverhagen J T, Peters A A, Huber A T, Hoppe H, Mougiakakou S and Ebner L 2023 Artificial intelligence and interstitial lung disease: diagnosis and prognosis *Invest. Radiol.* **58** 602–9
[25] Yasmin F *et al* 2021 Artificial intelligence in the diagnosis and detection of heart failure: the past, present, and future *Rev. Cardiovasc. Med.* **22** 1095–113
[26] Sharma Y and Singh B K 2020 Prediction of specific language impairment in children using speech linear predictive coding coefficients *2020 First Int. Conf. on Power, Control and Computing Technologies (ICPC2T)* (Piscataway, NJ: IEEE) 305–10
[27] Zakaria M Y, Djamal E C, Nugraha F and Kasyidi F 2020 Speech emotion identification using linear predictive coding and recurrent neural *2020 3rd Int. Conf. on Computer and Informatics Engineering (IC2IE)* (Piscataway, NJ: IEEE) 63–8
[28] Ali Y M, Noorsal E, Mokhtar N F, Saad S Z M, Abdullah M H and Chin L C 2022 Speech-based gender recognition using linear prediction and mel-frequency cepstral coefficients *Indones. J. Electr. Eng. Comput. Sci.* **28** 753–61
[29] Hammami I, Salhi L and Labidi S 2020 Voice pathologies classification and detection using EMD-DWT analysis based on higher order statistic features *IRBM* **41** 161–71
[30] Mehmood R M and Lee H J 2016 A novel feature extraction method based on late positive potential for emotion recognition in human brain signal patterns *Comput. Electr. Eng.* **53** 444–57
[31] Yang Y, Wu Q J, Zheng W L and Lu B L 2017 EEG-based emotion recognition using hierarchical network with subnetwork nodes *IEEE Trans. Cogn. Dev. Syst.* **10** 408–19
[32] Khare S K and Bajaj V 2020 A facile and flexible motor imagery classification using electroencephalogram signals *Comput. Methods Programs Biomed.* **197** 105722
[33] Taran S and Bajaj V 2019 Emotion recognition from single-channel EEG signals using a two-stage correlation and instantaneous frequency-based filtering method *Comput. Methods Programs Biomed.* **173** 157–65
[34] Khare S K, Bajaj V and Sinha G R 2020 Adaptive tunable Q wavelet transform-based emotion identification *IEEE Trans. Instrum. Meas.* **69** 9609–17
[35] Khare S K and Bajaj V 2020 An evolutionary optimized variational mode decomposition for emotion recognition *IEEE Sens. J.* **21** 2035–42

[36] Vicente J, Laguna P, Bartra A and Bailón R 2016 Drowsiness detection using heart rate variability *Med. Biol. Eng. Comput.* **54** 927–37
[37] Taran S and Bajaj V 2018 Drowsiness detection using adaptive Hermite decomposition and extreme learning machine for electroencephalogram signals *IEEE Sens. J.* **18** 8855–62
[38] Dutta A, Kour S and Taran S 2020 Automatic drowsiness detection using electroencephalogram signal *Electron. Lett.* **56** 1383–6
[39] Sharma S, Khare S K, Bajaj V and Ansari I A 2021 Improving the separability of drowsiness and alert EEG signals using analytic form of wavelet transform *Appl. Acoust.* **181** 108164
[40] Khare S K, Bajaj V and Sinha G R 2020 Automatic drowsiness detection based on variational non-linear chirp mode decomposition using electroencephalogram signals *Modelling and Analysis of Active Biopotential Signals in Healthcare, Volume 1* (Bristol: IOP Publishing) p 5–1
[41] Bajaj V, Taran S, Khare S K and Sengur A 2020 Feature extraction method for classification of alertness and drowsiness states EEG signals *Appl. Acoust.* **163** 107224
[42] Taran S and Bajaj V 2019 Motor imagery tasks-based EEG signals classification using tunable-Q wavelet transform *Neural Comput. Appl.* **31** 6925–32
[43] Baali H, Khorshidtalab A, Mesbah M and Salami M J 2015 A transform-based feature extraction approach for motor imagery tasks classification *IEEE J. Transl. Eng. Health Med.* **3** 1–8
[44] Taran S, Bajaj V, Sharma D, Siuly S and Sengur A 2018 Features based on analytic IMF for classifying motor imagery EEG signals in BCI applications *Measurement* **116** 68–76
[45] Kardam V S, Taran S and Pandey A 2023 Motor imagery tasks based electroencephalogram signals classification using data-driven features *Neurosci. Inform.* **3** 100128
[46] Taran S, Khare S K, Bajaj V and Sinha G R 2020 Classification of motor-imagery tasks from EEG signals using the rational dilation wavelet transform *Modelling and Analysis of Active Biopotential Signals in Healthcare, Volume 2* (Bristol: IOP Publishing)
[47] Loh H W, Ooi C P, Seoni S, Barua P D, Molinari F and Acharya U R 2022 Application of explainable artificial intelligence for healthcare: a systematic review of the last decade (2011–2022) *Comput. Methods Programs Biomed.* **226** 107161
[48] Chaddad A, Peng J, Xu J and Bouridane A 2023 Survey of explainable AI techniques in healthcare *Sensors* **23** 634
[49] Band S S, Yarahmadi A, Hsu C C, Biyari M, Sookhak M, Ameri R and Liang H W 2023 Application of explainable artificial intelligence in medical health: a systematic review of interpretability methods *Inform. Med. Unlocked* **40** 101286
[50] Khare S K, March S, Barua P D, Gadre V M and Acharya U R 2023 Application of data fusion for automated detection of children with developmental and mental disorders: a systematic review of the last decade *Inf. Fusion* **99** 101898

Chapter 2

Recent advancements in emerging technology for healthcare management systems

Bhawna Sachdeva, Jeebananda Panda and Sachin Taran

The healthcare industry is a significant application area that has experienced rapid growth in the use of Internet of Things (IoT), artificial intelligence (AI), and blockchain technology (BT). These technologies have become distinct areas of academic and professional interest in recent years. Many individuals' health has improved because of recent innovations in healthcare delivery that have made enhanced customized healthcare accessible to them. The amalgamation of healthcare technology with new technologies like BT, AI, and wearable sensor devices supported by IoT is very attractive and important to well-being. It is astonishing that the old core model of the healthcare management system (HMS) is being replaced by a new one that incorporates wearable smart sensors, IoT, and AI-enabled technologies. Concurrently deploying BTs, accurate IoT, AI, and smart sensors in HMS continues to be a big challenge. To get a better understanding of the accomplishments made so far, this chapter provides a thorough examination of how these emergent technologies (smart sensors, IoT, AI and BT) have been used by HMS. To be more precise, the utilization of these novel innovations in healthcare, together with crucial enabling factors and key uses, is discussed as a consequence of their examination of recent research. In this chapter, we emphasize the greatest challenges that BT, AI, and the IoT often face, and discuss the most pressing issues that need to be addressed so that these new technologies can be better used in HMSs.

2.1 Introduction

In the modern, globalized world, only 50% of people have access to universal health care. Effective, secure, and transparent access to exceptional health services (diagnosis, treatment, and prevention) must be provided to everyone [1]. To achieve this, new technologies are always under development; without them, hospitals would be unable to meet patient needs and would eventually lose their reputation [2, 3].

doi:10.1088/978-0-7503-5964-1ch2

For many forms of healthcare and medical treatment (telemedicine, for example), smart devices' capacity to store and send data is crucial [4]. While there are many uses for wearable sensors in HMSs, tracking patients' vitals and medical status is one of the most popular uses. To put it plainly, the vital signs track the patient's progress toward improving their condition, their physiological status, and the operation of their organs. The examination of these markers has a significant influence on diagnosis, sickness prevention, and nursing care [5]. These medical records can be a useful tool for providing timely, high-quality care if they are properly and promptly assessed. Many smart gadgets, IoT, and AI-based novel technologies have been developed and designed to enhance the quick and continuous assessment of patients' health status and pertinent healthcare sub-systems.

Because of this, the goal of this section is to perform a thorough review of the appropriate use of these emerging technologies (BT, internet of medical things (IoMT), AI, and sensors) in HMS, both separately and collectively, since development and research is crucial. This chapter is divided into eight sections. Section 2.2 provides an overview of HMS. In section 2.3, the previous research aimed at creating technology for HMSs is covered. Sections 2.4–2.7 cover the use of AI, BT, IoMT, and detectors for HMS as well as the challenges and facilitators associated with each of these application areas. Section 2.8 presents a thorough summary of the chapter's findings.

2.2 Healthcare management systems

An HMS can be used to fulfill all medical needs. Health records for patients, staff, and dependents are kept in such systems. For example, the usual 'Inventory Management of Materials' management module tends to patients' medicine supplies and their distribution. There are certain fundamental, one-time master data records that are often altered to standardize the program [6].

All patient records must be entered into the healthcare system using the master data. By just providing the registration number, the necessary information from the patient's, employee's, or dependent's master data stored in the system can immediately be retrieved. Figure 2.1 depicts the system for managing healthcare.

2.2.1 The healthcare system in India

A discussion of the healthcare system in India is included in this part of the chapter. A diagram illustrating the structure of the healthcare system in India is shown in figure 2.2.

2.2.2 Traditional healthcare systems in India

The World Health Organization (WHO) has identified and recorded hundreds of distinct traditional medicinal practices worldwide. A few instances of the many and interrelated traditional medical systems around the world are shiatsu in Japan, herbal medicine in Sweden, magnetic therapy in France, acupuncture in China, and Sowa Rig-pa in Tibet and Bhutan [8]. The most important well-known alternative medical practices include yoga, homeopathy, naturopathy, Siddha, Unani, and

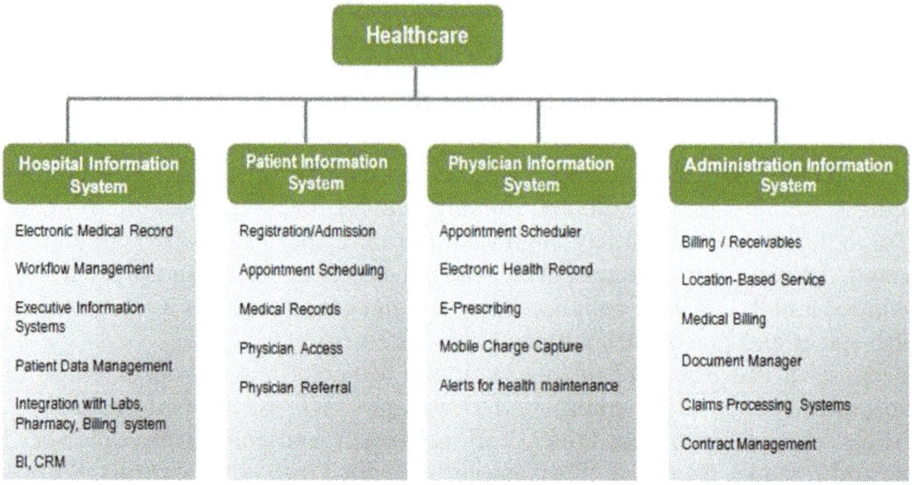

Figure 2.1. Healthcare management system.

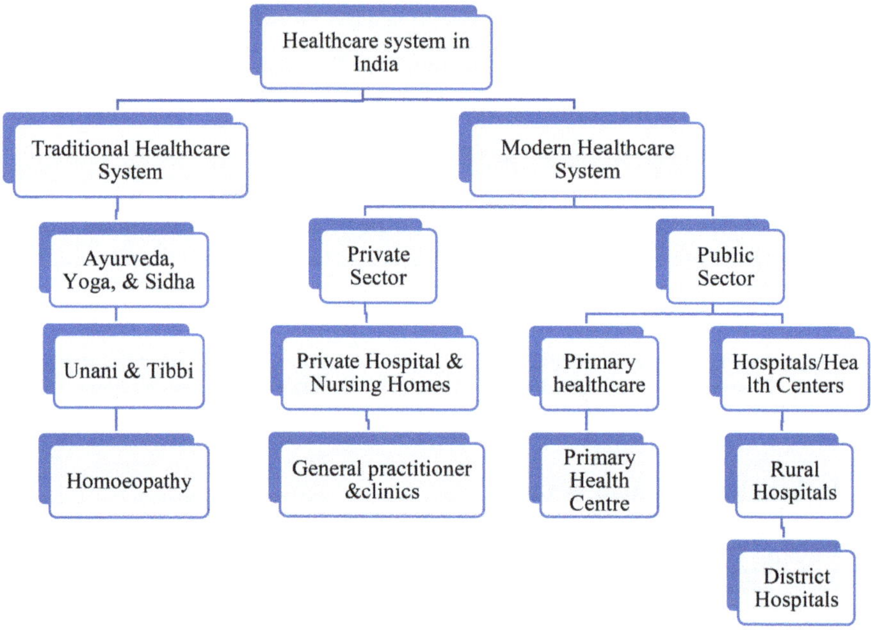

Figure 2.2. Healthcare system in India [7].

Ayurveda. Among the many organic conventional healthcare systems that developed on the Indian subcontinent and are still highly successful in treating both historical and contemporary issues are naturopathy, ayurveda, and siddha [9].

- **The Ayurveda** (literally, 'science of life') technique takes into account all aspects of one's wellness (mental illness, physical, and spiritual) when addressing triggers, symptoms, diagnosis, and therapy. Most of the time, these experts inherited their skills from their forebears. But since education was introduced, a number of institutions have begun to provide instruction in native medical practice.

- **The Siddha system** characterizes illness as a condition in which human beings' natural equilibrium of the five components is upset, leading to a variety of forms of pain. The Siddha medical system's diagnostic instruments place greater emphasis on the clinical judgment of the doctor following patient observation, assessment, diagnosis, and medical history.
- **Naturopathy** is mentioned multiple times in the Vedas and other ancient literature, indicating that these treatments were extensively used in ancient India. Naturopathy holds that all ailments are caused by a build-up of unhealthy matter in the body and that removing it offers a cure or alleviation. It also claims that the human body has innate self-building and healing abilities. Naturopathy distinguishes itself from other medical systems by its holistic approach, rejecting the notion of a singular cause or treatment for ailments. Instead, it embraces a comprehensive perspective, acknowledging the collective impact of various factors on health. These encompass not only individual lifestyle choices—like diet, mental patterns, occupational habits, sleep patterns, and relaxation practices—but also external influences such as environmental conditions that can disrupt the body's innate balance and functioning [10].

2.2.3 Modern (allopathic) healthcare systems in India

India's contemporary allopathic healthcare system is made up of a mix of the public and private sectors as well as an unofficial network of healthcare providers. Total compliance with the numerous well-meaning guidelines and directives was impeded by the size, reach, and distribution of the country.

In actuality, the industry functions in a mostly uncontrolled setting, with few restrictions on who can provide what services, how they can be delivered, or how much they can cost. As a consequence, there are significant variations in the availability, affordability, quantity, and quality of healthcare throughout the nation.

The field of public health encompasses both the science and the art of societally coordinated efforts to improve health, reduce the prevalence of illness, and increase the average lifespan [11]. The aim of public health, a social and physical concept, is to enhance health conditions, life expectancy, and quality of life for entire populations via promoting health, avoiding illness, and other forms of health intervention [12]. India's private healthcare sector has developed into a formidable force, receiving recognition on a worldwide level. The burgeoning middle class in India is driving exponential growth in the private healthcare sector by driving demand for advanced technology, better devices, and dependable surgical procedures [13].

2.3 Literature review

In this section, the literature on the use of BT, AI, IoMT, and sensors in HMS is cited and discussed.

Pawar *et al* [14] introduced eHealthChain, a personal health information management system (PHIMS) built on BT that can be used to manage health data provided by linked apps and IoMT devices. Unlike conventional systems, eHealthChain gives users complete control over the collection, sharing, and management of their personal health information. In addition, this paper describes a robust implementation of an eHealthChain proof of concept (PoC) prototype, meticulously crafted on the Hyperledger Fabric platform.

Minopoulos *et al* [15] suggested a new healthcare system design that integrates many emerging technologies. To create a smart healthcare system that can be implemented in healthcare facilities, it is necessary to specify the combination of many new technologies with sophisticated networks. Such a system would give medical professionals access to up-to-the-minute, accurate data, allowing for more targeted patient diagnosis and treatment.

Efthymiou *et al* [16] addressed the importance of AI in improving healthcare and other sectors. They also explored the importance of AI in transforming several healthcare industries.

Nahavandi *et al* [17] studied the present uses of AI-based wearable sensors. Research on medical analysis using machine learning (ML) methods is reviewed in the literature. Moreover, scenarios involving the integration of IoT and wearable sensors into HMS were deliberated.

Manickam *et al* [18] examine how AI stands poised to enhance the functionalities of IoMT devices and point-of-care (POC) technologies within advanced healthcare sectors, such as cardiac monitoring, cancer identification, and diabetes management. This study also covers the technical and engineering aspects of building efficient POC biomedical systems that are compatible with the intelligent healthcare of the future, as well as the possibilities and obstacles associated with AI-based cloud-integrated customized IoMT devices.

Kamruzzaman *et al* [19] examined healthcare delivery in ubiquitous contexts to be enhanced via the use of AI, IoMT, and edge computing. They hypothesized that the mentioned technology could assist with healthcare system administration and monitoring. Medical professionals are finding it very challenging to provide sufficient care to individuals with related medical difficulties, according to reports, because of the alarming increase in both the population and illnesses. Additionally, they contended that these growing problems could be resolved by the use of new technology, such as AI approaches.

Jabbar *et al* [20] explained BiiMED, a blockchain-based approach to improve data integrity and compatibility in electronic health record (EHR) sharing. Two suggested remedies are a dispersed trusted third-party auditor (TTPA) to ensure the integrity of data and a system for controlling access to permit various healthcare providers to share EHRs. This work lays the groundwork for future research on decentralized integrity verification and dynamic data interoperability.

Table 2.1. Comparison of literature review.

		Emerging technology			
Authors [reference]	Year	Blockchain	IoMT	Sensor	AI
Pawar *et al* [14]	2022	■			
Minopoulos *et al* [15]	2022				■
Efthymiou *et al* [16]	2020				■
Nahavandi *et al* [17]	2021			■	
Manickam *et al* [18]	2022		■		
Kamruzzaman *et al* [19]	2022		■		
Jabbar *et al* [20]	2020	■			
Giri *et al* [21]	2019		■		
Karthick *et al* [22]	2020			■	
Amin *et al* [23]	2020	■			■

Giri *et al* [21] examined the extent and prospective uses of IoMT in India's healthcare system, as well as how the IoMT might increase the effectiveness of healthcare administration. Their study used two statistical techniques, namely multiple regression and exploratory factor analysis (EFA).

Karthick *et al* [22] summarized the state of human healthcare IoT (H2IoT) deployment; looked at data transmission methods and sensing devices used in H2IoT; and discussed system problems, privacy difficulties, security threats, and vulnerabilities.

Amin *et al* [23] studied how edge computing environments are used in the healthcare IoT (H-IoT). Their research was centered on assessing edge computing's potential to provide universally accessible healthcare in the present and the future, as well as determining the advantages and disadvantages of various use cases. In their research, the most advanced AI-based techniques for computing at the edge were also examined in great detail. A comparison of the literature reviewed is shown in table 2.1.

2.4 Artificial intelligence (AI)

Determining, researching, and developing intelligent systems is the aim of AI research and development. AI incorporates ideas from computer science, philosophy, and mathematics, among other disciplines [24]. AI has a huge potential to advance both medical and public health. Many specific healthcare applications are presently utilizing or planning to use AI platforms. These include non-communicable disease (NCD) risk screening, medical diagnosis, patient monitoring, early problem detection, and health system learning [25]. These are leading to better care that is both more efficiently delivered and more effectively administered.

AI is a general term for computer programs that can learn and do tasks often associated with human intellect, such as reasoning, sensory comprehension, deep learning, adaptability, and interaction [26]. Modern computers' dramatically increased processing capability is largely responsible for the current increase in interest and development of AI applications for health. There is a lot of evidence that AI could enhance clinical therapy by making diagnoses and treatments more accurate. Medical imaging, health information systems, epidemic and syndromic monitoring, predictive modeling and decision assistance, and geo-coding of health data are just a few areas where AI applications have helped physicians and health professionals [27].

2.4.1 Key applications of AI in healthcare

Here we outline some of the most significant applications of AI in health care domains. A diagram depicting the use of AI in healthcare can be seen in figure 2.3.

2.4.1.1 AI in clinical practice

- **Radiology and imaging**

  Radiology is an area of medicine that has recently seen remarkable AI improvements. Radiologists have discovered that imaging AI tools make it easier for them to categorize medical images. Segmentation with minimal or no human intervention has been made possible, for example, by deep network models that can autonomously identify and define the borders of lesions or anatomical structures [29–31]. The use of AI in radiography has generated much speculation. Radiologists should expect their profession to be significantly transformed by the arrival of AI, which is anticipated to take place gradually over the next decade [28].
- **Pathology**

  A lot of interest is currently being shown in AI for pathology, which may be affected by the development of whole-slide digital scanners and the advent of digital pathology [32]. Algorithms for pattern recognition are being developed by numerous groups for use in digital pathology. The forecasting of disease development, including metastasis and recurrence, and the examination of tissue features would both benefit from these techniques. AI

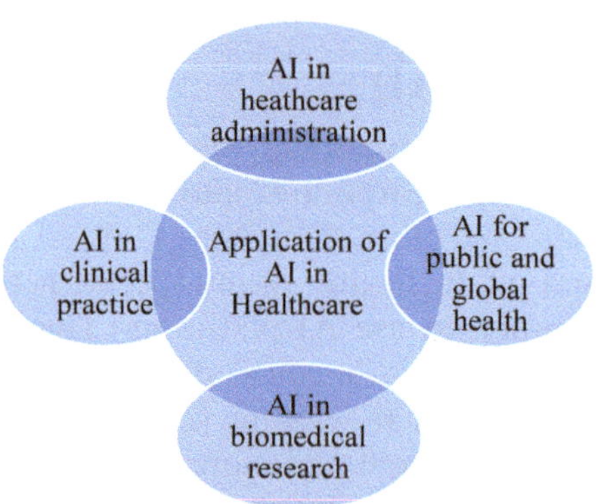

Figure 2.3. AI applications in healthcare [28].

software could identify symptoms of cancer, particularly those related to staging, grading, and differential diagnosis [33, 34].

2.4.1.2 AI in biomedical research

- **Clinical research**

  Recent studies showing unique uses of AI in medical data retrieval suggest that AI solutions are more useful for biological inquiry than for clinical applications. Traditional MIRs, for example, are beginning to incorporate ML approaches to sort search results through algorithms that continuously learn from consumers' search activity [35].
- **Clinical trials**

  While randomized controlled trials (RCTs) are often considered the most precise means of assessing the risks and benefits of medical interventions, conducting them is frequently impractical. Ineffective RCTs commonly arise due to challenges such as suboptimal patient selection, inadequate randomization, small sample sizes, and biased result interpretation. Integrating data-driven methodologies with advanced statistical techniques present an opportunity. Through training AI models to refine participant selection and accurately interpret study outcomes, AI holds the potential to enhance execution and statistical power beyond the capabilities of traditional RCTs [36].

2.4.1.3 AI for public and global health

- **Public health**

  AI may be used to identify a population that has a record of risky behavior or a high sickness prevalence. Numerous AI systems also enable the monitoring of diseases. Methods of concern verification can be examined by combining detectors, digital evidence, information and online media, smartphones, social networks, case-and-event-based monitoring, medical reports, and digital epidemiological surveillance. AI has been used by early warning systems for drug side effects and air pollution [37, 38].
- **Global health**

  Problems with health care in countries with low- or medium-income levels might be addressed with AI. A serious lack of qualified medical professionals and insufficient public health monitoring systems are two examples of these problems. These problems are not exclusive to these nations, but they are particularly pressing for low- and middle-income nations because of the correlation between them and illness and death [39]. As a result, various research on the use of AI-based technologies in health care is now being carried out (table 2.2).

2.4.2 Challenges of AI in healthcare

Note that there are a lot of obstacles to overcome when employing AI, including ethical difficulties, privacy and data protection, social gaps, medical consultation, empathy, and compassion [41–43].

Table 2.2. Applications of AI in healthcare [40].

Technology	Application scheme	Application area
Robotics	Provide high-quality care by enhancing the precision and accuracy of surgical operations.	Medical device, health information (IT)
Digital secretary	Determine the optimal time for appropriate action by continually monitoring patient condition indicators and informing the nurse as needed.	Medical device, health IT
ML	Predict and evaluate trends based on data that influence treatment outcomes. Reduce confusion in medical treatment decisions by analyzing vast amounts of diagnostic medical imagery using self-learning.	Diagnostic medical image, health IT
Natural language processing	Transform lengthy, unstructured text files (like medical records) into a format that is easy to read and understand.	Medical device, health IT
Big data analysis	Process the massive volumes of data kept by healthcare facilities to provide patients with individualized suggestions for therapies.	Medical device, health IT

2.4.2.1 Data privacy and security

- **The importance of data security**
  Patient data protection is crucial in the healthcare industry. The application of AI requires robust data security procedures. A breach that results in the release of confidential patient data could erode trust in medical professionals.
- **Challenges in maintaining patient privacy**
  Data anonymization and de-identification are challenges that arise from the fact that AI systems need access to large datasets. An ongoing difficulty is finding a balance between protecting patient privacy and making data useful for AI.
- **Regulatory compliance (e.g. HIPAA)**
  The Health Insurance Portability and Accountability Act (HIPAA) regulations must be followed by all medical professionals. These regulations impose stringent requirements for data protection and management. Getting AI systems to follow these guidelines is not a simple task.

2.4.2.2 Ethical concerns

- **The ethical imperative**
  Several moral challenges arise with using AI in healthcare, such as concerns about bias, fairness, and responsibility. Problems with transparency

and fairness in decision-making arise when algorithms are biased, and healthcare inequities are likely to continue as a result.

- **Bias and fairness**
  Biases that AI systems inherit through their training data can lead to disparities in healthcare. It is a significant ethical conundrum to face such biases. The goal of current research is to create algorithms that are impartial and capable of reducing biases.
- **Transparency and accountability**
  Transparency in AI decision-making is crucial. A better understanding of how AI systems reach their recommendations is crucial for both patients and healthcare providers. Equally critical is the establishment of transparent channels for investigation and punishment of mistakes caused by AI. IoMT has the potential to completely transform the healthcare industry by opening previously unheard-of possibilities for individualized and effective patient carc [44].

2.4.2.3 Regulation and compliance

- **Regulatory landscape**
  Given the rapid pace at which technology is advancing, it is not easy to regulate AI in healthcare. Regulators are required to balance privacy and patient safety against innovation.
- **Adapting regulations**
  The modification of extant regulations for new AI technology is problematical. Regulators and stakeholders need to come up with frameworks that recognize AI while addressing its unique advantages and disadvantages.
- **International standards**
  Healthcare is global in nature thus a universal standard on AI healthcare should be established. Therefore, use of AI globally can be attained easily when national legislations are aligned together.

2.4.2.4 Integration with existing systems

- **Integrating AI solutions**
  When incorporating AI systems into the current healthcare system, there are technological and practical challenges to be solved. In order to guarantee that legacy systems are completely compatible with AI technology, significant alterations might be required.
- **Interoperability challenges**
  Interoperability is crucial for the movement of patient data between various healthcare systems. Ensuring AI-enhanced systems can interact using past technologies and other applications is one of the primary challenges.
- **Successful integration stories**
  Many hospitals and clinics have already begun using AI systems. To better understand how to use AI in healthcare, case studies that focus on these successful examples might be quite helpful.

2.4.3 Advantages of AI

- AI is expected to make the time-consuming process of managing healthcare records much more efficient and streamlined.
- Illnesses would be detected more quickly and accurately than by a doctor, allowing for quicker treatment.
- With the help of AI and real-time data, clinical decision-making would be much simpler.
- Data about individual patients can be easily monitored with the use of AI, which would facilitate therapy.
- AI would make humans' jobs easier, freeing them up to focus on more meaningful projects, such as the crucial task of caring for patients' mental health [45].
- Administrative tasks are responsible for 30% of healthcare costs; but, with the aid of AI, these tasks can be completed far more quickly and efficiently, resulting in cost savings.
- AI in wearable healthcare electronic devices can spot issues quicker than traditional methods.
- AI would lower healthcare costs, allowing everyone to afford basic health services.
- AI would shorten the time it takes to diagnose and cure medical conditions.

2.5 Blockchain technology (BT)

BT has created a new kind of database. Information is stored differently than in a traditional database; blockchains use interconnected blocks to store data. BT is a revolutionary healthcare technology because it does not rely on a single administrator. The reason for this is that people still think of databases as physical objects composed of bits and bytes. Furthermore, there is a very high risk of data loss, abuse, or inadvertent deletion from manual documentation due to the physical nature of the data [46]. Securing the network infrastructure at all levels is a major concern for blockchain healthcare applications. Everyone who takes part has their identities verified. Authorization is regularly required for access to EHRs. Figure 2.4 shows the application of BT in healthcare.

More than 88% of business executives and more than 94%–95% of chief information officers include BT in their strategic plans. This is the primary rationale behind the importance of comprehending the real-world uses of BT in the field of healthcare [48]. Some consumers are wary of disclosing personal health information to a dispersed network, and some medical facilities are wary of giving insurance companies information about their patients' medicines. As demonstrated in table 2.3, BT has the potential to address several security concerns within the medical sector, in addition to those related to diagnosis and treatment [49].

As demonstrated in figure 2.4, blockchain offers a variety of uses in the healthcare industry. BT helps healthcare researchers discover genetic codes by controlling the medication supply chain, allowing safe transfer of medical information about patients, and facilitating the secure exchange of patient medical data [52, 53].

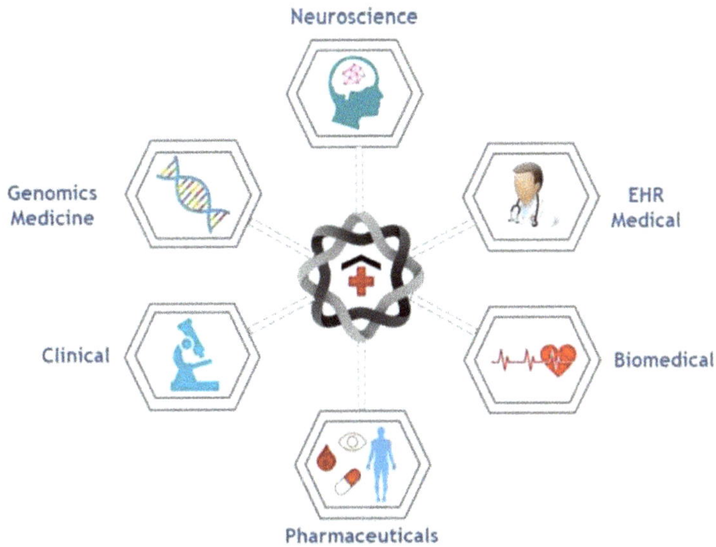

Figure 2.4. Application of blockchain in healthcare [47].

Table 2.3. Addressing healthcare issues with blockchain [50, 51].

Issues addressed	Blockchain-based healthcare approach	Advantages	Disadvantages
Security attacks, data privacy	Managing healthcare records	To decrease healthcare system assaults	High bandwidth and high computing power
Security attacks	Patient monitoring/ ERH	Integrating IoT solves security concerns	Mining incentives and certain blockchain assaults are irrelevant
Data leakage	Drug traceability	Privacy and data authentication increase system flexibility	Complex drug traceability
Real-time patient data monitoring security	Real-time patient monitoring/ERH	Systematic data protection and more appropriate patient data usage	Time delay during block verification
Access control, data tampering	Medical records and data management	Ensure patient data is lawful, transparent, and secure	Poor transaction time
Data security	Medical records and data management	Interoperable Healthcare IoT Trust Model	Unable to identify wearable symptom patterns

Data management	Data management and medical records	Secure paperwork	It cannot address IoT security/attacks
Monitoring and managing patient data	Patient monitoring/ ERH/data management in real time	Medical gear read and share patient vital signs with approved physicians and hospitals in a safe blockchain network	Server-device communication issues

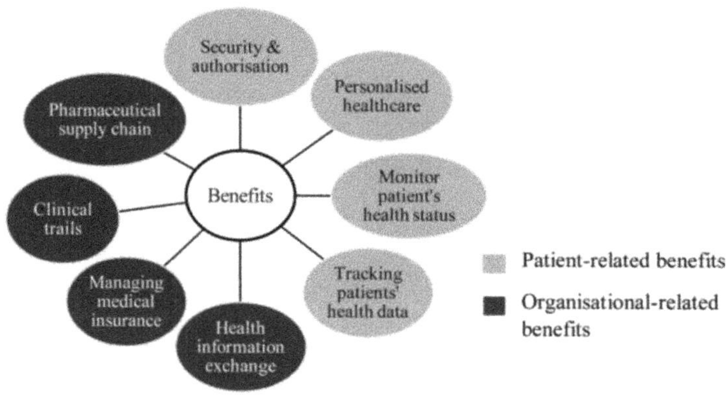

Figure 2.5. Benefits of BT [54].

Figure 2.5 presents eight benefits of BT. The benefits were divided into two categories: benefits to the patients and benefits to the organization.

2.5.1 Need for blockchain in healthcare

There is an increasing and concerning need for advancements in the field of healthcare. Strong healthcare facilities backed by state-of-the-art technology are in high demand these days. Under these circumstances, BT would be important in transforming the healthcare system. Furthermore, healthcare is shifting toward a patient-centered model that prioritizes two essentials: sufficient healthcare resources and services that are constantly available. When it comes to healthcare institutions and the speed of patient treatment, BT could transform the traditional HMS. BT has the potential to quickly tackle another painful and repeated task that adds to the high cost of healthcare. Using BT, patients can take part in health research projects. Additionally, most people's treatment could be improved by sharing data about public well-being and making educated judgments [55–57].

2.5.2 Blockchain use cases in healthcare

Here, we highlight the most relevant research organized by several use scenarios, including electronic medical records (EMRs), remote patient monitoring (RPM), pharmaceutical supply chains, and health insurance claims. Table 2.1 summarizes the papers that were considered. It has come to our attention that most of these applications are built on well-known blockchain platforms like Hyperledger Fabric and Ethereum.

- **Electronic medical records**

  Many individuals use the names interchangeably—EHRs are also frequently referred to as EMRs [58]. The medical history of a person was originally contained in a written document that has been digitally converted. Patient EHRs are started, managed, and kept up to date by healthcare facilities. They are private and only visible to medical professionals who are actively treating patients. A medical record that is editable and managed by the patient is referred to as a personal health record (PHR). PHRs are not protected by the HIPAA, a federal law [59].
- **Remote patient monitoring**

  RPM systems are meant to gather several kinds of physiological information from patients. Electrocardiogram, or (ECG), electroencephalogram (EEG) readings, levels of oxygen in the blood (pulse oximetry), heart rate, breathing rate, stress, temperature of the skin, blood glucose levels, and signals from the neurological system are among the most common types of data. Furthermore, information regarding the patient's weight, degree of activity, and sleeping habits is occasionally gathered [60].
- **Pharmaceutical supply chain (PSC)**

  A PSC is categorized as a difficult supply chain by a number of stakeholders. Important stakeholders include pharmaceutical companies, distributors, wholesalers, regulatory agencies, and data service providers [61]. Furthermore, it takes into account a network of companies involved in medicine distribution and supply as a factor in evaluating the effectiveness of the pharmaceuticals supply [62]. PSC management has numerous challenges, one of which is ordering drugs at multiple locations [63]. Figure 2.6 shows a PSC diagram.

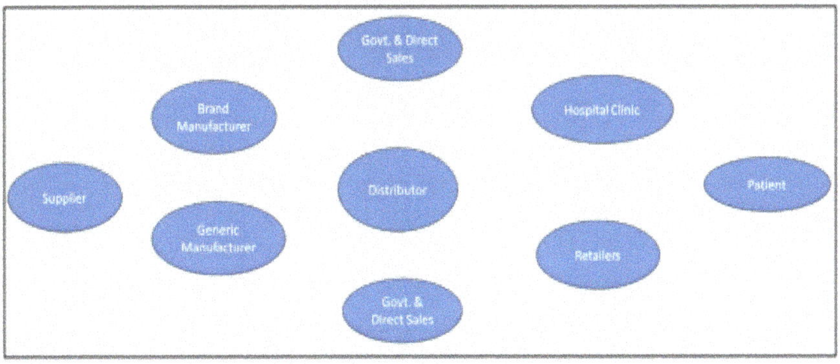

Figure 2.6. The PSC [64].

- **Health insurance claims**

  Medical coverage that a person or organization pays for in advance in the form of a premium is known as health insurance. To get the medical care and benefits that their health insurance covers, one needs to file a claim with one's insurer. Both cashless claims (sometimes called direct claim settlement) and claims for reimbursement of medical expenditure are possible. Table 2.4 indicates the use cases of BT in healthcare.

Table 2.4. Key contributions by use case [65].

Use cases	Framework	Data storage	Contribution	References
EMR	Ethereum	Off-chain	Create a patient-centric system to display medical history.	[66]
	Ethereum	Off-chain	Present a cloud-based medical data-sharing platform.	[67]
	Specific	Off-chain	PHR distributed model for latency solutions.	[68]
	Ethereum	Hybrid	Provide a blockchain-based EMR application that fulfills Office of the National Coordinator (ONC) requirements.	[69]
	Proprietary	Off-chain	Delivers EMR management solutions built on the blockchain.	[70]
	Proprietary	Off-chain	Integrating off-chain data storage with on-chain verification in a healthcare system.	[71]
	Ethereum	Hybrid	Offers an EHR system that safeguards personal health information.	[72]
RPM	Hyperledger Fabric	Off-chain	A mobile health blockchain-based solution for cognitive behavioral.	[73]
	Ethereum	Hybrid	Analyzing data in real-time using smart contracts built on the blockchain.	[74]
	—	—	Create a system that uses patient-recorded IoT sensor data in conjunction with blockchain technology.	[75]
PSC	Ethereum	Off-chain	Ensures that medication temperature data are accessible during transit.	[76]
	Hyperledger Fabric	On-chain	Create a blockchain-based medication turnover control system.	[77]
Health insurance claims	Ethereum	On-chain	Propose blockchain-based medical insurance storage.	[78]

2.6 IoMT

An IoMT-based smart healthcare system is a network of linked smart medical devices that use the internet to provide patient care [79]. There are various sorts of smart healthcare based on IoMT architecture. Using smart sensors integrated into wearable or implanted medical devices, the initial step is to collect health information from the patient's body. A body sensor network (BSN) or wireless sensor network (WSN) can be used to connect these devices [80]. The component that manages analysis and prediction would then get the data via the internet. After receiving the medical data, an appropriate AI-based method for transforming information and interpretation can be applied for analysis [81]. In the case of serious problems, clever AI-based smartphone applications can be utilized to get in touch with doctors or additional healthcare providers [82]. Figure 2.7 [83] illustrates the three fundamental components of the IoMT architecture: application, perceptual, and network layers.

The perceptual layer at the base of the hierarchy is responsible for obtaining data from its source and deriving important inferences from it. The network layer and intermediary layer are responsible for handling various kinds of data transmission and providing services relating to platforms and interfaces. The application layer, that utilizes information from the network layer to perform various applications, is in charge of managing the medical record. A few instances of IoT-based healthcare applications and use cases are displayed in table 2.5 [85].

2.6.1 Challenges of IoMT in healthcare

A number of current issues and their repercussions need to be addressed before IOMT is widely used. These consist of cost-effectiveness, interoperability, scalability and upgrades, data administration, privacy and security, and law (figure 2.8):

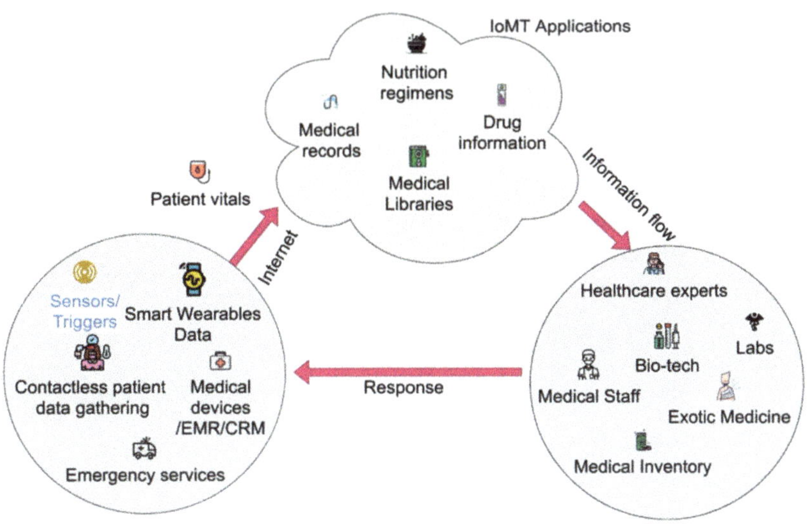

Figure 2.7. IoMT architecture. Reproduced from [84]. CC BY 4.0.

Table 2.5. Applications of IoT in healthcare and precise use cases [86].

Applications	Details	Technology	References
Electrocardiogram (monitoring, detection)	A wireless ECG testing device for IoT purchase.	IoT framework anomaly detection	[87]
Glucose level sensing (monitoring)	A non-invasive gadget that measures blood sugar levels includes an accumulator.	IoT, IPv6	[88]
Body temperature (monitoring)	A thermometer and IoT channel are used in this application.	Thermometer, IoT system, sensors	[89]
Blood pressure (monitoring)	A mobile smartphone and BP KIT meter are integrated to produce an IoT-based BP monitor.	IoT frameworks, pressure sensor	[90]
Smart devices (monitoring, detection	In real time, data is collected, analyzed, and sent.	IoT, Big Data	[91, 92]
Imminent healthcare (monitoring, prevention)	Practitioners are assisted by mobilized IoT-based services, designs, and apps.	IoT net framework, Intelligent security model	[93, 94]
Medicine management (monitoring, detection)	Using I2Pack and the iMed-Box, a medicine management system examines the authenticity of machines.	RFID, IoT	[95]

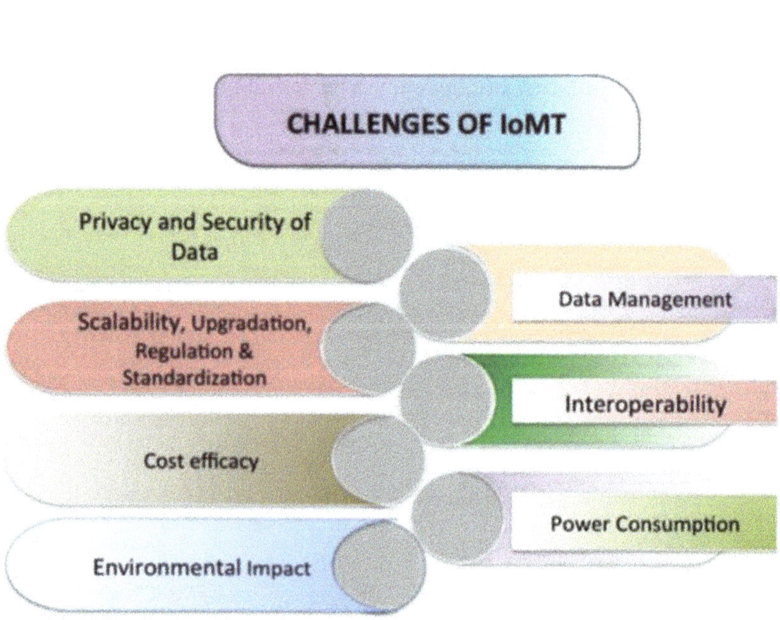

Figure 2.8. Schematics of healthcare IoMT challenges [96].

- **Privacy and security of data**

  Ensuring appropriate cyber safety inside healthcare monitoring systems is one of the primary problems and challenges in the deployment of IoMT. There is still no solution to the problem of how to ensure the security of the massive amounts of PHR that people transmit across different platforms.
- **Interoperability of data**

  If data cannot be processed and aggregated to provide outcomes that are both therapeutically appropriate and valuable, then there is little point in gathering information from many IoMT devices. Every IoMT device needs to be able to talk to other IoMT devices and exchange data with all parties, such as payers and providers [97].
- **Cost efficacy**

  Financial strain in the context of COVID-19 has spread to many individuals, companies, and even organizations, impeding the widespread adoption of IoMT. Ensuring cost-effectiveness is therefore of utmost importance. For the IoMT system to be developed, implemented, and run, a suitable budget is needed.
- **Environmental impact**

  The IoMT systems have been shown to be outfitted with an array of biological detectors that allow them to perform their functions. These are a blend of many semiconductors, including potentially hazardous materials that could affect the environment and earth metals. Regulatory organizations supervise and manage the manufacture of sensors in this way. Further research is necessary to optimize the design and fabrication of biodegradable material sensors [98].

2.6.2 Advantages of IoMT in healthcare

In the healthcare industry, connecting items can yield further benefits. In one way or another, IoMT is meant to help patients, healthcare providers, and insurers.

- **Accessibility**

  Real-time patient data retrieval is one of the main advantages of IoT-based medical equipment. Instead of wasting time asking the nurse or physically visiting the patient's room, physicians can simply take a few moments out of their hectic schedule to see how their patients are doing.

  Insurance companies can access patient records more quickly with the aid of IoMT, which speeds up the claims processing process without sacrificing accuracy. Once again, there are patient portals that allow people to access their own medical records.
- **Improved efficiency**

  One of the well-known advantages of IoMT is the improvement of efficiency via cost savings. Patients often express frustration about the length of time they have to wait for medical appointments. One way in which the adoption of IoMT devices could boost efficiency is by shortening the time it takes for clinicians to diagnose and treat patients. This bodes well for IoMT's ability to provide a superior experience for patients [99].

- **Faster implementation**
  IoMT devices are developed quickly and are easy to deploy. Patients can use these compact devices to track their vital signs and overall health.
- **Lower cost**
  Using IoMT, the healthcare business can save almost $300 billion, according to statistics from Goldman Sachs. With IoMT, there will be quicker access to patient data, which would improve operational efficiency. As a consequence, nurses should be able to focus on more productive duties, rather than having to transmit patient information to the visiting physician.

2.7 IoT-assisted wearable sensor devices

IoT-assisted worn sensor devices are a novel and fascinating field of healthcare technology. The healthcare sector needs data that can be easily monitored and controlled, as well as doorstep diagnostics. In the end, they hope to integrate IoT into emergency services, linked homes, smart hospitals, EHRs, and more [100]. Using information gathered from smart devices and an intelligent hospital, it can monitor symptoms of patients in real time. This could help us find new information about medications, vaccines, healthcare, and pharmaceuticals. The aim is to make certain that the information is secure and accessible to those who are permitted by utilizing technologies like cloud computing and fog computing, among others [101]. Figure 2.9 illustrates how the IoT is being used to monitor healthcare.

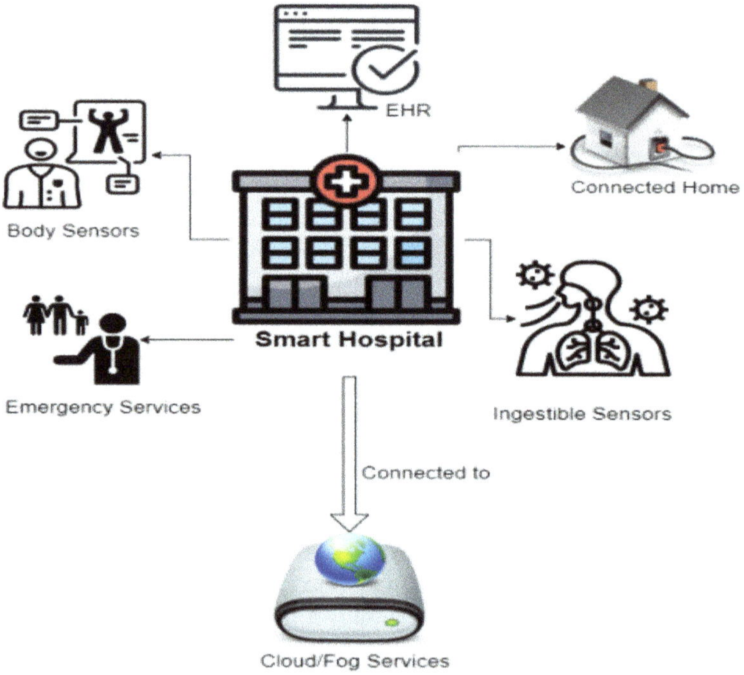

Figure 2.9. IoT-assisted hospital healthcare monitoring outlook [102].

2.7.1 Challenges of IoT-assisted wearable sensor devices in healthcare

The following subsections provide a quick overview of a few of the challenges that are faced by technology using wearable sensing.

- **Data transmission**

  An energy-efficient method of conveying data (gathered by sensors) for further processing must be provided. Although advancements in connection, like 5G and beyond, would allow for quicker data transfer, they could also lead to an explosion in data production, necessitating careful and sufficient preparation for processing and storage. It is not an option to depend only on a central data storage system because of the delays in processing data and the strain on network performance.
- **Security and privacy**

  There are still concerns about sensors that are worn privacy, security, and enforcement of trustworthiness [103]. Wearables' main characteristic is its capacity to continuously perceive and collect data.

  According to [102], the majority of modern wearables can track the user's location, amount of physical activity, and psychological well-being. This information could be considered sensitive by the user, thus it is important to keep their privacy protected. Wearable sensors provide a unique set of security and privacy challenges, and no existing solution solves them completely. Therefore, wearable device security and privacy must be further researched and developed.
- **Resource constraints**

  Improving wearable functionality is crucial for expanding service offerings and connecting with more people. However, wearables with limited resources already have a high battery consumption rate, and adding more functionality only makes things worse. Limited resources could make it so that the finished wearable product falls short in quality. Consequently, achieving the required performance with minimal energy consumption is one of the primary challenges of wearable sensors.

2.8 Conclusion

Recent years have seen the broad adoption of sensors, BT, AI, and the IoMT in a variety of areas. The healthcare industry is utilizing these advancements to improve HMSs. As a result, both consumers and academics are keeping a close eye on the introduction of these technologies into healthcare. This chapter investigates the use cases and challenges associated with research into the use of sensors, the IoMT, AI, and BT in HMSs. The research literature shows that sensors and IoT frameworks have successfully been integrated with different HMSs. Furthermore, in the information technology (IT) and healthcare sectors, AI and BT are increasingly material to the General Data Protection Regulation (GDPR). In particular, AI and BT provide a fundamental mechanism for storing, visualizing, and analyzing data that is very important for the effective functioning of HMSs. AI provides more complex methodologies that could use detailed information from health data for current needs and even for the near future if utilized in HMSs.

One additional BT is that doctors could build their own, distributed repositories in which personal patient records are stored with no one able to access the data other than those to whom sufficient rights are assigned. There are many conceivable applications of BT in healthcare but several barriers of BT to be widely adopted in healthcare from regulatory concerns including data privacy and ethics, practical issues such as cost and user /patient acceptability. More details about HMS technical specifications of sensors–IoT–AI–BT could be given to researchers at the end of it all. Furthermore, there are obvious avenues for future research given the unresolved problems described in this section.

References

[1] World Health Organization 2022 *Universal Health Coverage* (Geneva: World Health Organization)

[2] Villarreal E R D, García-Alonso J, Moguel E and Alegría J A H 2023 Blockchain for healthcare management systems: a survey on interoperability and security *IEEE Access* **11** 5629–52

[3] Aggelidis V P and Chatzoglou P D 2009 Using a modified technology acceptance model in hospitals *Int. J. Med. Inform.* **78** 115–26

[4] Da Costa C A, Pasluosta C F, Eskofier B, Da Silva D B and da Rosa Righi R 2018 Internet of health things: toward intelligent vital signs monitoring in hospital wards *Artif. Intell. Med.* **89** 61–9

[5] Fan Y, Xu P, Jin H, Ma J and Qin L 2019 Vital sign measurement in telemedicine rehabilitation based on intelligent wearable medical devices *IEEE Access* **7** 54819–23

[6] Khatoon A 2020 A blockchain-based smart contract system for healthcare management *Electronics* **9** 94

[7] Sidhu R K 2015 Health care in India: critical analysis *Int. J. Med. Health Sci.* **4** 264–8 https://ijmhs.net/journals-aid-254.html

[8] Kala C P 2017 Traditional health care systems and herbal medicines *Eur. J. Environ. Public Health* **1** 03

[9] Kala C P, Dhyani P P and Sajwan B S 2006 Developing the medicinal plants sector in northern India: challenges and opportunities *J. Ethnobiol. Ethnomed.* **2** 1–15

[10] Sheeba A and Seilan A 2010 Health care system in India: an overview *International Issues on Health Economics and Management* (New Delhi: TISSL International Publications) pp 215–8

[11] Singh M and Jyani G Indian health system & healthcare financing *A Handbook of Health System Costing* (Chandigarh and New Delhi: HTA Regional Resource Centre, Department of Community Medicine and School of Public Health, PGIMER and HTA in India, Department of Health Research, Ministry of Health and Family Welfare) pp 17–26

[12] Chauhan L S 2011 Public health in India: issues and challenges *Indian J. Public Health* **55** 88–91

[13] Preetha G S 2019 *Private Healthcare Sector—A Vibrant Force in Indian Healthcare Industry* (New Delhi: IIHMR) https://iihmrdelhi.edu.in/uploads/articles/pdf/private-health-care-sector.pdf

[14] Pawar P, Parolia N, Shinde S, Edoh T O and Singh M 2022 eHealthChain—a blockchain-based personal health information management system *Ann. Telecommun.* **77** 1–13

[15] Minopoulos G M, Memos V A, Stergiou C L, Stergiou K D, Plageras A P, Koidou M P and Psannis K E 2022 Exploitation of emerging technologies and advanced networks for a smart healthcare system *Appl. Sci.* **12** 5859

[16] Efthymiou-Egleton I-P, Sidiropoulos S, Kritas D, Vozikis A, Rapti P and Souliotis K 2020 AI transforming healthcare management during COVID-19 pandemic *HAPSc Policy Briefs Ser* **1** 130–8

[17] Nahavandi D, Alizadehsani R, Khosravi A and Acharya U R 2022 Application of artificial intelligence in wearable devices: opportunities and challenges *Comput. Methods Programs Biomed.* **213** 106541

[18] Manickam P, Mariappan S A, Murugesan S M, Hansda S, Kaushik A, Shinde R and Thipperudraswamy S P 2022 Artificial intelligence (AI) and internet of medical things (IoMT) assisted biomedical systems for intelligent healthcare *Biosensors* **12** 562

[19] Kamruzzaman M M, Alrashdi I and Alqazzaz A 2022 New opportunities, challenges, and applications of edge-AI for connected healthcare in internet of medical things for smart cities *J. Healthc. Eng.* **2022** 2950699 (retracted)

[20] Jabbar R, Fetais N, Krichen M and Barkaoui K 2020 Blockchain technology for healthcare: enhancing shared electronic health record interoperability and integrity *2020 IEEE Int. Conf. on Informatics, IoT, and Enabling Technologies (ICIoT)* (Piscataway, NJ: IEEE) pp 310–7

[21] Giri A, Chatterjee S, Paul P, Chakraborty S and Biswas S 2019 Impact of smart applications of IoMT (internet of medical things) on health-care domain in India *Int. J. Recent Technol. Eng.* **8** 1–15

[22] Karthick G S and Pankajavalli P B 2020 A review on human healthcare internet of things: a technical perspective *SN Comput. Sci.* **1** 198

[23] Amin S U and Hossain M S 2020 Edge intelligence and internet of things in healthcare: a survey *IEEE Access* **9** 45–59

[24] Panch T, Szolovits P and Atun R 2018 Artificial intelligence, machine learning and health systems *J. Glob. Health* **8** 020303

[25] Basatneh R, Najafi B and Armstrong D G 2018 Health sensors, smart home devices, and the internet of medical things: an opportunity for dramatic improvement in care for the lower extremity complications of diabetes *J. Diabetes Sci. Technol.* **12** 577–86

[26] de Kleijn M, Siebert M and Huggett S 2019 Artificial intelligence: how knowledge is created, transferred and used *IFLA WLIC 2019* https://library.ifla.org/id/eprint/2814/1/s02-2019-dekleijn-en.pdf

[27] Tran B X, Vu G T, Ha G H, Vuong Q-H, Ho M-T, Vuong T-T, La V-P *et al* 2019 Global evolution of research in artificial intelligence in health and medicine: a bibliometric study *J. Clin. Med.* **8** 360

[28] Alaskar K M, Tamboli F A, Memon S A, Gulavani S S, Mudalkar P K, Desai V V, Rasal P R, Tandale P G and Gaikwad D T 2022 Artificial intelligence (AI) in healthcare management *J. Pharmaceut. Neg. Res.* **13** 1011–20

[29] Gillies R J, Kinahan P E and Hricak H 2016 Radiomics: images are more than pictures, they are data *Radiology* **278** 563–77

[30] Hatt M, Tixier F, Visvikis D and Cheze Le Rest C 2017 Radiomics in PET/CT: more than meets the eye? *J. Nucl. Med.* **58** 365–6

[31] Krittanawong C, Tunhasiriwet A, Zhang H J, Wang Z, Aydar M and Kitai T 2017 Deep learning with unsupervised feature in echocardiographic imaging *J. Am. Coll. Cardiol.* **69** 2100–1
[32] Janowczyk A and Madabhushi A 2016 Deep learning for digital pathology image analysis: a comprehensive tutorial with selected use cases *J. Pathol. Inform.* **7** 29
[33] Mobadersany P, Yousefi S, Amgad M, Gutman D A, Barnholtz-Sloan J S, Velázquez Vega J E, Brat D J and Cooper L A D 2018 Predicting cancer outcomes from histology and genomics using convolutional networks *Proc. Natl. Acad. Sci.* **115** E2970–9
[34] Corredor G, Wang X, Zhou Y, Lu C, Fu P, Syrigos K, Rimm D L *et al* 2019 Spatial architecture and arrangement of tumor-infiltrating lymphocytes for predicting likelihood of recurrence in early-stage non-small cell lung cancer *Clin. Cancer Res.* **25** 1526–34
[35] Fiorini N, Leaman R, Lipman D J and Lu Z 2018 How user intelligence is improving PubMed *Nat. Biotechnol.* **36** 937–45
[36] Lee C S and Lee A Y 2020 How artificial intelligence can transform randomized controlled trials *Transl. Vis. Sci. Technol.* **9** 9
[37] Mooney S J and Pejaver V 2018 Big data in public health: terminology, machine learning, and privacy *Annu. Rev. Public Health* **39** 95–112
[38] Maharana A and Nsoesie E O 2018 Use of deep learning to examine the association of the built environment with prevalence of neighborhood adult obesity *JAMA Netw. Open* **1** e181535
[39] Schwalbe N and Wahl B 2020 Artificial intelligence and the future of global health *Lancet* **395** 1579–86
[40] Park C-W, Seo S W, Kang N, Ko B S, Choi B W, Park C M, Chang D K *et al* 2020 Artificial intelligence in health care: current applications and issues *J. Korean Med. Sci.* **35** e379
[41] Farhud D D and Zokaei S 2021 Ethical issues of artificial intelligence in medicine and healthcare *Iran. J. Public Health* **50** i
[42] Varkey B 2021 Principles of clinical ethics and their application to practice *Med. Princ. Pract.* **30** 17–28
[43] Farhud D 2019 Epigenetic and ethics: how are ethical traits inherited ? *Int. J. Ethics Soc.* **1** 1–4 https://ijethics.com/article-1–53-en.html
[44] Matheny M E, Whicher D and Israni S T 2020 Artificial intelligence in health care: a report from the National Academy of Medicine *JAMA* **323** 509–10
[45] Sharma A 2021 Artificial intelligence in health care *Int. J. Humanit. Arts Med. Sci.* **5** 106–9
[46] Huang G and Foysal A A 2021 Blockchain in healthcare *Technol. Invest.* **12** 168–81
[47] Siyal A A, Junejo A Z, Zawish M, Ahmed K, Khalil A and Soursou G 2019 Applications of blockchain technology in medicine and healthcare: challenges and future perspectives *Cryptography* **3** 3
[48] Hölbl M, Kompara M, Kamišalić A and Nemec Zlatolas L 2018 A systematic review of the use of blockchain in healthcare *Symmetry* **10** 470
[49] Idrees S M, Nowostawski M, Jameel R and Mourya A K 2021 Security aspects of blockchain technology intended for industrial applications *Electronics* **10** 951
[50] Haleem A, Javaid M, Singh R P, Suman R and Rab S 2021 Blockchain technology applications in healthcare: an overview *Int. J. Intell. Networks* **2** 130–9
[51] Tariq N, Qamar A, Asim M and Khan F A 2020 Blockchain and smart healthcare security: a survey *Procedia Comput. Sci.* **175** 615–20

[52] Kamruzzaman M M, Yan B, Sarker M N I, Alruwaili O, Wu M and Alrashdi I 2022 Blockchain and fog computing in IoT-driven healthcare services for smart cities *J. Healthc. Eng.* **2022** 9957888
[53] Wenhua Z, Qamar F, Abdali T-A N, Hassan R, Jafri S T A and Nguyen Q N 2023 Blockchain technology: security issues, healthcare applications, challenges and future trends *Electronics* **12** 546
[54] Abu-Elezz I, Hassan A, Nazeemudeen A, Househ M and Abd-Alrazaq A 2020 The benefits and threats of blockchain technology in healthcare: a scoping review *Int. J. Med. Inform.* **142** 104246
[55] Varshney A, Garg N, Nagla K S, Nair T S, Jaiswal S K, Yadav S and Aswal D K 2021 Challenges in sensors technology for industry 4.0 for futuristic metrological applications *Mapan* **36** 215–26
[56] Farouk A, Alahmadi A, Ghose S and Mashatan A 2020 Blockchain platform for industrial healthcare: vision and future opportunities *Comput. Commun.* **154** 223–35
[57] Mamun Q 2022 Blockchain technology in the future of healthcare *Smart Health* **23** 1–9 (retracted)
[58] Torrey T 2011 Electronic health records and electronic medical records—EHRs and EMRs. Patient empowerment at About.com—teaching patients to take charge for their health and medical care http://patients.about.com/od/electronicpatientrecords/a/emr.htm (accessed 20 February 2012)
[59] Seymour T, Frantsvog D and Graeber T 2012 Electronic health records (EHR) *Am. J. Health Sci.* **3** 201–10
[60] Malasinghe L P, Ramzan N and Dahal K 2019 Remote patient monitoring: a comprehensive study *J. Ambient Intell. Humaniz. Comput.* **10** 57–76
[61] Singh R K, Kumar R and Kumar P 2016 Strategic issues in pharmaceutical supply chains: a review *Int. J. Pharm. Healthc. Mark.* **10** 234–57
[62] Goodarzian F, Wamba S F, Mathiyazhagan K and Taghipour A 2021 A new bi-objective green medicine supply chain network design under fuzzy environment: hybrid metaheuristic algorithms *Comput. Ind. Eng.* **160** 107535
[63] George S and Elrashid S 2023 Inventory management and pharmaceutical supply chain performance of hospital pharmacies in Bahrain: a structural equation modeling approach *SAGE Open* **13** 21582440221149717
[64] Kapoor D, Vyas R B and Dadarwal D 2018 An overview on pharmaceutical supply chain: a next step towards good manufacturing practice *Drug Des. Int. Prop. Int. J.* **1** 107
[65] Ben Fekih R and Lahami M 2020 Application of blockchain technology in healthcare: a comprehensive study *The Impact of Digital Technologies on Public Health in Developed and Developing Countries: 18th Int. Conf., ICOST 2020 (June 24–26, 2020, Hammamet, Tunisia)* (Cham: Springer International Publishing) pp 268–76
[66] Ekblaw A, Azaria A, Halamka J D and Lippman A 2016 MedRec: using blockchain for medical data access and permission management *2016 2nd International Conference on Open and Big Data (OBD)* (Piscataway, NJ: IEEE) pp 25–30
[67] Xia Q I, Sifah E B, Asamoah K O, Gao J, Du X and Guizani M 2017 MeDShare: trustless medical data sharing among cloud service providers via blockchain *IEEE Access* **5** 14757–67
[68] Roehrs A, Da Costa C A and da Rosa Righi R 2017 OmniPHR: a distributed architecture model to integrate personal health records *J. Biomed. Inform.* **71** 70–81

[69] Zhang P, White J, Schmidt D C, Lenz G and Rosenbloom S T 2018 FHIRChain: applying blockchain to securely and scalably share clinical data *Comput. Struct. Biotechnol. J.* **16** 267–78

[70] Fan K, Wang S, Ren Y, Li H and Yang Y 2018 Medblock: efficient and secure medical data sharing via blockchain *J. Med. Syst.* **42** 1–11

[71] Jiang S, Cao J, Wu H, Yang Y, Ma M and He J 2018 Blochie: a blockchain-based platform for healthcare information exchange *2018 Int. Conf. on Smart Computing (Smartcomp)* (Piscataway, NJ: IEEE) pp 49–56

[72] Dagher G G, Mohler J, Milojkovic M and Marella P B 2018 Ancile: privacy-preserving framework for access control and interoperability of electronic health records using blockchain technology *Sustain. Cities Soc.* **39** 283–97

[73] Ichikawa D, Kashiyama M and Ueno T 2017 Tamper-resistant mobile health using blockchain technology *JMIR Mhealth Uhealth* **5** e7938

[74] Griggs K N, Ossipova O, Kohlios C P, Baccarini A N, Howson E A and Hayajneh T 2018 Healthcare blockchain system using smart contracts for secure automated remote patient monitoring *J. Med. Syst.* **42** 1

[75] Ray P P, Dash D, Salah K and Kumar N 2020 Blockchain for IoT-based healthcare: background, consensus, platforms, and use cases *IEEE Syst. J.* **15** 85–94

[76] Bocek T, Rodrigues B B, Strasser T and Stiller B 2017 Blockchains everywhere-a use-case of blockchains in the pharma supply-chain *2017 IFIP/IEEE Symp. on Integrated Network and Service Management (IM)* (Piscataway, NJ: IEEE) pp 772–7

[77] Bryatov S R and Borodinov A A 2019 Blockchain technology in the pharmaceutical supply chain: researching a business model based on hyperledger fabric *Proc. of the Int. Conf. on Information Technology and Nanotechnology (ITNT)* vol 10 *(Samara, Russia)* pp 1613–0073 https://ceur-ws.org/Vol-2416/paper18.pdf

[78] Zhou L, Wang L and Sun Y 2018 MIStore: a blockchain-based medical insurance storage system *J. Med. Syst.* **42** 149

[79] Islam M M, Rahaman A and Islam M R 2020 Development of smart healthcare monitoring system in IoT environment *SN Comput. Sci.* **1** 1–11

[80] Sundaravadivel P, Kougianos E, Mohanty S P and Ganapathiraju M K 2017 Everything you wanted to know about smart health care: evaluating the different technologies and components of the internet of things for better health *IEEE Consum. Electron. Mag.* **7** 18–28

[81] Anjali K, Anand R, Prabhu S D and Geethu R S 2021 IoT based smart healthcare system to detect and alert covid symptom *2021 6th Int. Conf. on Communication and Electronics Systems (ICCES)* (Piscataway, NJ: IEEE) pp 685–92

[82] Ahmad S, Abdeljaber H A M, Nazeer J, Uddin M Y, Lingamuthu V and Kaur A 2022 Issues of clinical identity verification for healthcare applications over mobile terminal platform *Wirel. Commun. Mob. Comput.* **2022** 1–10

[83] Khan H A, Abdulla R, Selvaperumal S K and Bathich A 2021 IoT based on secure personal healthcare using RFID technology and steganography *Int. J. Electr. Comput. Eng.* **11** 3300

[84] Razdan S and Sharma S 2021 Internet of medical things (IoMT): overview, emerging technologies, and case studies *IETE Tech. Rev.* **39** 775–88

[85] Subhan F, Mirza A, Su'ud M B M, Alam M M, Nisar S, Habib U and Iqbal M Z 2023 AI-enabled wearable medical internet of things in healthcare system: a survey *Appl. Sci.* **13** 1934

[86] Islam S M R, Kwak D, Kabir M D H, Hossain M and Kwak K-S 2015 The internet of things for health care: a comprehensive survey *IEEE Access* **3** 678–708
[87] Alshamrani M 2022 IoT and artificial intelligence implementations for remote healthcare monitoring systems: a survey *J. King Saud Univ.-Comput. Inf. Sci.* **34** 4687–701
[88] Kang J J and Larkin H 2017 Intelligent personal health devices converged with internet of things networks *J. Mob. Multimed.* **12** 197–212
[89] Lizhong Z 2014 Patient body temperature monitoring system and device based on Internet of Things *China Patent Specification* CN103577688A
[90] Milacski Z Á, Ludersdorfer M, Lőrincz A and van der Smagt P 2015 Robust detection of anomalies via sparse methods *Neural Information Processing (ICONIP 2015)* (Cham: Springer International Publishing) pp 419–26
[91] Nazir S, Ali Y, Ullah N and García-Magariño I 2019 Internet of things for healthcare using effects of mobile computing: a systematic literature review *Wirel. Commun. Mob. Comput.* **2019** 1–20
[92] Green M S, Mathew J J, Venkatesh A G, Green P and Tariq R 2018 Utilization of smartphone applications by anesthesia providers *Anesthesiol. Res. Pract.* **2018** 8694357
[93] Qadri Y A, Nauman A, Zikria Y B, Vasilakos A V and Kim S W 2020 The future of healthcare internet of things: a survey of emerging technologies *IEEE Commun. Surv. Tutor.* **22** 1121–67
[94] Okazaki K, Okazaki K, Uesugi M, Matsusima T and Hataya H 2022 Evaluation of the accuracy of a non-invasive hemoglobin-monitoring device in schoolchildren *Pediatr. Neonatol.* **63** 19–24
[95] Laranjo I, Macedo J and Santos A 2013 Internet of things for medication control: e-health architecture and service implementation *Int. J. Reliab. Qual. E-Healthc.* **2** 1–15
[96] Dwivedi R, Mehrotra D and Chandra S 2022 Potential of internet of medical things (IoMT) applications in building a smart healthcare system: a systematic review *J. Oral Biol. Craniofac. Res.* **12** 302–18
[97] Kumar S, Tiwari P and Zymbler M 2019 Internet of Things is a revolutionary approach for future technology enhancement: a review *J Big Data* **6** 111
[98] Pradhan B, Bhattacharyya S and Pal K 2021 IoT-based applications in healthcare devices *J. Healthc. Eng.* **2021** 1–18
[99] Joyia G J, Liaqat R M, Farooq A and Rehman S 2017 Internet of medical things (IoMT): applications, benefits and future challenges in healthcare domain *J. Commun.* **12** 240–7
[100] Rashmi I R, Sahana M K, Sangeetha R and Shruthi K S 2020 IOT based patient health monitoring system to remote doctors using embedded technology *Int. J. Eng. Res. Technol.* **8** 230–3
[101] Vahdati M, Gholizadeh HamlAbadi K and Saghiri A M 2021 IoT-based healthcare monitoring using blockchain *Applications of Blockchain in Healthcare. Studies in Big Data* (Singapore: Springer) pp 141–70
[102] Mamdiwar S D, Shakruwala Z, Chadha U, Srinivasan K and Chang C-Y 2021 Recent advances on IoT-assisted wearable sensor systems for healthcare monitoring *Biosensors* **11** 372
[103] Majumder S, Mondal T and Deen M J 2017 Wearable sensors for remote health monitoring *Sensors* **17** 130

Chapter 3

The role of high-performance computing in processing electronic healthcare records

Govind Prasad, Ayan Banerjee and Khushboo Rani

In recent years, the integration of electronic health records (EHRs) and Internet of Things (IoT) devices has transformed healthcare worldwide. This development is particularly promising for rural areas, where access to quality healthcare remains a major challenge. Research shows that patients in rural India could benefit from using IoT devices to improve healthcare, and EHRs can improve the quality of care in these areas. Indian physicians are more satisfied with EHR use than those in developed countries, highlighting an important area of technological development. This study is a valuable resource for EHR designers and organizations implementing EHRs, as it discusses the management of data flows in healthcare environments. Because provider satisfaction with EHR systems is primarily related to the systems' ability to facilitate communication with patients and care teams, it is imperative that designers and vendors focus on creating user-centered systems. Interoperability and connectivity should be seen not only as challenges but also as innovative design opportunities. The study also found that greater satisfaction is associated with the positive impact of EHRs on patient access to and management of care information flows [1–6]. Future research should seek to improve the development and implementation of electronic charts to increase efficiency, reduce errors, and achieve optimal satisfaction among participants in the healthcare process. This motivation underscores the need for continuous EHR technology improvement to better serve healthcare providers and patients, particularly in underserved rural communities.

3.1 Introduction

In the 1960s, the problem-oriented medical record (POMR) developed by Larry Weed introduced the use of electronic methods to record patient information, leading to the creation of the first electronic medical record (EMR) in 1972 at the Institute of Records [1–5]. This innovation marked the beginning of change in

doi:10.1088/978-0-7503-5964-1ch3

healthcare, paving the way for the widespread adoption of advanced technological tools such as EHR, telehealth services, health analytics, and patient-centered innovations. These systems have fundamentally changed the healthcare landscape, enabling seamless data exchange, optimizing treatment protocols, and providing actionable insights for patients and healthcare providers. In particular, EHRs have become essential for healthcare professionals, facilitating access to comprehensive patient information and improving clinical decision-making and care coordination in a variety of settings [6–10]. Telehealth and telecare services have further revolutionized healthcare by overcoming geographic barriers and providing convenient access to medical knowledge, especially in underserved communities. In addition, the integration of healthcare analytics and big data has improved decision-making processes, enabling healthcare organizations to identify trends, predict outcomes, and allocate resources more effectively. Patient-centric innovations, such as mobile health apps and wearables, promote collaboration and personalized care and enable people to actively participate in their healthcare [7–12]. Despite these advances, several challenges remain, including data interoperability, security, and privacy. Addressing these challenges is critical to the safe and effective implementation of electronic health systems. This chapter mainly addresses existing research spaces by examining factors influencing healthcare provider satisfaction with EHR systems, particularly in rural and urban settings, and exploring the broader impact on patient outcomes and organizational effectiveness [9, 13–17]. Motivated by the imperative to enhance healthcare in underserved regions, this chapter offers a thorough examination of current technologies, tackles persistent obstacles, and showcases case studies illustrating the profound changes brought about by these advancements. In addition, it delves into forthcoming trends in health informatics, including artificial intelligence (AI), precision medicine, and the IoT, which hold the potential to establish a more interconnected and patient-focused healthcare ecosystem. By addressing these elements, this chapter aims to inform EHR designers and healthcare organizations about best practices for the effective implementation and continuous improvement of eHealth systems [18–25].

3.2 Foundation of electronic healthcare systems

Electronic health systems are built on a framework of technology, infrastructure, and procedures that facilitate the collection, storage, and exchange of EHRs and other important patient data. These systems are designed primarily to improve the quality and efficiency of healthcare, simplify administrative tasks, and strengthen decision-making based on evidence [26]. At the core of electronic health systems is the adoption of EHRs, which serve as a digital platform for storing and retrieving patient information. These EHR systems replace traditional paper-based systems, improving the efficiency, accuracy, and accessibility of patient information. Electronic health systems are based on the principles of technology and information management [27]. They seamlessly integrate patient data, clinical documentation, and management functions to streamline healthcare workflows and improve patient outcomes.

3.2.1 State of electronic health records

The adoption of EHR has experienced a notable surge in recent years, primarily fueled by governmental initiatives and regulations aimed at fostering the integration of technology within the healthcare sector. EHRs function as a centralized hub for storing and accessing patient data, streamlining communication among healthcare professionals, and assisting in clinical decision-making [4, 5]. Their implementation has become pervasive across healthcare institutions, with the majority transitioning from traditional paper-based records to electronic formats.

Beyond merely streamlining communication among healthcare providers, EHRs have also played a pivotal role in augmenting patient involvement and their ability to access personal health information. Essentially, EHRs now serve as the cornerstone of contemporary healthcare systems, offering a comprehensive overview of a patient's medical history and treatment strategies. Nonetheless, challenges such as interoperability and obstacles in data exchange persist, impeding the full realization of EHRs' potential [28–31].

3.2.2 Optimization of care delivery

Electronic health systems represent a change in the field of medicine and offer a versatile approach to optimizing care. These systems are a cornerstone in improving communication and coordination between healthcare providers and are revolutionizing the landscape of patient care [6–8]. The integration of EHR and other digital platforms enables healthcare organizations to streamline clinical workflows, minimize errors, and promote collaboration between different healthcare facilities. One of the main advantages of electronic healthcare systems is their ability to facilitate seamless operations and communication between health professionals and patients. By centralizing patient information in an electronic database, these systems allow clinicians to access critical information in real time, regardless of their location [26]. The rapid exchange of information fosters informed decision-making and guarantees that every member of the care team possesses the latest patient information. In addition, electronic health systems play a key role in reducing medical errors—a long-standing challenge in the healthcare industry.

EHR systems contribute to minimizing adverse events and enhancing patient safety by offering functionalities such as automated drug reporting and reminders for preventive care. These systems aid in identifying potential risks associated with medications through automated reporting, thus reducing the occurrence of adverse drug events. In addition, they prompt healthcare providers with reminders for preventive care measures, ensuring timely interventions and follow-ups, which further contribute to patient safety by preventing complications and medical errors. Overall, EHR systems play a crucial role in improving patient safety by leveraging features such as automated drug reporting and preventive care reminders. Such systems also help to standardize care protocols and further minimize errors through the standardization of documentation practices and the introduction of clinical decision support tools. In addition, eHealth systems enable healthcare organizations to identify and capitalize on opportunities and improve quality and nursing effectiveness. Using

Table 3.1. Utilization of EHRs in different hospitals.

EHR utilization	Hospital A ($n = 70$)		Hospital B ($n = 60$)		Hospital C(n=50)		Total ($n = 180$)		Chi-square	p-value
	NO.	%	NO.	%	NO.	%	NO.	%		
Chart review										
Obtain and review lab results	66	96	59	87.2	29	65	152	63	16.99	0.002
Obtain and review radiology results	50	87	53	46	26	25	120	0.40	23	0.817
Obtain and review other test results	36	74	35	57	25	77	114	25	12.64	0.000
Create and review scanned documents	67	56.2	44	86	32	78	95	82	3.25	0.512
Decision support										
Receive drug interaction alerts	40	65	52	102	60	50	109	60	15	0.35
Clinical guidelines	45	72	31	20	52	25	96	46	6	0.005
Order entry										
Enter lab orders	57	86	13	20	65	50	22.35	92	50	0.000

data analytics and performance metrics, these systems allow providers to identify areas for improvement and implement evidence-based initiatives. Whether optimizing resource allocation, implementing best practices, or identifying trends in public health, eHealth systems are invaluable tools for continuous quality improvement. Indeed, effective eHealth systems are the cornerstone of modern healthcare, leveraging technology to optimize patient care levels. By simplifying communication, reducing errors, and promoting quality improvement efforts, these systems can transform the way healthcare is delivered, ultimately leading to better patient outcomes and treatment efficiency. The utilization of EHRs in different hospitals is reported in table 3.1 [2].

3.2.3 Economic and quality incentives

The adoption of electronic health systems is often driven by a combination of financial and quality incentives that lead healthcare organizations to embrace technological advances. These incentives include a variety of goals, such as reducing healthcare costs, improving patient outcomes, and improving overall patient satisfaction. When healthcare providers understand the potential financial benefits, such as reduced costs, increased revenue, and the promise of improved quality, they are more inclined to invest in and use advanced eHealth systems.

By streamlining administrative processes, minimizing documentation errors, and improving operational efficiency, these systems can bring significant savings to healthcare organizations. In addition, electronic systems facilitate better management of resources, reduce unnecessary expenses, and optimize budget allocation. At the same time, improving the quality of care serves as a compelling incentive for healthcare organizations to adopt electronic health systems. With features such as EMRs, clinical decision support tools, and telemedicine capabilities, these systems enable healthcare providers to provide more accurate diagnoses, personalized treatment plans, and timely interventions [15]. As a result, the adoption of electronic health systems has been associated with improved clinical outcomes, such as reduced medical errors, hospital readmissions, and patient safety. Furthermore, electronic health systems are pivotal in enhancing patient satisfaction, an aspect increasingly acknowledged as integral to healthcare. By offering convenient access to patient information, facilitating communication with healthcare providers, and enabling remote monitoring and telehealth services, these systems empower patients to take a more proactive role in managing their healthcare. As a result, healthcare organizations are increasingly motivated to adopt electronic systems that can track and improve patient outcomes, improve care coordination, and demonstrate value to payers and patients. By leveraging advanced technology, healthcare providers can achieve cost savings, improve clinical outcomes, and improve patient satisfaction, ultimately contributing to the delivery of high-quality, value-based care [9–12].

3.2.4 Data interoperability and exchange

Data interoperability and exchange play essential roles in eHealth systems, facilitating the smooth transfer of patient data among various healthcare providers and systems. Interoperable data can enhance care coordination, bolster patient safety, and contribute to population health initiatives. Interoperability of health information is crucial for the smooth communication and exchange of patient information between different healthcare providers, as reported in table 3.2. Electronic health systems need to be meticulously designed to guarantee data

Table 3.2. EHR adoption across healthcare settings.

Data source	Sample size	References
Single psychiatric unit	310 511	8396
Specialized center/clinic	2 537 909,773	1845
Prison network	477–48,565	9
Centralized anonymized repository	8 709 233 844	39 101
Multiple primary care practices	7 925 345 143	2283
Multiple hospitals	923–5 244 402	4473
Single hospital	467–55 492	7600
Consortium	7 820 320 133	1000

interoperability, facilitating secure and efficient sharing of patient information. Interoperability and data exchange are critical facets of electronic health systems, allowing for the smooth transfer of patient data across diverse healthcare settings. Standards such as HL7 and Fast Healthcare Interoperability Resources (FHIR) facilitate data exchange, leading to more coordinated and personalized care. High-performance computing (HPC) in the field of EHR data interoperability and exchange has enormous potential to revolutionize healthcare, as follows:

1. Speed and efficiency: HPC enables rapid processing and analysis of massive EHR data, enabling healthcare providers to quickly access critical information. This speed is important in emergencies where timely decisions can save lives.
2. Interoperability: HPC promotes interoperability by establishing standard data formats and protocols, enabling smooth communication and data exchange among various healthcare systems. This interoperability is crucial for providing coordinated care across health services and enhancing patient outcomes.
3. Data integration: HPC can be used to integrate and jointly analyze different sources of EHR data, such as clinical notes, laboratory results, imaging scans, and genomic data. This comprehensive review of patient data empowers healthcare professionals to make more informed decisions and tailor care to individual patient needs.
4. Advanced analytics: HPC facilitates the application of sophisticated analytics methods, such as machine learning and AI, to extract valuable insights from EHR data. These insights play a pivotal role in guiding personalized medicine initiatives, identifying patterns in diseases, forecasting patient outcomes, and enhancing the efficient allocation of treatment resources.
5. Security and privacy: HPC systems have the capability to incorporate robust security protocols to safeguard sensitive EHR data from unauthorized access and cyber threats. Through the deployment of technologies such as encryption, access control, and anomaly detection, HPC systems contribute to maintaining compliance with data protection and healthcare regulations.
6. Scalability: HPC architectures are highly scalable, enabling healthcare organizations to efficiently process increasing amounts of EHR data. As healthcare demand grows and new data sources emerge, HPC systems can adapt and scale to meet these changing needs.
7. Research and Innovation: HPC enables healthcare researchers and innovators to conduct large-scale research and simulations using EHR data. By utilizing computing resources, researchers can accelerate the pace of medical discovery, develop new treatments, and streamline clinical workflows.

In general, the integration of HPC with EHRs can significantly advance data interoperability and exchange, thus improving patient care, healthcare, and medical research. However, it is important to address data standardization, data privacy issues, and resource constraints to fully benefit from HPC in healthcare.

3.2.5 Telehealth and remote care

Telehealth and remote care technologies are expanding access to healthcare services, allowing patients to receive care from anywhere at any time. These technologies can enhance patient convenience, reduce healthcare costs, and improve outcomes for patients with chronic conditions or limited mobility, as shown in figure 3.1. Telehealth and remote care have become increasingly popular with the rise of electronic healthcare systems. Telehealth platforms allow patients to receive healthcare remotely, decreasing the necessity for physical appointments and enhancing access to healthcare services. Particularly as a result of the COVID-19 pandemic, telehealth and remote care technologies have experienced notable growth. They facilitate remote consultations, monitoring, and treatment, thereby enhancing access to care and convenience for patients. Since the COVID-19 pandemic, telehealth and remote care have emerged as essential components of modern healthcare delivery.

By facilitating patients to receive virtual medical advice, monitoring, and support, these technologies decrease the necessity for in-person visits and enhance healthcare accessibility, especially in underserved or remote areas. Through the utilization of various technologies such as wearable devices, smartphone applications, and video conferencing, telehealth and remote care platforms facilitate seamless and instant communication between patients and healthcare providers. These advancements hold the potential to significantly enhance patient outcomes, boost operational

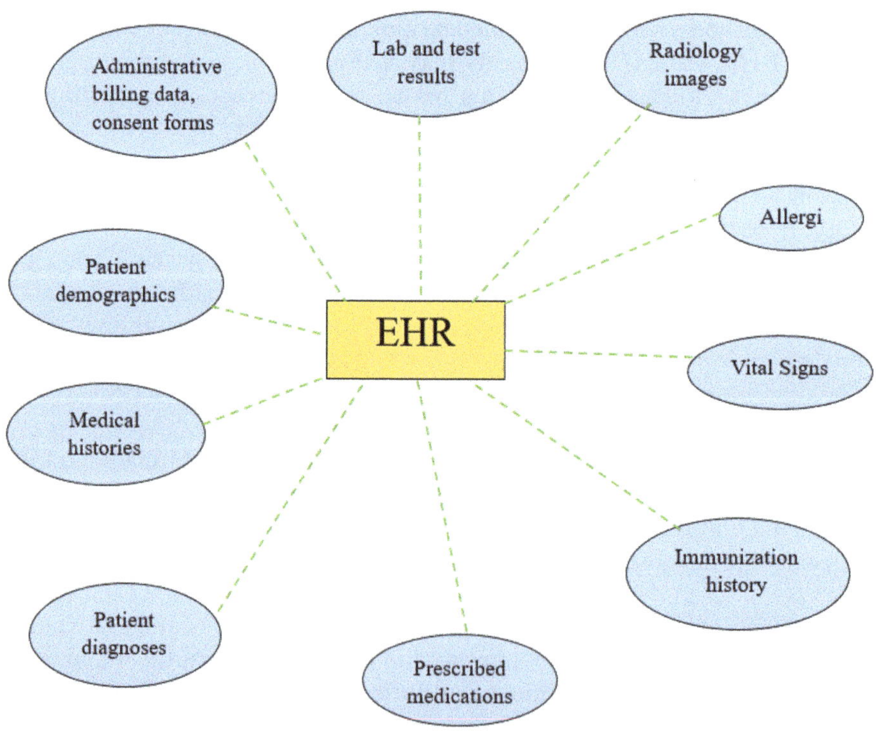

Figure 3.1. Tactics for enhancing EHR efficiency.

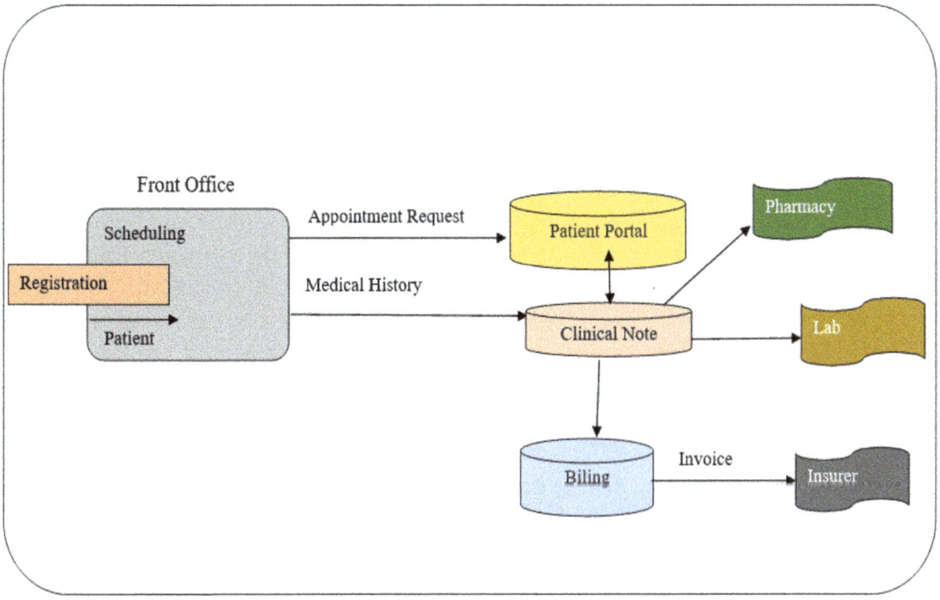

Figure 3.2. Schematic representation of an EHR system.

efficiency, and lower healthcare expenses by functioning outside traditional clinical environments. In addition, HPC has transformed the management and analysis of EHRs, empowering healthcare providers to process vast amounts of patient data swiftly and accurately.

By harnessing the computational power of HPC systems, healthcare organizations can obtain valuable insights from EHRs, ranging from identifying trends in patient care to predicting disease outcomes. This not only enhances patient care by facilitating more informed decision-making but also supports medical research and innovation. In addition, HPC plays a crucial role in advancing telehealth and remote care initiatives, enabling healthcare professionals to remotely monitor and provide care to patients in real time, regardless of geographic location. This fosters greater accessibility to healthcare services, especially for individuals in remote or underserved areas, while also promoting continuity of care and patient engagement. Through the convergence of HPC and healthcare, we are witnessing a transformative shift toward personalized, efficient, and equitable healthcare delivery. The diagram in figure 3.2 illustrates the workflow of an EHR system.

3.3 Healthcare analytics and big data

Healthcare analytics and big data represent powerful catalysts for transformation in healthcare and management. The exponential growth of data produced in the healthcare industry, ranging from EHRs to patient demographics and treatment outcomes, presents a huge opportunity to obtain valuable information that can revolutionize various aspects of healthcare. Integration is at the heart of this initiative. Thanks to healthcare analytics and big data, service providers can extract meaningful insights from huge data sets. This knowledge can be an invaluable tool in clinical decisions, improving population health strategies and optimizing the efficiency of health organizations [9, 10].

One of the most important areas where health analytics and big data will have a significant impact is eHealth systems. Using advanced analytics techniques, healthcare providers can gain a deep understanding of patient populations, identify trends in healthcare, and identify areas ripe for improvement. For example, analytics can help identify patterns in patient outcomes, allowing providers to more effectively tailor care and improve the overall quality of care. In addition, the power of big data analytics extends beyond the treatment of individual patients to the broader population. Using health trends obtained by analyzing large data sets, healthcare organizations can identify common health problems in certain populations, predict disease epidemics, and more effectively allocate resources to public health needs. In addition, healthcare organizations can optimize their performance using analytics and big data. A flow diagram of a backend database for EHRs is shown in figure 3.3.

By analyzing information about patient flows, staffing, and equipment usage, providers can identify inefficiencies and implement targeted actions to improve workflow and reduce costs. Finally, the integration of analytics and big data into healthcare systems enables organizations to make data-driven decisions, thereby improving ongoing maintenance. By leveraging the wealth of information available to them, healthcare providers can improve patient outcomes, improve population health, and ensure that resources are effectively allocated to meet the changing needs of their communities, as reported in table 3.3. A significant portion of the survey respondents (doctors) described in table 3.3 were aged 50 or above (70.32%), practiced as primary care specialists (54.34%), and operated within individual practice settings (47.03%) [7–12].

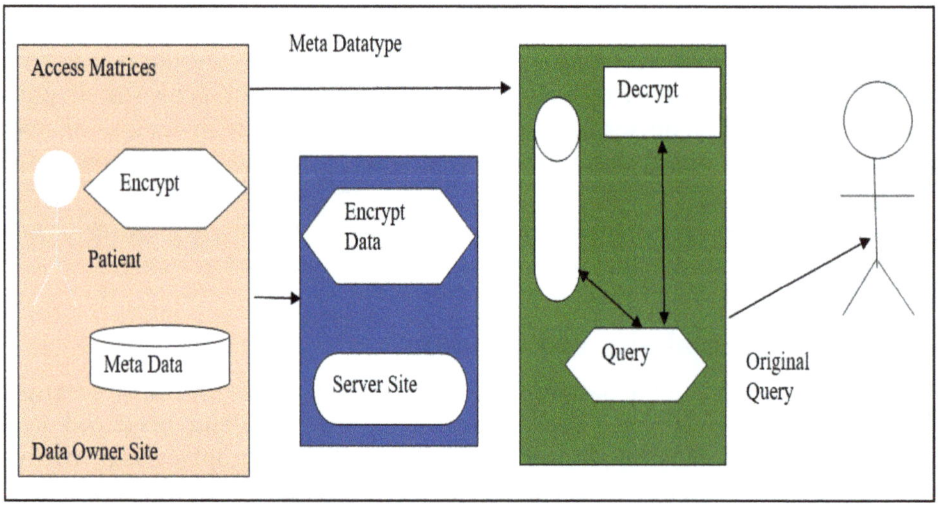

Figure 3.3. A backend database for EHRs.

Table 3.3. Characteristics of the respondents surveyed regarding EHRs.

	Variables	Percentage
Sex	Female	25%
	Male	75%
Age	< 50 yrs old	30%
	⩾ 50 yrs old	70%
Specialty	Primary care	54.34%
	Surgical specialty	20.55%
	Medical specialty	25.11%
Medical degree	MD	94%
	Do	6%
Practice size	2 practices	37%
	More than 2 physicians	63%

Table 3.4. Influence of characteristics of computerized systems on physicians' satisfaction with EHR systems.

Services included and characteristics	Satisfaction		Odds ratio (OR)		p-value
'Patient access feature?'	No	Yes (%)	No (%)	NA	0.128
Can patients download records?	Yes	41%	60%	3.68	0.0002
Does EHR allow patient data sharing?	No	22%	58%	NA	0.005
'Patient data upload?'	No	33%	66%	4.22	0.0004
EHR meaningful use compliance?	Yes	12.5%	87%	NA	0.13

Doctors' satisfaction with EHRs was notably influenced by particular service attributes. Their satisfaction levels were higher when EHR systems helped patients to access, download, and share their medical records online, along with the capability to upload health data from various devices or applications. Interestingly, compliance with certification standards did not significantly impact their satisfaction, as highlighted in table 3.4.

3.3.1 Patient-centered innovations

The field of eHealth systems is increasingly emphasizing patient-centered innovations that aim to change the way individuals participate in their health journey. These innovations are carefully designed not only to facilitate the active participation of patients in healthcare but also to promote better communication channels between patients and healthcare providers, as shown in figure 3.4. By prioritizing the patient's role in care delivery, these revolutionary technologies strive to elevate patient satisfaction and, ultimately, enhance health results. A pivotal avenue for

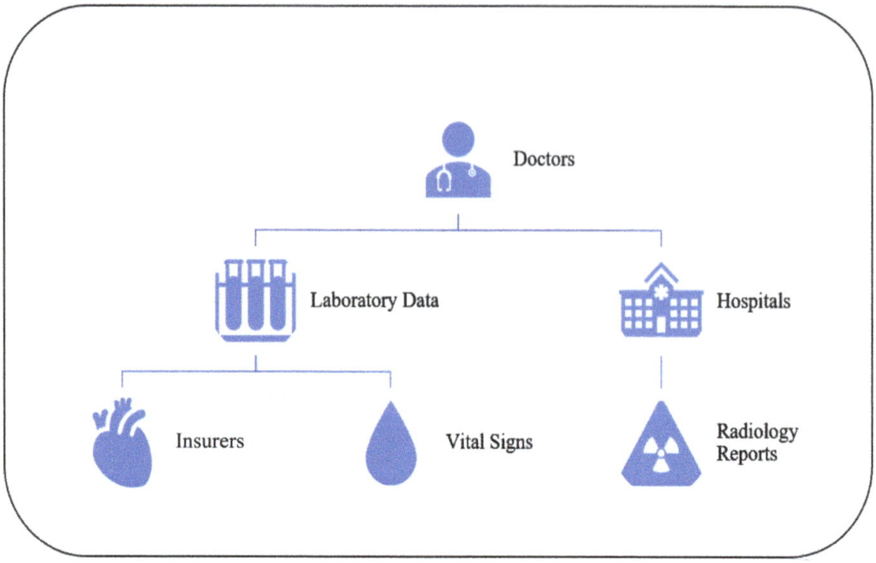

Figure 3.4. Flow diagram showing how a doctor can access all patient details using an EHR.

patient-centric innovation lies in the evolution of patient portals, mobile health applications, and remote monitoring solutions. These technological strides serve as indispensable assets, giving patients greater autonomy over their healthcare journeys. Patient portals enable individuals to retrieve their medical records, arrange appointments, and engage securely with their healthcare providers, fostering a streamlined and accessible approach to health management.

Similarly, mobile health apps give users instant access to key health resources, from medication reminders to symptom tracking, allowing patients to stay active and engaged in their wellness. In addition, remote monitoring devices provide real-time insights into important health indicators, allowing patients to actively monitor their progress and address rapidly emerging issues under the guidance of healthcare providers. Using these patient care innovations, patients are not only empowered to take care of their health but also equipped with the necessary tools to strengthen partnerships with their healthcare providers. With the improved communication channels provided by these technologies, patients can more effectively voice their concerns, actively participate in shared decision-making processes, and ultimately co-create individualized care plans tailored to their unique needs and preferences. Such a collaborative approach to healthcare not only increases patients' sense of empowerment and autonomy but also leads to deeper trust and satisfaction with the treatment process.

In essence, patient-centered innovations in electronic health systems represent a paradigm shift toward a more comprehensive and patient-centered care model. The different types of EHRs are shown in table 3.5. By prioritizing the needs, preferences, and desires of individuals, these transformative technologies can not only revolutionize healthcare but enable people to live healthier and more fulfilling

Table 3.5. Different types of EHRs.

Ambulatory Medical Records (AMRs)	**Computerized Medical Records** (CMRs)	EMRs	**Electronic Patient Records** (EPRs)	EHRs
Half of the data is generated through IT processes, while the remaining half relies on paper-based medical records. Retains certain aspects of automation already used for medical documentation such as order entry, result reporting, communication, and digital recording.	Medical record digitization involves scanning paper documents and importing digital files to replicate the structure and viewing experience of paper records, resulting in a paperless system. This process does not rely on optical character recognition (OCR) or intelligent character recognition (ICR) but utilizes a pure image system.	Digitized medical records, including data management, offer various perspectives on records, supporting clinical processes within IT-based organizational frameworks. These records, entirely generated by IT systems, incorporate decision support and interactive guidelines. They also establish connections with business and management data.	Encompass all pertinent patient health data, extending beyond institutional boundaries to regional levels, surpassing standard documentation requirements within a medical record. This longitudinal approach facilitates initiatives such as telemedicine and supports information systems research and data networks.	Encompass comprehensive health-related data for individuals, covering aspects such as wellness, nutrition, and other health-related information. This system operates beyond institutional boundaries, extending regionally, nationally, or globally and is web-based. It encourages citizen participation in record creation, fostering a collaborative approach to health management.

lives. Patient referrals pose a significant challenge within healthcare centers (HCs): in 27 out of 83 reported instances, patients returned for entirely different treatments. On average, each HC typically refers between five and ten patients per month to other HCs. However, in regions affected by fluctuating climates or endemic diseases, this number can rise to as high as 20 referrals per month.

Referrals primarily rely on documents, which account for 77% of cases, while the remainder occur via telephone. Regrettably, the accuracy of information flow suffers due to inadequate patient history records, particularly within paper-based referral systems. In telephone referrals, the accuracy heavily relies on the doctor's familiarity with the patient's medical background and the time available to convey this information. Given that doctors handle an average of 70 patients daily, conveying precise diagnostic information during referrals becomes challenging. Consequently, both paper-based and telephone referrals suffer from reduced quality, leading to repetitive or ineffective treatments at secondary HCs. This not only compromises healthcare quality but also escalates treatment costs.

3.3.2 Security and privacy considerations

In the realm of electronic health systems, emphasizing the significance of security and privacy is paramount. Due to the sensitive nature of patient information, stringent measures must be taken to safeguard it against unauthorized access or breaches. Healthcare entities bear the responsibility for establishing robust security frameworks to uphold the confidentiality and integrity of patient data. Encryption forms a cornerstone of these measures; it involves the encoding of sensitive data to permit interpretation solely by authorized entities or systems. Through encrypting data during transmission and storage, healthcare organizations mitigate the risks associated with eavesdropping or unauthorized data entry. Authentication mechanisms play a pivotal role in validating the identity of users accessing the system. The adoption of robust authentication protocols such as multifactor authentication is essential to ensure that only authorized individuals access patient records and sensitive medical data.

Access restrictions are another important aspect of eHealth security. Organizations can protect patient information by defining and enforcing access rights based on roles and responsibilities, ensuring that only those with legitimate needs can view it. This not only reduces the risk of unauthorized access but also helps maintain data integrity. Regular audits and monitoring are required to identify and correct system vulnerabilities or suspicious activity. By conducting periodic security assessments and audits, healthcare organizations can proactively identify and mitigate potential risks to patient data. Moreover, maintaining data backups is essential to guarantee the accessibility and retrievability of patient information in case of data breaches or system malfunctions. Consistently backing up data to off-site, secure locations is crucial for minimizing the consequences of unforeseen incidents and expediting the restoration of services. Finally, protecting the security and privacy of patient data is paramount in eHealth systems. By incorporating robust security protocols such as encryption, authentication, access control, and data backup, healthcare institutions can fulfill their obligation to safeguard sensitive data and uphold patient confidence.

3.3.3 Implementing high-performance systems

Establishing high-performance eHealth systems transcends mere technology acquisition; it entails a multifaceted business endeavor necessitating meticulous strategic planning and unwavering commitment from all involved stakeholders. To ensure success, healthcare organizations must take a holistic approach that includes several key elements. First, strategic planning is essential. This requires setting clear goals, understanding the needs of the organization, and adapting technical solutions to those goals. This requires consideration of factors such as workflow optimization, regulatory compliance, and budget constraints. In addition, stakeholder engagement throughout the implementation process is critical. This applies not only to healthcare professionals but also to patients, administrators, IT staff, and vendors. Effective communication and collaboration between these various stakeholders are essential to identify needs, solve problems, and support the new system. In addition, it is important to invest in training so that employees have the necessary skills to use it.

This includes not only initial training during implementation but also ongoing support and professional development to keep up with evolving technologies and best practices. In addition, infrastructure plays an important role in supporting high-performance eHealth systems. This includes not only the hardware and software components of the system but also aspects such as network infrastructure, data storage, and cybersecurity measures to protect patient data. Continuous improvement aims to maximize the benefits of eHealth systems over time. This requires monitoring performance metrics, soliciting user feedback, and implementing iterative changes to optimize usability, interoperability, and security. In summary, implementing effective eHealth systems requires a holistic approach that includes strategic planning, stakeholder engagement and training, infrastructure investments, and continuous improvement measures. By prioritizing these elements and fostering collaboration among all stakeholders, healthcare organizations can successfully navigate the complexities of implementing electronic systems and realize their full potential to improve patient care and organizational effectiveness.

3.3.4 Challenges and barriers to adoption

Electronic health systems offer many advantages, but their widespread adoption is associated with enormous challenges. These barriers include a variety of issues, from interoperability and privacy issues to resistance rooted in healthcare cultures. Organizations face a multifaceted barrier to adopting eHealth systems. First, interoperability issues are common, as different systems often find it difficult to communicate seamlessly with each other. Such fragmentation complicates the effective exchange of patient data and undermines the potential benefits of a unified digital infrastructure. Both patients and healthcare providers have legitimate concerns about the security of sensitive medical information stored in electronic systems.

Without strong safeguards and open protocols, these fears can stifle enthusiasm for digital transformation. Resistance to change is another major obstacle. Healthcare professionals accustomed to traditional paper-based workflows may resist the unfamiliar landscape of electronic systems. Overcoming this inertia requires not only technical training but also a cultural shift toward innovation and efficiency. Financial constraints complicate the equation. The substantial initial investment needed for implementing electronic health systems may deter organizations that lack the necessary resources from adopting them. In addition, financial pressures are compounded by ongoing maintenance costs and the need for regular updates. Control rules are both a driver for deployment and a potential stumbling block. While regulations are intended to protect patients' rights and ensure quality care, navigating the maze of compliance requirements can be daunting.

Failure to meet regulatory standards can result in severe penalties that complicate the implementation process. Addressing these challenges requires collaboration and a holistic approach. Healthcare organizations should initiate proactive dialog with stakeholders to identify and mitigate barriers to adoption. Innovations in both technology and processes are needed to overcome entrenched resistance and bring about meaningful change. In conclusion, while the benefits of eHealth systems are undeniable, their realization involves transcending a number of huge challenges. By fostering collaboration, embracing innovation, and prioritizing continuous improvement, healthcare organizations can overcome these barriers and unlock the full potential of healthcare digital transformation.

3.3.5 Scalable solutions for big data analytics in electronic health records

In the realm of modern healthcare, EHRs have become integral for documenting patient information, clinical encounters, and medical histories. With the exponential growth of data generated by these records, the need for efficient and scalable solutions for big data analytics has become paramount. Traditional methods of managing and analyzing EHR data are often limited by infrastructure constraints and the sheer volume and complexity of the data involved. Scalable solutions for big data analytics in EHRs aim to address these challenges by leveraging HPC technologies. These technologies empower healthcare organizations to efficiently process, store, and analyze extensive data sets within reasonable timeframes and costs. By harnessing the power of parallel processing and distributed computing, HPC systems can handle the massive data sets inherent in EHRs and perform complex analytics tasks with efficiency and speed.

A key aspect of scalable solutions for EHR analytics is the use of cloud computing platforms. Cloud-based HPC infrastructure provides healthcare organizations with the flexibility to adjust their computing resources according to workload demands, offering scalability on demand. This capability enables them to efficiently scale their computing resources up or down as needed, without the

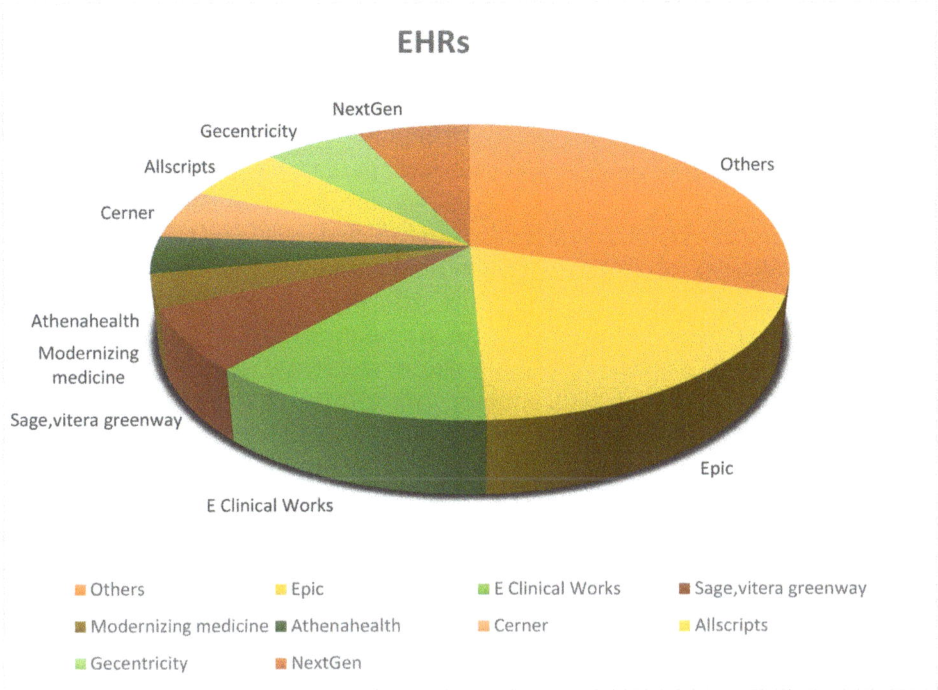

Figure 3.5. EHR systems utilized by survey-responding physicians.

constraints of fixed hardware infrastructure. This flexibility is particularly valuable for handling peak loads of data processing and analysis, such as those encountered during clinical trials or population health studies. Moreover, sophisticated data management techniques, including data partitioning and compression, are essential for maximizing the efficiency of HPC systems in EHR analytics. Physicians utilize diverse EHR systems, such as clinical tools, while other practitioners employ a variety of additional tools, as depicted in figure 3.5. These techniques help reduce storage requirements and improve data access times, enhancing the overall efficiency of data processing and analysis workflows.

In addition to improving the efficiency and scalability of EHR analytics, scalable solutions also facilitate advanced analytics techniques, such as machine learning and predictive modeling. These techniques enable healthcare organizations to derive valuable insights from EHR data, such as identifying patterns in patient outcomes, predicting disease progression, and personalizing treatment plans. Overall, scalable solutions for big data analytics in EHRs empower healthcare organizations to unlock the full potential of their data assets, leading to improved clinical outcomes, operational efficiency, and patient care. However, achieving these benefits requires careful consideration of factors such as data security, privacy compliance, and interoperability to ensure the responsible and ethical use of EHR data.

3.3.6 Clinical research and population health

HPC and the use of EHRs is revolutionizing both clinical research and population health. In the field of clinical trials, HPC facilitates rapid data processing and analysis, allowing researchers to identify meaningful cohorts and stratify patients based on a myriad of variables such as demographics, genetic markers, and medical history. By harnessing the power of HPC, researchers can undertake extensive cohort studies on a massive scale with unparalleled efficiency. This enables the generation of valuable insights that have the potential to drive the advancement of novel treatments and personalized medicine strategies.

In addition, HPC-enabled analytics in population health enables healthcare organizations to gain actionable insights from vast EHR data sets, as shown in figure 3.6. Using advanced data mining algorithms and predictive modeling techniques, healthcare providers can identify population health trends, detect disease in real time and implement targeted interventions to improve health outcomes at the community level. This combination of HPC and EHR not only accelerates the speed of clinical research but also improves the ability of health systems to deliver predictable, evidence-based care to diverse populations. As the amount and intricacy of EHR data grow, ethical and regulatory concerns become increasingly critical. Researchers and healthcare institutions must prioritize adherence to stringent privacy standards, comply with regulations such as the Health Insurance Portability and Accountability Act (HIPAA) and the General Data Protection Regulation (GDPR), and establish robust security protocols to safeguard patient confidentiality and maintain data integrity. If these ethical and regulatory challenges

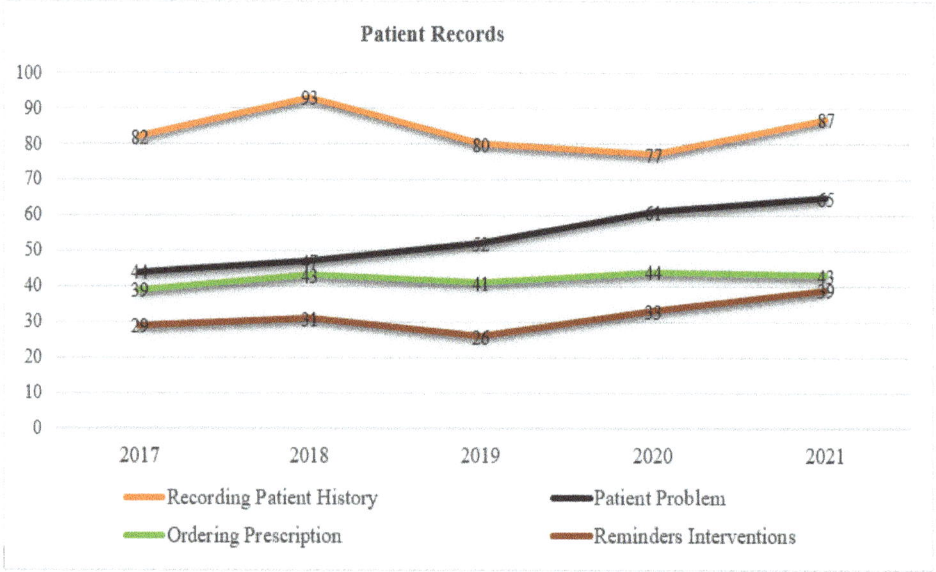

Figure 3.6. Analysis of patient records.

are effectively addressed, the integration of HPC into EHRs promises to transform healthcare and advance both clinical research and public health worldwide.

3.3.7 Ethical and regulatory considerations

In the realm of HPC as applied to EHRs, ethical and regulatory considerations are paramount to ensure the responsible and secure use of sensitive patient data. Ethical guidelines serve as the cornerstone of ethical research and clinical practice, guiding researchers and healthcare providers in their interactions with patient information. Leveraging HPC for processing and analyzing EHR data necessitates adherence to ethical principles such as beneficence, non-maleficence, respect for patient autonomy, and justice. This involves securing informed consent from patients for the utilization of their data in research endeavors, maintaining transparency in data management procedures, and placing utmost importance on safeguarding patient privacy and confidentiality throughout the research journey.

Furthermore, adherence to regulatory standards such as the HIPAA and the GDPR is crucial for safeguarding patient rights and minimizing the potential risks linked to unauthorized access or misuse of EHR data. These regulations mandate strict protocols for data security, access control, data sharing, and breach notification, thereby safeguarding patient privacy and ensuring the integrity and confidentiality of health information. In addition, responsible data stewardship practices play a pivotal role in promoting ethical conduct and regulatory compliance in the use of HPC-enabled EHRs. This encompasses implementing robust data governance frameworks, conducting regular audits and risk assessments, and fostering a culture of accountability and transparency within healthcare organizations. By upholding ethical principles and complying with regulatory requirements, the integration of HPC with EHRs can unlock transformative insights while safeguarding patient rights and promoting trust in the healthcare ecosystem.

3.4 Success stories and case studies

A wealth of success stories and case studies vividly illustrate the transformative impact of electronic healthcare systems on various facets of patient care, clinical outcomes, and operational efficiencies within healthcare organizations. These narratives not only serve as powerful testimonials but also provide invaluable insights and inspiration for other healthcare entities seeking to embark on similar journeys of technological advancement. One such compelling narrative revolves around healthcare organizations that have embraced high-performance electronic health systems with remarkable success. Through diligent implementation and utilization of cutting-edge technologies, these institutions have witnessed tangible improvements across multiple fronts, ranging from streamlined operational processes to enhanced quality of care and ultimately, better patient outcomes.

Examining these instances of success reveals a clear transformation brought about by the integration of electronic healthcare systems, reshaping the landscape of healthcare delivery and management. By leveraging innovative digital solutions, healthcare providers have been able to optimize various aspects of their operations, leading to greater efficiency and effectiveness in delivering care. Moreover, these case studies underscore the pivotal role played by electronic healthcare systems in driving clinical excellence [9–12]. Through the seamless integration of EMRs, decision support tools, and telehealth platforms, healthcare professionals are empowered to make more informed and timely decisions, thereby improving the overall quality of care delivered to patients.

Beyond clinical benefits, the implementation of high-performance electronic healthcare systems has also yielded significant operational advantages for healthcare organizations. From streamlining administrative tasks to automating routine processes, these systems have helped to alleviate burdensome workflows and enhance overall productivity within healthcare settings.

The study conducted in [19] by NCC Switzerland, looks at mechanical and biological aortic valve replacements. These replacements often do not last long and can cause compatibility issues because of irregular blood flow patterns. The flow patterns are affected by the design of the replacement valves, which has not changed much in recent years. We are using advanced computer simulations on powerful computers to understand how blood flows around these valves. By studying this, we hope to find new valve designs that can reduce or delay turbulent blood flow. Our findings suggest that even small changes to the valve design could make a big difference in reducing turbulence.

Perhaps most importantly, these success stories serve as beacons of hope and guidance for other healthcare organizations embarking on similar journeys of digital transformation. By demonstrating real-world examples of how electronic healthcare systems benefit patients and providers, these stories instill trust and offer practical guidance on navigating challenges and maximizing benefits. The numerous success stories and case studies underscore how advanced electronic healthcare systems can truly revolutionize the industry. As organizations learn from these experiences and adopt innovative approaches, the vision of a streamlined, patient-focused healthcare landscape draws nearer.

3.5 Future trends in health information technology

In the dynamic realm of health information technology (health IT), numerous trends are influencing the landscape of healthcare delivery, as depicted in figure 3.7. From AI to telemedicine and from wearables to precision medicine, the future holds enormous promise for transforming the way healthcare is managed and experienced. Looking ahead, it is increasingly clear that continuing these trends is not only affordable but essential for healthcare organizations striving to remain competitive and deliver optimal patient care. Artificial intelligence is one of the most transformative forces in healthcare IT.

Its capabilities range from streamlining administrative tasks to streamlining clinical decision-making processes. Using machine learning algorithms and predictive analytics, AI can examine vast amounts of patient data, identify patterns, predict outcomes, and ultimately facilitate more individualized and effective treatment strategies. Telemedicine has also emerged as a key form of the trend. Thanks to

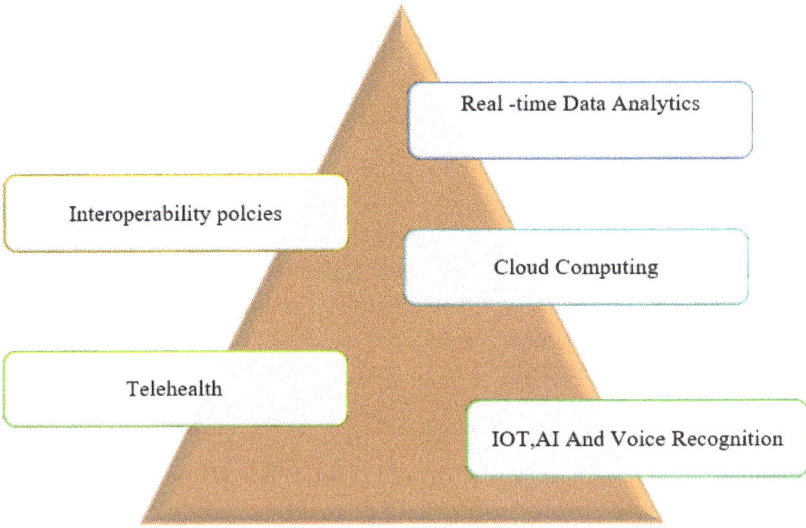

Figure 3.7. Future of EHR.

advances in communication technology, telemedicine overcomes geographic barriers and gives patients access to medical knowledge regardless of their physical location. This not only increases patient comfort but also facilitates timely intervention and reduces the burden on healthcare infrastructure. Wearable devices are another part of the healthcare IT landscape that is poised for explosive growth. From fitness trackers to continuous glucose monitors, these devices provide real-time health information and allow people to proactively monitor their well-being. In addition, the integration of wearable technology with AI algorithms enables a revolution in preventive medicine, which enables the early detection of health problems and preventive measures.

Precision medicine, which focuses on adapting treatment to the individual characteristics of each patient, represents a paradigm shift in healthcare. Utilizing genomic data, biomarkers, and other molecular insights, healthcare providers can offer highly targeted therapies that are remarkably effective and have fewer side effects. Precision medicine not only holds the potential to significantly enhance patient outcomes but also ensures more efficient use of resources within healthcare systems. Looking to the future, the convergence of AI, machine learning, blockchain technology, and telemedicine will continue to develop. Embracing these trends will not only increase the capabilities of eHealth systems but also promote a culture of innovation in the delivery of patient care. By staying ahead of these technological advances, healthcare organizations can deliver quality care that is both efficient and patient-friendly in an ever-evolving healthcare environment. Telehealth and telecare services have further revolutionized health delivery by overcoming geographic barriers and providing convenient access to medical expertise, especially in underserved communities. In addition, the integration of healthcare analytics and big data has enhanced decision-making processes, allowing healthcare organizations to identify trends, predict outcomes, and allocate resources more effectively. Innovations centered around patients, including mobile health apps and wearable devices, enable individuals to take an active role in managing their health. This promotes a collaborative and personalized approach to healthcare [27–31].

3.6 Conclusions

In recent years, the integration of electronic health systems has significantly transformed the delivery of medical services. This change has significantly impacted various aspects of healthcare, from operational efficiency to improving patient outcomes. Healthcare organizations have embraced the capabilities of advanced electronic systems and consistently aim to stay at the forefront of emerging trends in health information technology. The success of these efforts hinges on recognizing electronic health systems as catalysts for increased efficiency, higher quality standards, and ultimately, improved patient outcomes. By seamlessly integrating digital platforms, medical professionals can streamline their workflow, optimize resource allocation, and ensure timely treatment. In addition, thanks to the digitization of health records, doctors can quickly access comprehensive patient data, facilitating informed decision-making and personalized treatment strategies. Beyond enhancing operational efficiency, electronic health systems have revolutionized patient care. By leveraging advanced technology and data analytics, healthcare providers can tailor their services to meet the unique needs and preferences of individual patients. This emphasis on personalization fosters a deeper sense of patient engagement and empowerment, ultimately improving adherence and health outcomes. In addition, the emergence of eHealth systems has brought significant benefits in terms of cost containment and resource optimization. Healthcare organizations can achieve substantial savings and enhance the accuracy and efficiency of their operations by automating administrative processes, minimizing errors, and reducing dependence on paper-based documentation. Finally, high-performance electronic systems will be widely adopted in healthcare. Systems have enormous potential to revolutionize the delivery of medical services. By leveraging technology, data, and patient innovation, healthcare organizations can transcend traditional boundaries and create a more efficient, effective, and equitable healthcare system for all. These ongoing developments underscore the importance of remaining nimble and proactive in the face of emerging trends to ensure patients continue to receive high-quality care in an increasingly digital age.

References

[1] Waithe W E 2009 Healthy relationships: use and influence of community-based participatory approaches *J. Ambul. Care Manage.* **32** 295–8

[2] Shekelle P G, Morton S C and Keeler E B 2006 *Costs and benefits of health information technology* 132 Rockville (MD); Agency for Healthcare Research and Quality 1–71

[3] Ahmad A, Tariq A, Hussain H K and Gill A Y 2023 Revolutionizing healthcare: how deep learning is poised to change the landscape of medical diagnosis and treatment *J. Comput. Netw. Archit. High Perform. Comput.* **5** 458–71

[4] Minanton M, Agustina H S and Khoirunnisa N 2024 UI/UX design of the ENC application as electronic nursing care in clinical practice education for nursing students in hospitals *J. Comput. Netw. Archit. High Perform. Comput.* **6** 191–200

[5] Blumenthal D, DesRoches C M, Donelan K, Rosenbaum S J and Ferris T 2006 *Health information technology in the United States: the information base for progress* Robert Wood Johnson Foundation, Princeton, NJ; MGH Institute for Health Policy; George Washington University School of Public Health and Health Services The Health Law Information Project

[6] Guduri M, Chakraborty C and Margala M 2023 Blockchain-based federated learning technique for privacy preservation and security of smart electronic health records *IEEE Trans. Consum. Electron.* **70** 2608–17

[7] Roy C L, Poon E G, Karson A S, Ladak-Merchant Z, Johnson R E, Maviglia S M and Gandhi T K 2005 Patient safety concerns arising from test results that return after hospital discharge *Ann. Intern. Med.* **143** 121–8

[8] Song X, Waitman L R, Alan S L, Robbins D C, Hu Y and Liu M 2020 Longitudinal risk prediction of chronic kidney disease in diabetic patients using a temporal-enhanced gradient boosting machine: retrospective cohort study *JMIR Med. Inform.* **8** e15510

[9] Bates D W 2005 Physicians and ambulatory electronic health records *Health Aff.* **24** 1180–9

[10] Mamlin B W and Tierney W M 2016 The promise of information and communication technology in healthcare: extracting value from the chaos *Am. J. Med. Sci.* **351** 59–68

[11] Friedman C P, Wong A K and Blumenthal D 2010 Achieving a nationwide learning health system *Sci. Transl. Med.* **2** 57cm29

[12] Miraz M H, Ali M, Excell P S and Picking R 2015 A review on internet of things (IoT), internet of everything (IoE) and internet of nano things (IoNT) *2015 Internet Technologies and Applications (ITA)* **8** 219–24

[13] Tiwari A and Maurya H 2017 Challenges and ongoing researches for IOT (Internet of Things): a review *Int. J. Eng. Dev. Res.* **5** 57–60 https://rjwave.org/ijedr/viewpaperforall.php?paper=IJEDR1702008

[14] Persell S D, Kaiser D, Dolan N C, Andrews B, Levi S, Khandekar J, Gavagan T, Thompson J A, Friesema E M and Baker D W 2011 Changes in performance after implementation of a multifaceted electronic-health-record-based quality improvement system *Med. Care* **49** 117–25

[15] Pushpan A and Ali Akbar N 2017 Data mining applications in healthcare *IOSR J. Comput. Eng.* **1** National Conference On Discrete Mathematics & Computing (NCDMC-2017) 4–7 https://www.iosrjournals.org/iosr-jce/papers/Conf.17013-2017/Volume-1/2.%2004-07.pdf?id=7557

[16] Macias C G, Remy K E and Barda A J 2023 Utilizing big data from electronic health records in pediatric clinical care *Pediatr. Res.* **93** 382–9

[17] Sarwar M U, Hanif M K, Talib R, Mobeen A and Aslam M 2017 A survey of big data analytics in healthcare *Int. J. Adv. Comput. Sci. Appl.* **8** 355–9

[18] Elkefi S and Asan O 2022 Exploring doctors' satisfaction with electronic health records and their features: a nationwide survey study *2022 IEEE Int. Symp. on Systems Engineering (ISSE)* (Piscataway, NJ: IEEE) 1–5

[19] Elkefi S, Yu Z and Asan O 2021 Online medical record nonuse among patients: data analysis study of the 2019 health information national trends survey *J. Med. Internet Res.* **23** e24767

[20] Ben-Assuli O 2015 Electronic health records, adoption, quality of care, legal and privacy issues, and their implementation in emergency departments *Health Policy* **119** 287–97

[21] Singh H and Sittig D F 2016 Measuring and improving patient safety through health information technology: the health IT safety framework *BMJ Qual. Saf.* **25** 226–32

[22] Tanner C, Gans D, White J, Nath R and Pohl J 2015 Electronic health records and patient safety *Appl. Clin. Inform.* **6** 136–47

[23] Koppar A R and Sridhar V 2009 A workflow solution for electronic health records to improve healthcare delivery efficiency in rural India *2009 Int. Conf. on eHealth, Telemedicine, and Social Medicine* (Piscataway, NJ: IEEE) 227–32

[24] Qiao S, Li X, Olatosi B and Young S D 2024 Utilizing big data analytics and electronic health record data in HIV prevention, treatment, and care research: a literature review *AIDS Care* **36** 583–603

[25] Jung S Y, Lee K, Lee H Y and Hwang H 2020 Barriers and facilitators to implementation of nationwide electronic health records in the Russian far east: a qualitative analysis *Int. J. Med. Inform.* **143** 104244

[26] Zafar M H, Langås E F and Sanfilippo F 2024Oct1 Exploring the synergies between collaborative robotics, digital twins, augmentation, and industry 5.0 for smart manufacturing: a state-of-the-art review *Rob. Comput. Integr. Manuf.* **89** 102769

[27] Khare S K, Khan A M, Bajaj V and Sinha G R 2023 Introduction to smart healthcare and the role of cognitive sensors *Cognitive Sensors, Volume 2: Applications in Smart Healthcare* (Bristol: IOP Publishing) 1-1–1-21

[28] Khare S K, March S, Barua P D, Gadre V M and Acharya U R 2023 Application of data fusion for automated detection of children with developmental and mental disorders: a systematic review of the last decade *Inf. Fusion.* **99** 101898

[29] Yaacob H, Hossain F, Shari S, Khare S K, Ooi C P and Acharya U R 2023 Application of artificial intelligence techniques for brain-computer interface in mental fatigue detection: a systematic review (2011–2022) *IEEE Access* **11** 74736–58

[30] Khare S K, Blanes-Vidal V, Nadimi E S and Acharya U R 2023 Emotion recognition and artificial intelligence: a systematic review (2014–2023) and research recommendations *Inf. Fusion* **102** 102019

[31] El. Dahshan E S A, Bassiouni M M, Khare S K, Tan R S and Acharya U R 2024 ExHyptNet: an explainable diagnosis of hypertension using EfficientNet with PPG signals *Expert Syst. Appl.* **239** 122388

Chapter 4

Detection of attention deficit hyperactivity disorder using electroencephalogram signals: a review

Joseph Nixon Kiro, Bam Bahadur Sinha, Madhu Kumari and Shalini Mahato

Attention deficit hyperactivity disorder (ADHD) is a chronic physiological illness that affects children. Adolescents with ADHD encounter numerous kinds of issues in maintaining their attentiveness and regulating their behavior. It is the most prevalent neurological condition that affects a child's behavior, memory, and ability to learn. ADHD persists from childhood into adulthood. Electroencephalogram (EEG) signals play a crucial role in identifying ADHD, as they provide extensive information about mental abilities. Therefore, these signals have the potential to serve as a biomarker for ADHD identification. This chapter discusses how EEG signals can be used for the detection of ADHD using machine learning (ML) and/or deep learning (DL) techniques as well as state-of-the-art approaches.

4.1 Introduction

Children with ADHD suffer from a very prevalent neurodevelopmental disorder; its estimated global prevalence ranges from 2% to 7.2% [1]. ADHD is characterized by the presence of negligence, hyperactivity, or impulsivity that is inappropriate for a person's age, and it causes problems in their ability to perform well at home, at school, and in social situations [2]. ADHD is a neurobehavioral condition whose symptoms may potentially be broken down into three categories: changes of attention, emotion, and promptness of action, both mental and physical [3, 4]. Some of its most common symptoms are uncontrolled movement, problems in focusing on a particular thing, anxiety, nervousness, abrupt manners, excessive talking, daydreaming, etc [5]. Children with ADHD are generally careless, quickly flustered, and overactive and face problems in their studies. The origin of ADHD is often assumed to be brain injury, heredity, or natural causes [4, 6]. Figure 4.1 shows features and their characteristics that are seen in children diagnosed with ADHD.

doi:10.1088/978-0-7503-5964-1ch4

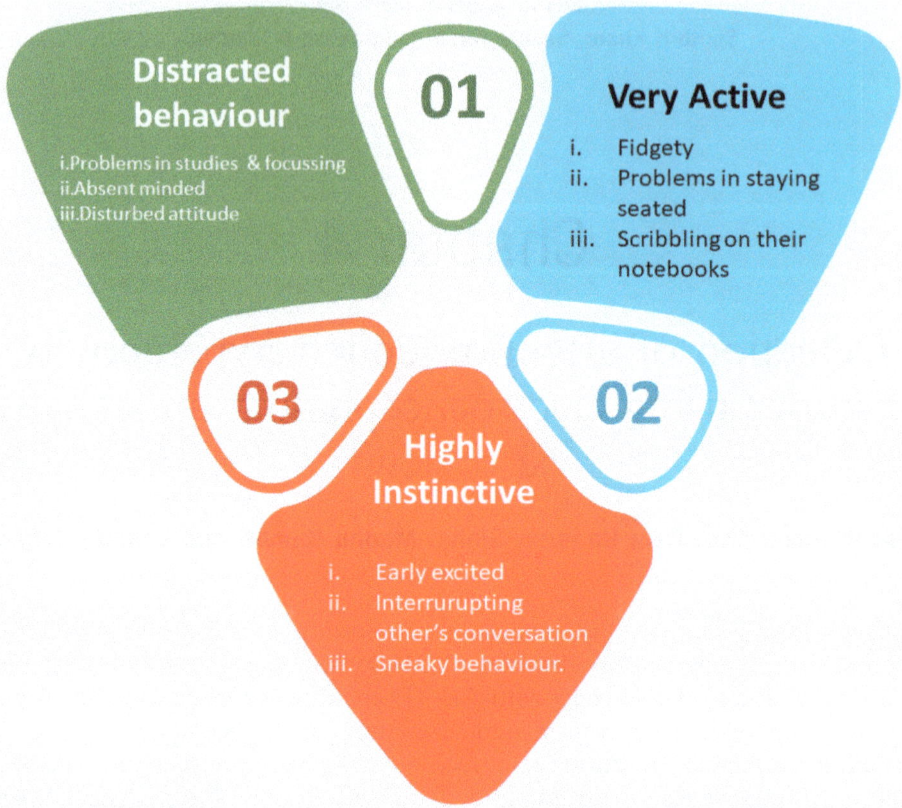

Figure 4.1. Notable features and their characteristics seen in ADHD children.

The early detection of ADHD is essential and plays an important role in avoiding issues in a child's social life. Since there is no characterized biomarker for the distinctive subtypes of ADHD, its detection is based upon information acquired from a few sources, looking for mental and neurological evidence in the components generally discernible from family and school bonds [3]. One of the most widely recognized approaches for analyzing ADHD is through the individual or those around them [6, 7].

EEG signals have been explored in research for the early diagnosis of many mental health disorders (such as depression, schizophrenia, and autism), hypertension, emotion detection, etc [8–11]. The EEG is a famous and broadly utilized estimation procedure for extracting data from the brain. EEG signals can be combined with computer aided tools to identify ADHD.

Functional connectivity can be used to detect ADHD. This examines the analytical connection between the functional behaviors of various parts of the brain over time and is based on analytical estimation of an EEG signal [12]. EEG signals allow a straightforward review of the brain's action, breaking down the brain's signals and thereby giving the possible location of disorders, i.e. differences between

between ordinary working and unusual working. For this reason, EEG signals are favored for the detection of ADHD. Another reason for the use of EEG signals is that the human brain has an extremely irregular dynamic framework and its activities exhibit unrestrained conduct; therefore, chaos theory is applied to EEG signal analysis to diagnose clinical disorders [4, 5]. Several popular ML algorithms for characterizing the EEGs of ADHD patients include support vector machine (SVM), *k*-nearest neighbors (*k*-NN), linear discriminant analysis (LDA), logistic regression (LR), and different sorts of neural networks. Convolutional neural networks (CNNs) are widely used in biomedical image signal processing [13]. Other ML tools used by researchers are wavelet techniques and neural networks (NNs), the radial basis function (RBF) neural network classifier, the correlation dimension, the Lyapunov exponent (LE), wavelet entropy variants of SVM types, approximate entropy (ApEn), LE, and others [7].

4.2 Introduction to the detection of ADHD using EEG signals

For the detection of ADHD, DSM-IV (or the updated version, DSM-V) criteria are used by the healthcare provider [2]. In this study, groups of ADHD patients and healthy controls (HCs) were included. A child's intelligence (age group 6–16 years) can be evaluated using the Korean Educational Developmental Institute–Wechsler Intelligence Scale for Children (KEDI-WISC-III). In general, expert therapists of children and teenagers diagnose them as having ADHD using the DSM-IV or DSM V rules.

The children are asked to do some mathematical calculations, for example various pictures are shown to them that incorporate various shapes or animated characters. Then they are asked to sum up the total of shapes shown in the lower and upper halves of the image. Finally, the children are told to declare the total. This task lasts for 30 s, during which, EEG signals are recorded using electrodes. Figure 4.2 shows the general steps employed for the prediction of ADHD using ML/DL.

4.2.1 Data set

The predictive factors used to distinguish between children with ADHD and healthy children are a medical history of major neurological issues (such as brain injury or epilepsy), a significant clinical sickness, learning or language impairment, other mental health conditions, and the use of barbiturate and benzodiazepine medications.

4.2.2 Preprocessing

When biological artifacts like electrooculograms (EOGs), electromyograms (EMGs), and electrocardiograms (ECGs) are analyzed, it is very important to clean the raw information in the preprocessing phase [7]. There are usually high-magnitude changes in EEGs because of eye activity, heart rate, movement of the muscles, and noise caused by electromagnetic fields. All these artifacts degrade the

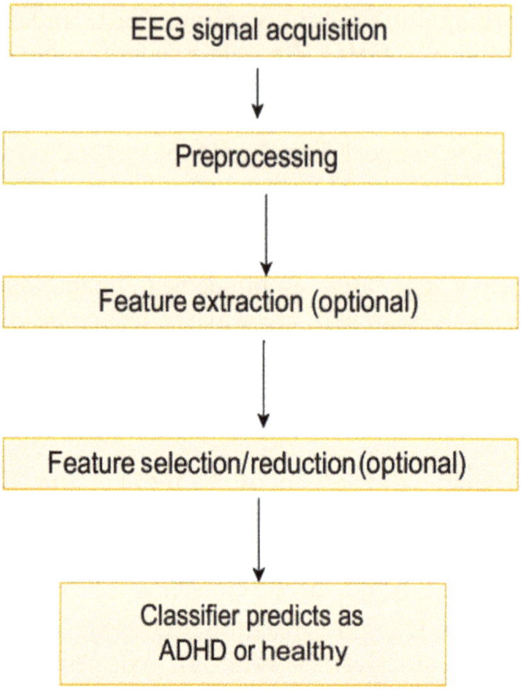

Figure 4.2. General steps employed for prediction of ADHD.

EEG signals. Thus, it is essential to remove such artifacts, which helps to increase the accuracy of detection [13]. Tools such as BrainVision Analyzer, EEGLAB, etc. can be used for EEG data preprocessing. Independent component analysis (ICA) has been used to discriminate between numerous sources and to eliminate artifacts from EEG signals over time. An automatic method can also be utilized to find artifacts based on the elimination criterion of $\pm$ 150 μV [14] in order to remove them. Noise in EEG signals can also be removed by visual inspection [15].

4.2.3 Feature extraction

Different frequency-domain, time-domain, and nonlinear features can be mined from EEG signals. Time-domain features include the standard deviation, variance, mean, median, kurtosis, skewness, etc. Frequency-domain features include δ (0.5–4 Hz), θ (4–8 Hz), α (8–13 Hz), and β (13–30 Hz), which are the most widely used. Nonlinear features include fractal dimension (FD)-based characteristics such as the approximate entropy Higuchi, LE, Katz, and Petrosian fractal dimensions. Some of the nonlinear features are discussed below:

(i) Katz fractal dimension—this algorithm is supposed to be a very successful strategy for active changes. The FD in this algorithm is calculated using the following equation:

$$\mathrm{FD} = \frac{\ln\,(A - 1)}{\ln\,(A - 1) - \ln \frac{b}{d}} \tag{4.1}$$

where d is the summation of the distance between consecutive points, A is the range of the data arrangement, and b is the broadness of data arrangement [7].

(ii) Largest Lyapunov exponent (LLE)—this algorithm is a measurement that evokes the disordered actions of a framework. At the points where the value of the LLE is positive, the framework has disordered behavior. The LLE of a period depends on the product of the contrasts between progressive tests. The LLE of a signal is estimated using the following equation:

$$\lambda = \frac{1}{n} \ln \left(\frac{d_m}{d_0} \right) \tag{4.2}$$

where d_m is the distance between successive samples separated by time m, and d_0 is the initial distance [5, 7, 16]

(iii) Approximate entropy (ApEn)—this is a technique for calculating the sum of the discipline or irregularity in a signal. This is calculated using the formula given below:-

$$\mathrm{ApEn}(k, r_f, n) = \phi^k(r_f) - \phi^{k+1}(r_f) \tag{4.3}$$

$$C_i^k(r_f) = \frac{\text{number of } j \text{ such that } d[x_k(i), x_k(j)] \leqslant (r_f)}{n - k + 1} \tag{4.4}$$

$$B[x_k(i), x_k(j)] = \text{maximum}\,(|\, p(i + t - 1) - (j + t - 1)|) \tag{4.5}$$

$$x_k = \{p(i), p(i + 1), \ldots, p(i + k - 1)\}; \;\; 1 \leqslant i \leqslant n - k + 1 \tag{4.6}$$

where k is range of the data, r_f is the level of filtering, n is the number of samples, and B is the distance between the two vectors $x_k(i)$ and $x_k(j)$[5, 7, 16].

(iv) Sample entropy (SampEn)—this method is based on ApEn and has two significant provisions. First, it is less complex than the ApEn calculation, since it is generally independent of the extent of record information and dispenses with oneself matches. Second, SampEn represents the rate of formation of new information. This methodology may be utilized to investigate the brief and chaotic timelines of signals [5].

(v) Fuzzy entropy (FuzzyEn)—FuzzyEn is utilized for assessing the pace of intricacy in a timeline. FuzzyEn works by recreating a vector utilizing the time delay estimation (TDE) technique by taking a timeline. It then estimates the greatest distance between two nearby states and gives a fuzzy result. It subsequently acquires the comparability degree between the two vectors, which is then used for calculating the FuzzyEn [5].

(vi) Correlation dimension (CD)—CD is another technique for measuring chaotic behavior to acquire data about the hidden elements of a chaotic cycle as a time series. The component of a signal can depict the idea of the framework. The CD can be used with the FD and identifies the topological component of its attractor (the number of data points). CD is interrelated with the correlation integral, $F(r)$ as:

$$F(r) = \lim_{n\to\infty} \frac{1}{M(M-1)} \sum_{i=0}^{M-1} \sum_{j=i+1}^{M-1} \theta(r - |x_i - x_j|) \tag{4.7}$$

where M is the length of the attractor, θ is the Heaviside function, r is the distance of the variable, and x_i and x_j are the two points. Then, $F(r)$ is the possibility that the range between the two points is not greater than r in the attractor.

(vii) Higuchi fractal dimension—this algorithm is another way of calculating the FD by producing a new timeline from the initial one $x(1)$, $x(2)$, …, $x(N)$, as shown in equation (4.7):

$$x_a^n = \left\{x(a),\ x(a+n),\ x(a+2n),\ \dots,\ x\left(a + \left[\frac{N-a}{n}\right]n\right)\right\} \tag{4.8}$$

for $a = 1, 2, \dots, n$

where a is the original test sample and N is the number of test samples [7, 16].

(viii) Petrosian fractal dimension—in this technique, tests of a timeline are subtracted sequentially and another time series is produced. At that point, positive and negative tests are assigned the values 1 and −1, respectively. In this way, the signals changed in the generated timeline become equivalent to the number of maximum signals in the main timeline. The equation used to calculate the FD in this algorithm is:

$$D = \frac{\log_{10^n}}{\log_{10^n} + \log_{10}\left(\frac{n}{n + 0.4N\Delta}\right)} \tag{4.9}$$

where n is the total number of tests and $N\Delta$ is the total number of changes in the signal in the binary timeline [16].

4.2.4 Feature selection

Many features can be extracted from EEG signals. The use of every feature results in the addition of improper or unsuitable features and diminishes classification accuracy. So, a feature selection or reduction method is used to select significant features or a combination of features. Since the data and the feature set are reduced, it is very important to use such a method, as it helps to enhance performance and speed.

The feature selection methods used in the research literature about ADHD detection include minimum redundancy maximum relevance (mRMR), double input symmetrical relevance (DISR), the non-dominated sorting genetic algorithm II (NSGA-II) (an evolutionary algorithm) and many more. DISR is a bilateral algorithm that assumes the shared data of a subset S and an objective variable Y has a minimum value which is equivalent to the total sum of all sub-subsets. This algorithm works by increasing the lower bound instead of the shared data.

mRMR works in two steps. First, a bunch of possible features is chosen; then, in the next step, a conservative feature is decided. This technique uses common data to categorize the features [16]. In another study, the NSGA-II evolutionary algorithm was used. The data was rearranged and the relevant parts of it used for preparation and validation. Then, an improvement cost function was characterized to boost the precision of approved data, namely:

$$\text{Cost} = 1 - \text{ACC}\,(\text{Data}_{\text{validation}}) \tag{4.10}$$

4.2.5 Classification

ML and DL algorithms, such as k-NN, SVM, NNs, and CNNs, have been used to detect ADHD, as described in the research literature.

k-NN is a widely used classification method which characterizes the samples according to their consonance with the k-nearest samples that have known classes. The range is determined by an algorithm commonly utilized in signal processing, known as dynamic time warping (DTW). DTW has the capability to evaluate waves that are not yet determined and have a unique scale, and it can locate the best match within a specified range. DTW has produced impressive outcomes when used in combination with k-NN classification [17]. SVM is another ML algorithm that is utilized for direct, non-deterministic data classification. SVMs are capable of positioning a hyperplane that effectively separates two distinct classes [17, 18]. SVM classifies linearly separable binary data sets using the following equation:

$$g(\vec{x}) = (\vec{\omega})^T\vec{x} + \omega 0 \tag{4.11}$$

where $g(\vec{x})$ is the hyperplane which differentiates the features, and ω is the weight factor [4].

NNs have great adaptability and the capacity to implement practically any function. As indicated by their abilities, NNs rapidly become advanced and have unique designs and learning algorithms. The architecture frequently employed for NNs is the multilayer perceptron (MLP) with back propagation learning. The system is composed of three separate layers: the input layer, the hidden layer, and the output layer. In one study, an MLP utilized one hidden layer together with five neurons for classification, achieving an accuracy of 92.28% [16].

Another popular data classifier is the CNN. CNNs are among the most exceptional algorithms in the field of machine vision and clinical image classification. In one study, EEG signals were turned into color pictures and were examined using the

CNN model [13]. The CNN accepted the images as input data and utilized convolution and pooling layers to output the features of the image. These features were then taken into the flattening and completely associated layers for classification. The CNN layers are:

(i) Convolutional layer: this accepts the image as the input and extracts the features using image processing techniques.
(ii) Pooling layer (downsampling): this layer decreases the proportion of the features.
(iii) Flattening layer: this process involves taking the output of the preceding layer and transforming the features matrix into a single-dimensional vector by flattening it.
(iv) Fully connected layer (dense layer): the output of the flattening layer is fed as an input to one or many neural layers to make predictions for classification [13].

4.3 Literature review

The detection of ADHD using EEG signals has been the subject of many studies and analyses described in the research literature [19]. A literature review based on the current state of the art is presented in table 4.1.

From table 4.1, it can be observed that EEG signals can act as tool for detecting ADHD, as a very high accuracy of 99.81% has been achieved [27]. Also, a very high accuracies were achieved using ELM (99.5%) [26] and CNN (99.46%) with $\beta1$, $\beta2$, and γ [24]. Thus, the results show that the higher frequency bands $\beta1$, $\beta2$, and γ are affected by ADHD. In addition, these results demonstrate that the frontal region has the highest explainability and interpretability [27].

However, the major issue with EEG signals is that it is immensely difficult to obtain noise-free data. Thus, for future research into the development of wearable devices for the detection of ADHD, not only should EEG signals be considered but also ECGs or photoplethysmography (PPG) should be used due to brain–heart communication. These are linked [11]. Thus, using combined data obtained from EEGs, PPGs, and ECGs could lead to better and more stable systems.

The results achieved from the model discussed in table 4.1 cannot be generalized, as the size of the data set is very small in each of the studies. Thus, testing must be done with much larger data sets collected from across the world, as the characteristic EEG signals may also differ from one geographic location to other. Also, gender acted as an important covariate in [28]. Thus, to arrive at a final stable system for the detection of ADHD, there is a requirement for a very large data set with global participation and not only EEG data but also data from other sensors (ECG/PPG).

4.4 Conclusions

The results cited in this chapter prove that an extremely high accuracy of almost 100% (99.81%) has been achieved. This implies that EEG-based detection of ADHD could act as a computer-aided tool for healthcare providers and could help to treat ADHD in early stages by accurate detection. Early and accurate detection would

Table 4.1. Literature review of different studies on the detection of ADHD using EEG signals.

Sl. No.	Reference	Methodology	Data set	No. of channels	Accuracy
1.	[7]	Within this research, EEG signals' frequency features, temporal features, and nonlinear features were obtained using filter banks and time windowing techniques along with a *k*-NN classifier.	Forty-six ADHD patients and 45 HCs; sampling rate 512 Hz	Nineteen channels	83.33%
2.	[4]	Band power features were extracted and analyzed using a using the minimum value of δ, θ, α, β, and γ band power. The signals were subjected to feature extraction and then classified using an SVM. The resulting classification was further examined.	Five ADHD patients and five HCs; recording was done in eyes-open and eyes-closed states at a 256 Hz sampling rate.	Sixteen channels	85.0%
3.	[13]	In this study, artifacts were removed from the EEG signals, then samples were segmented into many parts and after that four distinct frequency bands (θ, α, β and γ) were extracted and a red/green/blue image was created with three channels. Further images were input into a thirteen-layer CNN for feature extraction and classification.	Thirty-one ADHD patients and 30 healthy participants; sampling rate: 512 Hz	Nineteen channels	98.48%

(*Continued*)

Table 4.1. (*Continued*)

Sl. No.	Reference	Methodology	Data set	No. of channels	Accuracy
4	[5]	In this study, the nonlinear features such as the LE, fractal dimension, CD, SampEn, FuzzyEn, and ApEn were extracted from the frontal lobe (F4, FP1, Fz, F3, and FP2) and a further SVM was applied.	Fifty ADHD patients and 30 HCs; sampling rate: 512 Hz (eyes open, eyes closed, and performing cognitive tasks)	Nineteen channels	96.05%
5	[3]	Oddball paradigms were used and EEG signals from T6, Pz, F4, Cz, Fp1, T4, F3, and Fp2 were recorded. Morlet wavelet transform was applied. Band power (δ, θ, α, β) was computed and a further SVM (poly kernel and RBF) was applied.	Nine ADHD patients and ten HCs; sampling rate:1000 Hz	Five electrodes	94.74%
6	[20]	In this study, the EEG signals were recorded from 21 different regions of children with ADHC while their eyes were closed. The coherence of the wave shape was then assessed for a total of 16 electrodes, with eight electrodes located inside the same hemisphere and eight electrodes located in different hemispheres for different frequency bands i.e. δ, θ, α, β. Further statistical analysis (analysis of variance, ANOVA) was applied.	Total 102 (34 HCs, 34 ADHD patients with a 'typical' EEG profile, and 34 with excess beta activity)	Twenty-one channels.	Analysis showed increase in β power in children with ADHD and higher interhemispheric coherence compared to that of the control group.

7	[21]	In this study, The EEG signals' structural and functional characteristics were utilized. The functional-based features were extracted using graph learning (GL) techniques, while the structural-based features were extracted using graph signal processing (GSP). A further SVM classifier was applied.	Fifty ADHD patients and 58 HCs; sampling rate: 512 Hz	Thirty-two channels	93.47%
8	[22]	In this study, ADHD was detected utilizing audio and visual cognitive continuous performance tests (CPTs) and the EEG power and the cognitive function were detected in children with ADHD. The EEG power test used the comparative power of the ratios of different frequency bands i.e. α, β, θ, and θ/β and θ/α. Further statistical paired t-tests were applied.	Forty-four ADHD patients and 44 HCs; sampling rate: 512 Hz	Three electrodes (Cz, A1, and A2)	Patients with ADHD exhibited considerably higher θ relative power, lower β relative power, and a higher θ/β ratio ($p < 0.05$). Patients with ADHD exhibited a notably lower score on the auditory CPT ($p < 0.05$). The EEG power parameters exhibited a significant correlation with children's visual attention function in cases of ADHD ($p < 0.01$).

(Continued)

Table 4.1. (*Continued*)

Sl. No.	Reference	Methodology	Data set	No. of channels	Accuracy
9.	[16]	EEG signals were extracted from the participants while they had to do some tasks that required their attention. Nonlinear features (FD, ApEn, and LE) were extracted from the EEG signals. DISR and mRMR techniques were applied for selection and an MLP NN was used as the classifier.	Thirty ADHD patients and 30 HCs; sampling rate:256 Hz	Nineteen channels	92.28% (mRMR) and 93.65% (DISR)
10	[15]	In this study, the detection of ADHD was done using brain networks. The study used transfer entropy as the data transfer to identify pairwise data from EEG signals in different frequency bands. Further statistics and the receiver operating characteristic (ROC) curve were used for analysis.	Sixty-one ADHD patients and 60 HCs. Sampling rate:128 Hz	Nineteen channels	The graph metrics obtained from the estimated directed brain networks in the β-band exhibited the greatest differentiation between the control and ADHD groups.
11.	[18]	In this study, EEG signals were recorded during 'oddball paradigm' activity. Morlet wavelet transform was applied to the EEG records, yielding the energy and power variables, which were then used as inputs for an SVM algorithm.	Four hundred and seven ADHD patients and 310 HCs.	Eight electrodes	94.74%

12.	[14]	In this study, participants in the age range of 6–45 years suffering from ADHD were analyzed. EEG data was obtained with the eyes closed and open and during CPTs. General regression and as stepwise regression were applied. The band power (δ, θ, α, β) was also computed from the EEG channels Fz, Cz, and Pz. Different studies were performed to examine the influence of age, medication, and the conditions used to make the recording. Stepwise regression was also applied to examine the effects of data quality on the EEG band power.	Total 305 participants, 184 children with ADHD, 39 teenagers with ADHD, 57 adults with ADHD, and 325 HCs; sampling rate: 256 Hz	Twenty-two channels	Demographic factors, particularly age and signs of hyperactivity/ impulsivity, significantly influenced data quality. There was no effect due to methodological variations in the study design and analytical techniques discussed here. The results indicated that the delta, theta, and alpha power decreased with increasing age.
13	[23]	In this study, a neurocognitive assessment tool (NCAT) was developed for the detection of ADHD. Four measures were used in NCAT: (1) the Swanson, Nolan, and Pelham rating scale version IV(SNAP-IV), which includes subjective measures related to ADHD that may be influenced by parental biases or a desire for diagnosis; (2) NCAT-core, which consists of objective measurements	Total 214 participants, 53 ADHD patients and 161 healthy participants; sampling rate: 512 Hz	One channel (Fp1)	93.4% (Combined Model)

(*Continued*)

Table 4.1. (*Continued*)

Sl. No.	Reference	Methodology	Data set	No. of channels	Accuracy
		that do not specifically evaluate ADHD symptoms; (3) EEGs, which involve objective physiological measures; and (4) the combination of all three models. The EEG signal was recorded with eyes open, eyes closed, and with a focus task. To identify the continuous factors that distinguished between the control group and the ADHD group discriminant function analysis (DFA) was used. EO and FO (θ/β ratio, θ, δ, α, β power), β, δ, θ and α activation were used as features.			
14.	[24]	Used multiclass classification for inattentive ADHD (ADHD-I), combined ADHD (ADHCC), and normal patients. A deep convolutional neural network was used along with $\beta 1$, $\beta 2$, γ, δ, θ, α as features.	Twelve ADHD-I patients and 14 HCs; sampling frequency: 250 Hz	Twenty-one channels	99.46% ($\beta 1$, $\beta 2$, and γ along with CNN)
15	[25]	In this study, CNN feature maps from different layers were used as inputs to LR, SVM, and random forest (RF).	Sixty-one ADHD patients and 60 HCs; sampling frequency: 128 Hz	Nineteen channels	95.83% (CNN + LR)

16	[26]	This study introduced a novel technique called variational mode and Hilbert transform (HT)-based EEG rhythm separation (VHERS). The instantaneous frequency (IFE) and instantaneous amplitude (IA) were obtained by applying variational mode decomposition (VMD) and HT. The delta, theta, alpha, beta, and gamma rhythms were formed by the appropriate IFE and IA. Five entropy-based features, namely Tsallis entropy (TsEn), fuzzy entropy (FEN), Renyi entropy (REN), sample entropy (SEN), and permutation entropy (PEN) were obtained from the rhythms and then fed into the following classifiers: SVM, extreme learning machine (ELM), naive Bayes (NB), LDA, *k*-NN, and decision tree (DT).	Sixty-one ADHD patients and 60 healthy participants; sampling frequency: 128 Hz	Nineteen channels	99.5%(ELM)
17	[27]	In this study, a total of 41 statistical parameters (entropy measurements, statistical measures, and nonlinear measures), were retrieved, and further classification was done using the explainable boosted machine	Sixty-one ADHD patients and 60 healthy participants; sampling frequency: 128 Hz	Nineteen channels	99.81% (the frontal region's interpretability and explainability were at their highest).

(*Continued*)

Table 4.1. (*Continued*)

Sl. No.	Reference	Methodology	Data set	No. of channels	Accuracy
		(EBM) model. The model's interpretability was assessed using statistical analysis and performance measurement. The significance of the characteristics, channels, and brain areas was determined through the utilization of both the glass box and black box methodologies. The local and global explainability of the model was obtained using advanced techniques such as local interpretable model-agnostic Explanations (LIME), SHapley Additive exPlanations (SHAPs), partial dependence plots (PDPs), and Morris sensitivity analysis.			

thus lead to proper treatment and better quality of life for millions of individuals suffering ADHD across the world. However, to generalize the model and obtain a stable system, there is a requirement for a larger data set and different types of sensor data.

References

[1] Thomas R, Sanders S, Doust J, Beller E and Glasziou P 2015 Prevalence of attention-deficit/hyperactivity disorder: a systematic review and meta-analysis *Pediatrics* **135** e994–1001

[2] American Psychiatric Association 2013 *Diagnostic and Statistical Manual of Mental Disorders* 5th edn (Washington, DC: American Psychiatric Association)

[3] Gabriel B, Spendola M M, Mesquita A and Neto A Z 2017 Identification of ADHD cognitive pattern disturbances using EEG and wavelets analysis *Proc. 2017 IEEE 17th Int. Conf. on Bioinformatics and Bioengineering, BIBE 2017 (2018 January)* 157–62

[4] Joy R C, Thomas George S, Rajan A A and Subathra M S P 2019 Detection of attention deficit hyperactivity disorder from eeg signal using discrete wavelet transform *Proc. 2019 5th Int. Conf. on Computing, Communication Control and Automation, ICCUBEA* vol 2019 pp 3–7

[5] Boroujeni Y K, Rastegari A A and Khodadadi H 2019 Diagnosis of attention deficit hyperactivity disorder using non-linear analysis of the EEG signal *IET Syst. Biol.* **13** 260–6

[6] Sridhar C, Bhat S, Acharya U R, Adeli H and Bairy G M 2017 Diagnosis of attention deficit hyperactivity disorder using imaging and signal processing techniques *Comput. Biol. Med.* **88** 93–9

[7] Taghibeyglou B, Hasanzadeh N, Bagheri F and Jahed M 2020 ADHD diagnosis in children using common spatial pattern and nonlinear analysis of filter banked EEG *2020 28th Iranian Conf. on Electrical Engineering, ICEE* 2020 0–4

[8] Khadidos A O, Alyoubi K H, Mahato S, Khadidos A O and Mohanty S N 2023 Computer aided detection of major depressive disorder (MDD) using electroencephalogram signals *IEEE Access* **11** 41133–41

[9] Mahato S, Pathak L K and Kumari K 2021 Detection of schizophrenia using EEG signals *Data Analytics in Bioinformatics: A Machine Learning Perspective* ed S Choudhury, R Satpathy, S N Mohanty and X Zhang (New York: Wiley) pp 359–90 (SCOPUS Indexed)

[10] Khare S K, Blanes-Vidal V, Nadimi E S and Acharya U R 2024 Emotion recognition and artificial intelligence: a systematic review (2014–2023) and research recommendations *Inf. Fusion* **102** 102019

[11] El-Dahshan E S, Bassiouni M M, Khare S K, Tan R S and Acharya U R 2024 ExHyptNet: an explainable diagnosis of hypertension using EfficientNet with PPG signals *Expert Syst. Appl.* **239** 122388

[12] Shen M, Wen P and Song B 2021 Graph theoretical analysis based on EEG effective connectivity in ADHD children https://doi.org/10.21203/rs.3.rs-375557/v1

[13] Moghaddari M, Lighvan M Z and Danishvar S 2020 Diagnose ADHD disorder in children using convolutional neural network based on continuous mental task EEG *Comput. Methods Programs Biomed.* **197** 105738

[14] Kaiser A *et al* 2021 EEG data quality: determinants and impact in a multicenter study of children, adolescents, and adults with attention-deficit/hyperactivity disorder (ADHD *Brain Sci.* **11** 1–36

[15] Abbas A K, Azemi G, Amiri S, Ravanshadi S and Omidvarnia A 2021 Effective connectivity in brain networks estimated using EEG signals is altered in children with ADHD *Comput. Biol. Med.* **134** 104515
[16] Mohammadi M R, Khaleghi A, Nasrabadi A M, Rafieivand S, Begol M and Zarafshan H 2016 EEG classification of ADHD and normal children using non-linear features and neural network *Biomed. Eng. Lett.* **6** 66–73
[17] Alchalabi A E, Elsharnouby M, Shirmohammadi S and Eddin A N 2017 Feasibility of detecting ADHD patients' attention levels by classifying their EEG signals *2017 IEEE Int. Symp. on Medical Measurements and Applications, MeMeA 2017–Proc.* pp 314–9
[18] Gabriel R, Spindola M M and Chiaramonte M 2020 Wavelets and SVM analysis applied to signals responsive to auditory and visual stimulus captured by EEG in students with ADHD *Rev. Argent. Bioing.* **24** 73–9
[19] Khare S K, March S, Barua P D, Gadre V M and Acharya U R 2023 Application of data fusion for automated detection of children with developmental and mental disorders: a systematic review of the last decade *Inf. Fusion* **99** 101898
[20] Clarke A R, Barry R J, McCarthy R, Selikowitz M, Johnstone S J, Hsu C I, Magee C A, Lawrence C A and Croft R J 2007 Coherence in children with attention-deficit/hyperactivity disorder and excess beta activity in their EEG *Clin. Neurophysiol.* **118** 1472–9
[21] Einizade A, Mozafari M, Rezaei-Dastjerdehei M, Aghdaei E, Mijani A M and Hajipour Sardouie S 2020 Detecting ADHD children based on EEG signals using graph signal processing techniques *27th National and 5th Int. Iranian Conf. of Biomedical Engineering, ICBME (2020, November)* 264–70
[22] Shi T, Li X, Song J, Zhao N, Sun C, Xia W, Wu L and Tomoda A 2012 EEG characteristics and visual cognitive function of children with attention deficit hyperactivity disorder (ADHD) *Brain Dev.* **34** 806–11
[23] Johnstone S J, Parrish L, Jiang H, Zhang D W, Williams V and Li S 2021 Aiding diagnosis of childhood attention-deficit/hyperactivity disorder of the inattentive presentation: discriminant function analysis of multi-domain measures including EEG *Biol. Psychol.* **161** 108080
[24] Ahmadi A, Kashefi M, Shahrokhi H and Nazari M A 2021 Computer aided diagnosis system using deep convolutional neural networks for ADHD subtypes *Biomed. Signal Process. Control* **63** 102227
[25] TaghiBeyglou B, Shahbazi A, Bagheri F, Akbarian S and Jahed M 2022 Detection of ADHD cases using CNN and classical classifiers of raw EEG *Comput. Methods Programs Biomed. Update* **2** 100080
[26] Khare S K, Gaikwad N B and Bajaj V 2022 VHERS: a novel variational mode decomposition and hilbert transform-based EEG rhythm separation for automatic ADHD detection *IEEE Trans. Instrum. Meas.* **71** 1–10
[27] Khare S K and Acharya U R 2023 An explainable and interpretable model for attention deficit hyperactivity disorder in children using EEG signals *Comput. Biol. Med.* **155** 106676
[28] Orgo L, Bachmann M, Kalev K, Hinrikus H and Järvelaid M 2016 Brain functional connectivity in depression: gender differences in EEG *2016 IEEE EMBS Conference on Biomedical Engineering and Sciences (IECBES)* (Piscataway, NJ: IEEE) 270–3

IOP Publishing

Artificial Intelligence

A tool for effective diagnostics

Smith K Khare, Sachin Taran and Ankush D Jamthikar

Chapter 5

Artificial neural network-based classification of eye states using electroencephalogram signals: a comparative analysis of algorithms and artifact removal techniques

Pranjali Gajbhiye, Vineet Singh, Sandeep Saharan and Shyam Joshi

Electroencephalography offers a noninvasive approach for the study of brain activity patterns. This research explores the potential of electroencephalography for identifying eye states, a critical component of human–computer interaction (HCI) applications. We analyze electroencephalographic data recorded during various eye conditions to detect distinct brain activity signatures. Machine learning (ML) algorithms are employed to classify eye states based on the extracted electroencephalographic features. Our findings demonstrate high classification accuracy (96.79%) using random forests (RFs), which outperform the other algorithms investigated. This chapter emphasizes the significance of employing artifact removal techniques for robust electroencephalographic data analysis. This work contributes to the development of practical HCI applications utilizing EEG-based eye state detection.

5.1 Introduction

Electroencephalography is a noninvasive diagnostic test used to measure the electrical activity of the brain [1–3]. In the early 1920s, Hans Berger was the first to measure the brain's electrical activity by placing electrodes on the scalp [4]. Signals recorded using electrodes positioned on the scalp are called electroencephalograms (EEGs). Over the last few years, researchers have diligently studied EEGs to understand the cognitive process better [4]. Imaging techniques that produce two-dimensional or three-dimensional images of the human brain are costly. On the other hand, EEGs have high temporal resolution, and the cost of instruments that record EEGs is less than those of imaging instruments [3]. EEG signals are used for

doi:10.1088/978-0-7503-5964-1ch5

different applications, such as driver drowsiness detection [5], sleep stage classification [6], the detection of epileptic seizures [7], music therapy [8], tonic pain characterization [9], cognitive task recognition [10], etc. The clinical utility of EEG signals is important for the aforementioned neural information-processing applications. The magnitude of an EEG signal is normally in the micro-volt range, and it can be intermixed with potentials of non-cerebral origins, which are called artifacts [11]. For accurate analysis in EEG processing applications, removing artifacts from the signal is essential. Because of their low power usage, EEG machines have become increasingly important in recent years. Researchers have employed multiple methodologies to detect and eliminate artifacts. This chapter presents a thorough summary of notable techniques for reducing and ultimately removing artifacts from EEG data. Avoiding motions that may cause artifacts is the first step toward reducing their occurrence in EEG data. Numerous techniques have been employed to minimize artifacts; nevertheless, the exploration of eliminating multiple unwanted components seems to be a major challenge.

Extrinsic artifacts are caused by electric and electronic components, notably high electrode impedance and interference. The term 'intrinsic' describes a wide range of aberrations present in EEG signals, including bioelectric potentials produced by the heart and muscles, blinking, and eye movements. Artifacts are undesired components that come from external sources. These factors complicate the processing of the EEG data by distorting the true cerebral activity in the collected EEG data. Artifacts cause the original EEG signal to be distorted. Therefore, the most important task in the field of EEG signal processing is to separate clean EEG signals from contaminated EEG signals. Researchers can acquire a more accurate depiction of brain activity by eliminating artifacts from EEG readings. In order to reliably differentiate real EEG signals from artifacts, a number of strategies and algorithms have been developed, facilitating more accurate data analysis and interpretation. The contributions examined in this chapter are listed below:

- Exploration of diverse artifacts affecting EEG signals
- Examination of methodologies employed in the mitigation of physiological artifacts within EEG recordings, encompassing filtering and blind source separation (BSS) techniques
- Evaluation of an artificial neural network (ANN)-based approach for removing physiological artifacts from EEGs using both synthetic and real-world data
- Comparative analysis of decision trees, *k*-nearest neighbors (*k*-NN), support vector machine (SVM), and RF classifiers for the discrimination of eyes-open versus eyes-closed states in EEG data, aiming at discerning optimal algorithms for this classification task

5.1.1 Human brain

The telencephalon, referred to as the cerebrum, is the paramount segment of the human brain [12]. Comprising six lobes [13], the cerebrum houses the four primary lobes of the cerebral cortex in humans: the frontal, parietal, temporal, and occipital

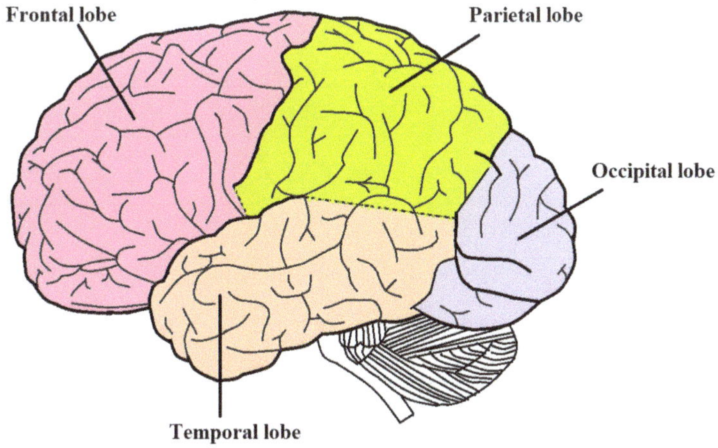

Figure 5.1. Various lobes of the brain (redrawn from [2]).

lobes [14]. The lobes of the human brain are shown in figure 5.1. The functions and locations of the human brain lobes are as follows:

- **Frontal lobe:** located at the front of the cerebral hemisphere near the forehead. It contains dopamine-sensitive neurons and controls important cognitive skills, such as attention, planning, motivation, and short-term memory tasks [15].
- **Parietal lobe:** the portion of the brain above the occipital lobe and behind the frontal lobe [16]. Sensory information of various kinds is processed and collected in this area, including the sensory input from the skin. The regions in the parietal lobe play a crucial role in language processing.
- **Temporal lobe:** the portion below the lateral fissure on both sides of the cerebral hemispheres is known as the temporal lobe [17]. Emotion, memory, and language comprehension are processed in the temporal lobe.
- **Occipital lobe:** acknowledged to be the central hub for visual processing within the brain due to its extensive coverage of the anatomical region known as the visual cortex [18]. Cognitive tasks such as perception and color differentiation are processed in the occipital lobe.

5.1.2 EEG rhythms

In general, five types of rhythms or bands are associated with EEG signals [7]. The rhythms are categorized according to their frequency range [6]. Plots of EEG rhythms such as a δ-wave, a θ-wave, an α-wave, a β-wave, and a γ-wave are depicted in figure 5.2. The frequency range and the presence of a rhythmic pattern in EEG signals during various cognitive tasks are shown in table 5.1.

The δ-wave patterns are seen in EEG signals during deep sleep and in the unconscious state [1]. Similarly, θ-wave patterns are observed in psychological events such as low-level alertness and problem-solving. α-wave patterns in EEG signals are observed during relaxed states or during meditation [19]. β-waves are seen in EEG

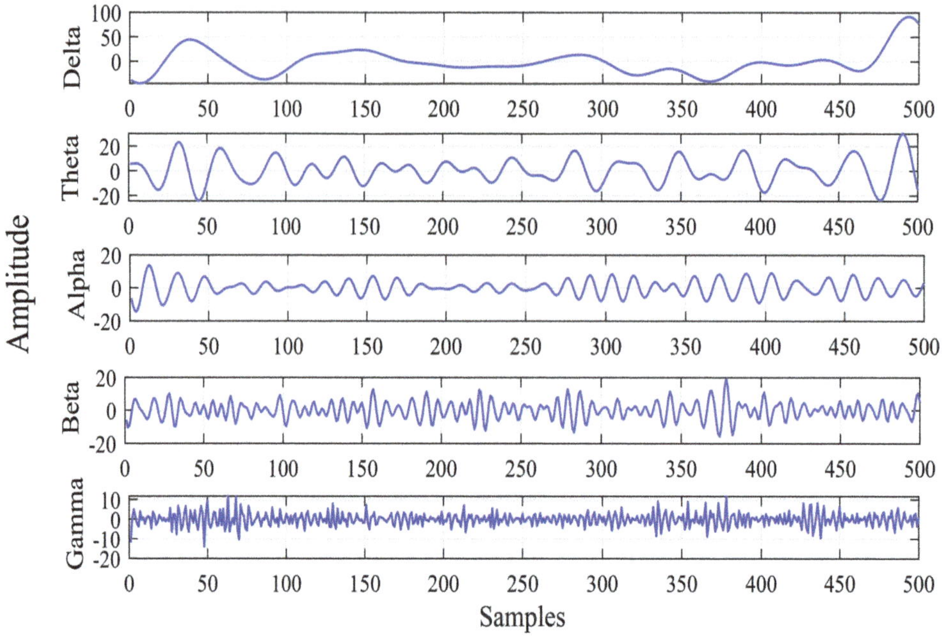

Figure 5.2. EEG brain rhythms corresponding to δ, θ, α, β, and γ-waves from low to high frequencies.

Table 5.1. Standard EEG frequency ranges [1].

Rhythm	Range (Hz)	Cognitive task
δ-Wave	0.5–4	Deep sleep and the unconscious state
θ-Wave	4–8	Relaxed and wakeful
α-Wave	8–13	Meditative and relaxed states
β-Wave	13–30	Active thinking
γ-Wave	30–75	Attention and information processing

signals during attentiveness, active thinking, and problem-solving tasks [1]. γ-waves have less amplitude, and these patterns are associated with various cognitive tasks such as information processing and attention [1].

5.1.3 EEG recording using the 10–20 electrode system

The 10–20 system is the globally accepted approach that defines the positions of the electrodes during EEG recording [20], as shown in figure 5.3. This system assigns specific locations to electrodes based on brain regions. Electrodes are positioned at distances of either 10% or 20% of the head circumference, measured front-to-back or left-to-right [1]. Each electrode location is denoted by a letter: central (C), parietal (P), temporal (T), occipital (O), frontal (F), and prefrontal (frontal pole, FP) [20].

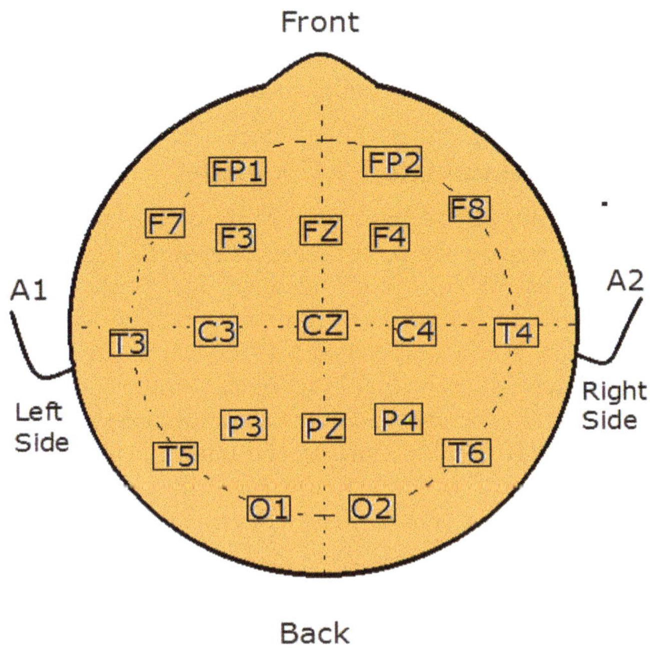

Figure 5.3. The 10–20 electrode placement system [3].

This standardized placement allows for consistent data collection and analysis across different studies. A block diagram of the 10–20 system for electrode placement on the scalp for the recording of EEG signals is shown in figure 5.3. In this recording system, the distances between the adjacent electrodes are 10% or 20% of the front-to-back or right-to-left dimensions of the skull [20]. The even numbers (2,4,6,8) correspond to the right hemisphere of the brain. Similarly, the odd numbers (1,3,5,7) denote the left hemisphere part in recordings of multichannel EEG signals. The symbol 'Z' corresponds to the placement of electrodes on the midline. The EEG signals recorded using electrodes reveal the sum of the electrical activity of thousands of neurons in the brain. This signal contains many slow waves if a person is in a relaxed state [21]. Similarly, fast waves appear in the EEG signal when the person is in an excited state [21]. The 10–20 system is used to record EEG signals in sleep studies [6], lab research [22], and other clinical studies such as epileptic seizure detection [23], the location of focal seizure areas [3], emotion recognition [24], brain–computer interfacing [10], and the diagnosis of various neurological disorders. The presence of artifacts during the recording of EEG signals may affect diagnostic performance. Therefore, the elimination of various artifacts using signal processing techniques is the primary task for EEG processing applications.

5.1.4 Ambulatory EEG recording systems

Ambulatory EEG monitoring systems allows for the continuous recording of the brain's electrical activity, even when the subject is in motion, thereby enhancing their effectiveness in the diagnosis of neurological disorders [25, 26]. These systems enable longer-duration EEG signal recordings and are comparatively more cost-effective than clinical EEG monitoring [27]. However, during recording, the EEG signals often suffer from contamination by various artifacts [28–30].

5.2 Artifacts that contaminate EEG signals

The International Federation of Clinical Neurophysiology defines an artifact as a potential difference due to an extra-cerebral source in an EEG signal [31]. The initial step in EEG signal processing is to identify the type of artifact [11]. A suitable filtering algorithm can then be applied to remove the artifact from the EEG recording. The artifacts associated with EEG signals are broadly categorized into two classes, namely those with physiological origins and those with non-physiological origins [32]. The methodology used to categorize EEG artifacts is shown in figure 5.4. Motion, ocular, cardiac, and muscle artifacts are interpreted as EEG artifacts of physiological origin [33]. Similarly, the non-physiological artifacts in EEG signals are due to improper electrode placement, power line interfaces, and other environmental factors [33].

- **Motion artifacts:** these mainly occur in EEG signals during ambulatory recording [34]. Electrode movement during the recording and involuntary patient movements are responsible for the presence of motion artifacts in the EEG signal [35]. An EEG signal with motion artifacts is shown in figure 5.5.

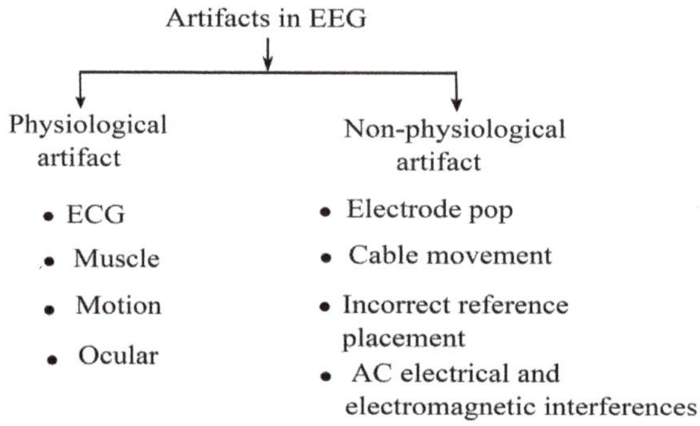

Figure 5.4. Physiological and non-physiological artifacts in EEGs.

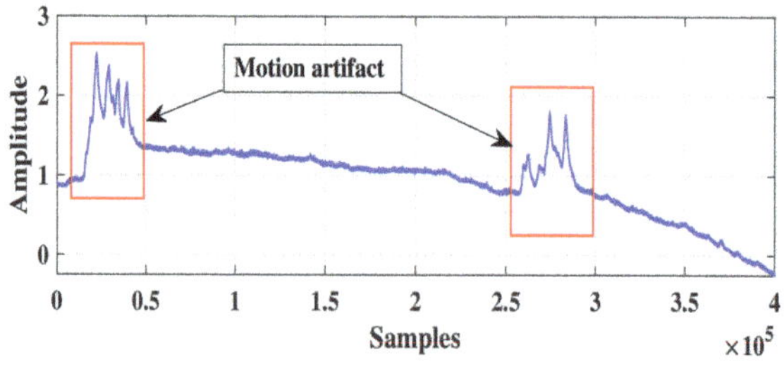

Figure 5.5. EEG signal with motion artifacts.

- **Ocular artifacts:** these artifacts, a common occurrence in EEG signals, stem from voltage changes during corneal–retinal dipole and eyelid movement [36]. These movements disrupt electric fields around the eye and scalp, resulting in ocular artifacts in the EEG signals. Typically, these artifacts manifest within a frequency range of 0–5 Hz, primarily affecting frontal lobe EEG channels such as FP1–F7 and FP2–F8 [37, 38]. Eyeblink artifacts similarly corrupt EEG signals across all channels, often exhibiting higher amplitudes than artifact-free EEG signals [36]. For a visual representation of EEG signals with ocular artifacts, please refer to figure 5.6.

- **Electrocardiogram (ECG) artifacts:** cardiac or ECG artifacts often resemble spikes in recorded EEG signals [39]. Typically, the electrical field distribution of the heart across most patients' scalps remains consistent, allowing for the removal of residual ECG artifacts through bipolar montage in the recorded EEG signal [40]. However, if a unipolar montage is employed, the ECG artifact might be prominently visible in the EEG signal [39]. See figure 5.7 for an example of an EEG signal affected by an ECG artifact.
- **Muscle artifacts:** these artifacts appear in EEG signals due to muscle activity, namely activity in the muscles associated with the neck, face, and jaw [41]. The broad spectral distribution of muscle artifacts causes interference in the visual inspection of the EEG components. These artifacts are more predominant in the EEG signals acquired from the temporal channels (T7–P7 and T8–P8) [42]. An EEG signal with a muscle artifact is shown in figure 5.8.

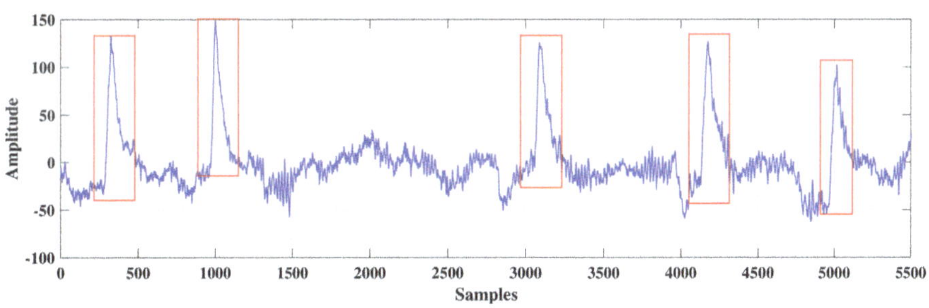

Figure 5.6. EEG signal with ocular artifacts.

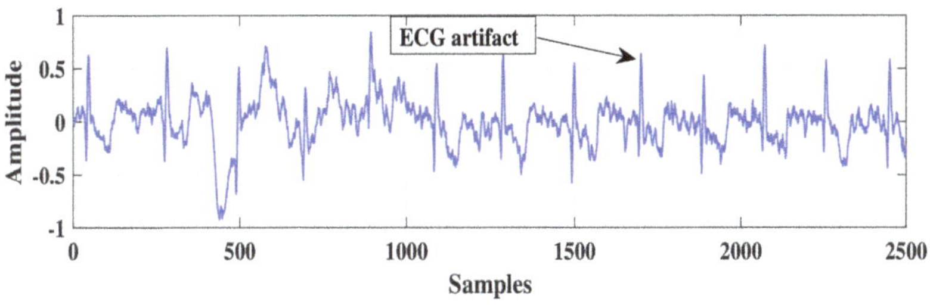

Figure 5.7. EEG signal with ECG artifacts.

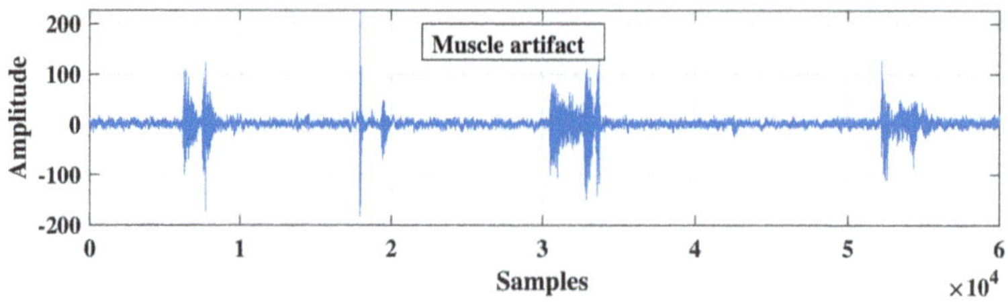

Figure 5.8. EEG signal with a muscle artifact.

The diagnostic quality of EEG signals is compromised by the presence of various artifacts, which pose a significant challenge in biomedical signal processing. Recent research has focused on developing methods to effectively filter motion and ocular artifacts from EEG signals [43, 44]. These approaches incorporate diverse multiscale analysis techniques such as discrete wavelet transform (DWT) [38], empirical mode decomposition [45], ensemble empirical mode decomposition (EEMD) [46], and singular spectrum analysis (SSA) [47], among others. In addition, dimension reduction techniques such as independent component analysis (ICA) [48], canonical correlation analysis [46], and principal component analysis (PCA) [49] have been employed for artifact filtering in EEG signals. Some studies have explored adaptive noise cancellation (ANC) in combination with multiscale analysis methods such as DWT and SSA to mitigate artifacts in EEG recordings [47]. However, these techniques often exhibit limited denoising performance and high computational complexity. Thus, there is a need for the development of novel methods that offer superior denoising capabilities while maintaining computational efficiency in filtering various artifacts from EEG signals. A detailed analysis of the proposed algorithms is given in the following sections.

5.3 Existing methods for eliminating various artifacts

In the last two decades, various algorithms have been proposed to remove ocular artifacts from EEG signals [50]. These algorithms employ different techniques including regression [38, 51], DWT [52, 53], ICA [48, 54], and PCA [49, 55] for artifact filtering.

Khatun *et al* [52] explored combining DWT with thresholding techniques (universal and statistical) for single-channel EEG artifact removal. Their findings suggested that the combination of stationary wavelet transform (SWT) and statistical thresholding outperforms other wavelet-based methods [52]. Similarly, Patel *et al* [55] investigated a combination of EEMD and PCA for ocular artifact filtering. They evaluated the filtered EEG signal by selecting principal components from the intrinsic mode function (IMF) matrix, achieving a mean absolute error in power spectral density (MAE-PSD) of 0.669 dB Hz^{-1} for the alpha band in the filtered signal [55]. These authors also explored a combination of EEMD and kernel PCA, achieving a lower MAE-PSD value of 0.583 dB Hz^{-1} for the alpha band [55].

Peng *et al* [36] proposed a framework that combined DWT and ANC for the elimination of ocular artifacts. The reference artifact component for ANC was derived using the DWT of the contaminated EEG signal. Their work resulted in an MAE-PSD value of 0.416 dB Hz^{-1} for the alpha band [36]. Another study by Maddirala and Shaik [47] combined SSA and ANC for electrooculogram (EOG) artifact removal from single-channel EEG signals. SSA was used to extract the ocular artifact component, which was then fed into the ANC stage for artifact elimination. This SSA-ANC approach achieved an MAE-PSD value of 0.167 dB Hz^{-1} for the alpha band [47].

Further research explored the combination of DWT and ICA [56] and regression techniques with ICA [57] for ocular artifact removal. Recent studies have examined deep learning-based approaches [58]. These approaches require rigorous training using gradient descent to obtain optimal weight parameters for artifact filtering within deep neural networks [59]. Deep learning approaches require a fixed EEG signal length during training for optimal weight parameter evaluation, unlike ICA-based methods that depend on selecting independent components (ICs) for artifact removal and regression approaches that require simultaneous EEG and EOG recordings. In addition, wavelet-based approaches necessitate careful selection of the decomposition level and basis function for effective artifact elimination.

These observations highlight the need for ongoing research and the development of novel signal processing techniques to further enhance ocular artifact removal from EEG recordings.

5.3.1 Independent component analysis

ICA is a signal processing method used to decompose a multivariate signal into its ICs. Its application proves especially beneficial in the context of filtering EEG signals. This method operates using the premise that the observed signal is a linear amalgamation of independent sources. The objective is to identify the ICs that most accurately depict the observed signal. This pursuit involves maximizing the non-Gaussian nature of the estimated sources, which are conventionally assumed to exhibit non-Gaussian characteristics.

The algorithm for correcting the EEG signal using the ICA method can be outlined as follows:
The ICA algorithm typically involves the following steps:

1. Preprocessing: to prepare the EEG signal for analysis, unwanted noise and artifacts are removed through filtering.
2. Mixing model: the EEG signal is represented as a linear mixture of independent components.
3. Unmixing: the ICs are estimated by maximizing the non-Gaussian character of the sources.
4. Separation: the ICs are separated from the observed signal.

The ICA algorithm can be mathematically represented as follows:

$$\mathbf{X}_i = \mathbf{A}\mathbf{S}_i$$

where $\mathbf{X}_i$ is the observed signal, $\mathbf{A}$ is the mixing matrix, and $\mathbf{S}_i$ is the IC matrix. The goal is to find the unmixing matrix $\mathbf{W}$ such that

$$\mathbf{S}_i = \mathbf{W}\mathbf{X}_i.$$

The unmixing matrix $\mathbf{W}$ is typically estimated using an optimization algorithm that maximizes the non-Gaussian character of the estimated sources. ICA has been used to remove various types of artifacts from EEG signals, including muscle artifacts. For example, in the study by Maddirala and Shaik [47], a hybrid approach combining SSA and ANC was used to eliminate EOG artifacts from single-channel EEG signals. SSA was used to evaluate the ocular artifact component in the contaminated EEG signal, and then the ocular artifact component was used as the reference signal for the ANC stage to eliminate ocular artifacts from the EEG recording. ICA has been compared with other techniques for EEG artifact removal, such as DWT and regression. For example, in [60], a hybrid framework combining DWT and ANC was used to eliminate ocular artifacts from EEG recordings. DWT was used to decompose the EEG signal into different frequency bands, and then ANC was applied to each frequency band to remove ocular artifacts. ICA has several advantages, including its ability to handle nonstationary signals and its robustness to noise. However, it also has some limitations, such as its sensitivity to the choice of the mixing model and the unmixing algorithm.

5.3.2 Principal component analysis

PCA is a technique that minimizes a data set's complexity by finding a smaller set of features that capture the most important information. This makes it easier to identify patterns and visualize high-dimensional data. PCA achieves this by transforming the data into a new set of uncorrelated variables, called principal components, ordered by their explanatory power. In essence, PCA aims to find the directions in the data that show the most variation.

The algorithm for correcting the EEG signal using the PCA method can be outlined as follows:

The PCA algorithm typically involves the following steps:

1. Preprocessing: standardize the data by subtracting the mean from each feature and then dividing by its standard deviation. This ensures all features are on a similar scale.
2. Covariance analysis: calculate the covariance matrix to capture the relationships between features.
3. Dimensionality Reduction: perform eigenvalue decomposition on the covariance matrix. This identifies new directions (eigenvectors) that capture the most variance (eigenvalues) in the data.
4. Component selection: choose the most informative principal components based on their corresponding eigenvalues. Components with higher eigenvalues represent greater variance.
5. Data projection: transform the original data into the newly created principal component space.

The PCA algorithm can be mathematically represented as follows:

$$\mathbf{X} = \mathbf{U}\boldsymbol{\Lambda}\mathbf{V}^T$$

where **X** is the original data, **U** is the matrix of eigenvectors, **Λ** is the diagonal matrix of eigenvalues, and **V** is the matrix of principal components.

PCA is often used to visualize high-dimensional data in lower dimensions. Peng *et al* used PCA to visualize EEG signals in the frequency domain. The EEG signals were segregated into different frequency bands using PCA, and then the frequency range was visualized using a bar chart. The resulting bar chart showed the distribution of the EEG signal in the frequency domain, which helped to identify the dominant frequency bands. PCA has been compared with other techniques for dimensionality reduction, such as ICA and largest Lyapunov exponent (LLE). Li *et al* proposed a method where PCA was compared with ICA and LLE to reduce the dimensionality of EEG signals. The results showed that PCA performed better than ICA and LLE in terms of retaining the most important features in the data. PCA has several advantages, including its ability to handle high-dimensional data and its simplicity. However, it also has some limitations, such as its sensitivity to the choice of the number of principal components and its inability to handle nonlinear relationships in the data.

5.3.3 Singular spectrum analysis–adaptive noise cancellation

SSA and ANC are two techniques that have been combined to effectively remove artifacts from EEG signals. The hybrid of these approaches, known as SSA-ANC, leverages the strengths of both methods to achieve better denoising performance and computational efficiency. SSA is a time-series analysis method that decomposes a signal into its constituent components, often referred to as IMFs. Each IMF represents a specific frequency band in the signal. SSA is particularly useful for identifying and removing artifacts from EEG signals because it can separate the signal into its different frequency components, allowing for targeted filtering. SSA consists of two main stages: decomposition and reconstruction.

Decomposition:

1. **Embedding:** the embedding step transforms the one-dimensional time series $\{x_t\}_{t=1}^{N}$ into a multidimensional series by creating lagged vectors. Define the embedding dimension L (window length) and construct the trajectory matrix **X**:

$$\mathbf{X}_s = \begin{pmatrix} x_s1 & x_s2 & \cdots & x_sK \\ x_s2 & x_s3 & \cdots & x_sK+1 \\ \vdots & \vdots & \ddots & \vdots \\ x_sL & x_sL+1 & \cdots & x_sN \end{pmatrix},$$

where $K_s = N_s - L_s + 1$.

2. **Singular value decomposition (SVD):** perform SVD on **X** as follows:

$$\mathbf{X}_s = \sum_{i=1}^{L} \sqrt{\lambda_i} \mathbf{U}_i \mathbf{V}_i^\top,$$

where λ_i are the eigenvalues and $\mathbf{U}_i$ and $\mathbf{V}_i$ are the left singular vectors, respectively.

Reconstruction:

1. **Grouping:** group the SVD components into a smaller number of components that represent the original signal and the noise/artifacts.
2. **Diagonal averaging:** reconstruct the time series from the grouped components by averaging along the anti-diagonals of the trajectory matrix.

Adaptive noise cancellation for artifact removal

ANC is a signal processing technique that uses a reference signal to cancel out noise from a primary signal. In the context of EEG artifact removal, ANC is used to eliminate artifacts by using the artifact component as the reference signal. ANC is effective in removing artifacts because it can adapt to the changing characteristics of the artifact over time. The ANC process involves the following steps:

1. **Primary input:** the contaminated EEG signal $x(t)$.
2. **Reference input:** the reference signal $d(t)$ containing the noise to be canceled.
3. **Adaptive filter:** a filter $w(t)$ that adjusts its coefficients to minimize the error signal $e(t)$.

   The adaptive filter's output, represented by $y(t)$, is subtracted from the primary input.

   $$e(t) = x(t) - y(t).$$

   The coefficients are updated using an adaptive algorithm, such as the least mean squares (LMS) algorithm:

   $$w_n(p + 1) = w_n(p) + \mu e(p)d(p),$$

   where μ is the step size.

Singular spectrum analysis–adaptive noise cancellation hybrid approach

The SSA-ANC hybrid approach combines the strengths of both techniques to achieve better denoising performance and computational efficiency. The SSA stage is used to decompose the EEG signal into its different frequency components, and then the ANC stage is used to eliminate the artifact components from each frequency band.

The algorithm for correcting the EEG signal using the SSA method can be outlined as follows:

1. **SSA decomposition:** decompose the EEG signal into its frequency components using SSA.

2. **Artifact identification:** identify the artifact components using SSA.
3. **ANC processing:** use the identified artifact components as reference signals in the ANC stage to remove artifacts from the EEG signal. Maddirala and Shaik [47] used a hybrid approach combining SSA and ANC to eliminate EOG artifacts from single-channel EEG signals.

To remove ocular artifacts from EEG recordings, the SSA stage first isolated the ocular artifact component from the contaminated signal. This isolated component then served as the reference signal for the subsequent ANC stage, effectively eliminating ocular artifacts from the EEG data. The results showed that the SSA-ANC hybrid approach achieved an MAE-PSD value of 0.167 dB Hz^{-1} for the α-band, which is significantly better than the results obtained by other methods.

The SSA-ANC hybrid approach has several advantages, as follows:

- **Improved denoising performance**: by combining the strengths of SSA and ANC, the SSA-ANC hybrid approach can achieve better denoising performance than either technique alone.
- **Computational efficiency**: the SSA–ANC hybrid approach can be computationally efficient because it uses a reference signal to cancel out artifacts, reducing the computational complexity of the algorithm.

However, the SSA-ANC hybrid approach also has some limitations, including:

- **Complexity**: The SSA-ANC hybrid approach can be complex to implement because it requires the signal to be decomposed into its different frequency ranges and the use of a reference signal for ANC.
- **Parameter selection**: The SSA-ANC hybrid approach requires the selection of effective factors for both the SSA and ANC stages, which can be challenging.

5.3.4 Fourier–Bessel series expansion empirical wavelet transform-based linear periodic time variation approach

Fourier–Bessel series expansion (FBSE) and empirical wavelet transform (EWT) are two techniques that have been combined to effectively process EEG signals. This hybrid approach, known as FBSE–EWT-based linear periodic time variation (LPTV) [61], leverages the strengths of both methods to achieve better efficiency. FBSE is a signal processing technique that separates a multivariate signal into its constituent sources based on their frequency characteristics. FBSE is particularly useful for EEG signal processing because it can effectively separate the signal into its different frequency components, allowing for targeted filtering. FBSE represents a signal $x(t)$ as the sum of the frequency-based components:

$$x(t) = \sum_{k=1}^{K} s_k(t),$$

where $s_k(t)$ are the separated source components, each representing a distinct frequency band.

Empirical wavelet transform for EEG signal processing
EWT is a time–frequency analysis method that decomposes a signal into its constituent components, known as wavelet sub-bands. Each sub-band represents a specific frequency band in the signal. EWT is particularly useful for EEG signal processing because it can effectively decompose the signal into its different frequency components, allowing for targeted filtering.

Mathematical representation of empirical wavelet transform
EWT constructs wavelet filters in the Fourier domain and applies them to the signal:

$$x(t) = \sum_{n=1}^{N} w_n(t),$$

where $w_n(t)$ are the wavelet sub-band components obtained through EWT.

Fourier–Bessel series expansion–empirical wavelet transform-based linear periodic time variation hybrid approach
The FBSE–EWT-based LPTV approach combines the strengths of both techniques to achieve better denoising performance and computational efficiency. The FBSE stage is used to separate the EEG signal into its different frequency components, and then the EWT stage is used to decompose each frequency component into its constituent wavelet sub-bands. The LPTV stage is used to filter out the artifacts from each sub-band, resulting in a denoised EEG signal.

Mathematical representation
Let $x(n)$ be the contaminated EEG signal, $y(n)$ be the corrected EEG signal, and W be the LPTV weights. The LPTV for EEG artifact removal can be mathematically represented as follows:

$$y(n) = \sigma\left(\sum_{i=1}^{N} W_i \cdot x(n)\right),$$

where σ is the activation function, W_i are the LPTV weights, and N is the number of layers or components in the model.

Algorithm

1. Preprocess the EEG signal $x(n)$ by normalizing and segmenting it into frames.
2. Apply FBSE to separate the EEG signal into its frequency components.
3. Use EWT to decompose each frequency component into wavelet sub-bands.
4. Apply the LPTV filter to remove artifacts from each sub-band.
5. Reconstruct the denoised EEG signal $y(n)$ from the processed sub-bands.

Advantages and limitations
The FBSE-EWT-based LPTV approach has several advantages, including:

- Improved denoising performance: by combining the strengths of FBSE and EWT, this approach can achieve better denoising performance than either technique alone.
- Computational efficiency: the FBSE-EWT-based LPTV approach is computationally efficient because it uses adaptive filtering techniques to cancel out artifacts, reducing the computational complexity of the algorithm.

However, the FBSE-EWT-based LPTV approach also has some limitations, including:

- Complexity: the FBSE-EWT-based LPTV approach can be complex to implement because it requires the EEG signal to be decomposed into its different frequency components and the use of adaptive filtering for artifact removal.
- Parameter selection: the FBSE-EWT-based LPTV approach requires the selection of appropriate parameters for both the FBSE and EWT stages, which can be challenging.

5.4 Existing artificial neural network-based methods

ANN-based methods represent a significant advancement in EEG artifact reduction, offering improved accuracy and robustness over traditional techniques. By leveraging the power of convolutional neural networks (CNNs), recurrent neural networks (RNNs), and hybrid models, researchers can obtain cleaner EEG signals, facilitating more accurate neural signal analysis and interpretation. A detail explanation of each method is given here.

5.4.1 Wavelet neural network method

The wavelet neural network (WNN) method involves decomposing contaminated EEG signals into wavelet coefficients, passing low-frequency wavelet sub-band coefficients through a trained neural network, and correcting the EEG signals. This technique does not rely on reference EOG signals or visual inspection, making it a robust and efficient method of EEG artifact removal.

The mathematical representation of the WNN method can be described as follows:

Let $x(n)$ be the contaminated EEG signal, $w(n)$ be the wavelet coefficients, and (n) be the corrected EEG signal. The WNN method can be mathematically represented as follows:

$$y(n) = \sum_{i=1}^{N} w_i \cdot \phi_i(n) \tag{5.1}$$

where $\phi_i(n)$ are the wavelet basis functions, w_i are the weights, and N is the number of wavelet coefficients.

The algorithm for correcting the EEG signal using the WNN method can be outlined as follows:

1. Decompose the EEG signal $x(n)$ into wavelet coefficients $w(n)$ using a wavelet transform (e.g. DWT).
2. Pass the low-frequency wavelet sub-band coefficients through a trained neural network to obtain the weights w_i.
3. Combine the wavelet basis functions $\phi_i(n)$ with the weights w_i to obtain the corrected EEG signal $y(n)$.

5.4.2 Federated learning with matching optimization-based algorithm

The federated learning with matching (FLM) optimization-based learning algorithm utilizes a neural-network-enhanced adaptive filtering approach for EEG artifact removal. This method combines a learning algorithm with adaptive filtering to enhance artifact removal efficiency. It is based on a neural network model and optimization techniques for effective artifact removal from EEG signals.

Mathematical representation

Let $x(n)$ be the contaminated EEG signal, (n) be the corrected EEG signal, and $w(n)$ be the adaptive filter weights. The FLM optimization-based learning algorithm can be mathematically represented as follows:

$$y(n) = x(n) - w(n) \cdot x(n) \tag{5.2}$$

where $w(n)$ is updated using an optimization algorithm (e.g. LMS) to minimize the error between the original and corrected signals.

Algorithm

1. Initialize the adaptive filter weights $w(n)$.
2. Calculate the error between the original and corrected signals using the LMS algorithm.
3. Update the adaptive filter weights $w(n)$ based on the error.
4. Repeat steps 2–3 until convergence occurs.

5.4.3 Hybrid blind source separation–support vector machine algorithm

The hybrid BSS-SVM algorithm combines BSS and SVM to remove artifacts from EEGs. This hybrid approach enhances the accuracy and efficiency of artifact removal by integrating the advantages of both BSS and SVM algorithms. By utilizing a hybrid model, this method aims to improve the quality of EEG signal analysis by effectively eliminating unwanted signals and artifacts.

The mathematical representation of the BSS-SVM method can be described as follows:

Let X be the EEG signal matrix, S be the source signal matrix, and A be the mixing matrix. The hybrid BSS-SVM algorithm can be mathematically represented as follows:

$$X = AS$$

where S is separated using BSS and then classified using SVM.

The algorithm for correcting the EEG signal using the BSS-SVM method can be outlined as follows:

1. Use BSS to separate the source signals S from the EEG signal matrix X.
2. Classify the separated source signals S using SVM.
3. Combine the classified source signals S to obtain the corrected EEG signal $y(n)$.

5.4.4 Convolutional neural network approach for EEG artifact removal

The CNN approach for EEG artifact removal leverages the powerful feature extraction capabilities of CNNs to identify and remove various types of artifacts, such as eye blinks, muscle movements, and power-line interference. This method has shown promising results in improving the quality of EEG signals by effectively removing a wide range of artifacts.

The mathematical representation of the CNN for EEG can be described as follows:

Let $x(n)$ be the contaminated EEG signal, $y(n)$ be the corrected EEG signal, and W be the CNN weights. The CNN for EEG artifact removal can be mathematically represented as follows:

$$y(n) = \sigma\left(\sum_{i=1}^{N} W_i \cdot x(n)\right) \tag{5.3}$$

where σ is the activation function, W_i are the CNN weights, and N is the number of convolutional layers.

Algorithm

1. Preprocess the EEG signal $x(n)$ by normalizing and segmenting it into frames.
2. Apply convolutional and pooling layers to extract features from the EEG signal.
3. Use fully connected layers to classify the features and remove artifacts.
4. Combine the classified features to obtain the corrected EEG signal $y(n)$.

5.4.5 Recurrent neural network with long short-term memory architecture for EEG artifact removal

An RNN with long short-term memory (LSTM) architecture has been employed for EEG artifact removal. This method exploits the temporal dependencies in EEG signals and the ability of LSTM to capture long-term dependencies, enabling effective identification and removal of artifacts. The RNN-LSTM approach has improved performance in preserving the underlying EEG signal characteristics while eliminating various artifacts.

The mathematical representation of the RNN-LSTM for EEG can be described as follows:
Let $x(n)$ be the contaminated EEG signal, $y(n)$ be the corrected EEG signal, and W be the RNN-LSTM weights. The RNN-LSTM for EEG artifact removal algorithm can be mathematically represented as follows:

$$y(n) = \sigma\left(\sum_{i=1}^{N} W_i \cdot x(n)\right) \tag{5.4}$$

where σ is the activation function, W_i are the RNN-LSTM weights, and N is the number of recurrent layers.

Algorithm

1. Preprocess the EEG signal $x(n)$ by normalizing and segmenting it into frames.
2. Apply recurrent layers to capture temporal dependencies in the EEG signal.
3. Use LSTM units to capture long-term dependencies and remove artifacts.
4. Combine the classified features to obtain the corrected EEG signal $y(n)$.

5.5 Database

We utilized a publicly available data set from the UCI Machine Learning Repository [62] for eye state classification. This data set contains EEG recordings collected from participants wearing a headset with 14 electrodes positioned on the scalp. These electrodes captured the electrical activity of the brain with the participants' eyes open and closed. It is important to note that the original data set had an uneven distribution of classes, with over 50% of instances belonging to one eye state. To ensure balanced training, the data was filtered to create a data set with 2000 samples for each eye state (open and closed). While [13] provides additional details about decision tree algorithms for eye state prediction, the focus here is on the characteristics of the data set itself.

5.6 Proposed algorithm

Analysis of the RF algorithm revealed several key insights about eye state prediction using EEG signals. First, the decision tree achieved a high level of accuracy (96.79%) in classifying eye states using only ten specific EEG channels. These channels, namely P7, AF4, T8, O1, AF3, F8, F4, FC6, T7, and FC5, were found to be the most informative for this task. Second, sensor P7 played a particularly important role in the classification. This indicates that P7 provided the most critical information for differentiating between open and closed eyes.

Figure 5.9 outlines a comprehensive workflow for classifying EEG eye state data from the UCI EEG Eye State Database. Initially, the raw EEG data undergoes preprocessing, which includes steps such as checking for missing data, data normalization, and noise reduction through artifact removal. Following preprocessing, the clean data is labeled for further classification. Four different ML algorithms—

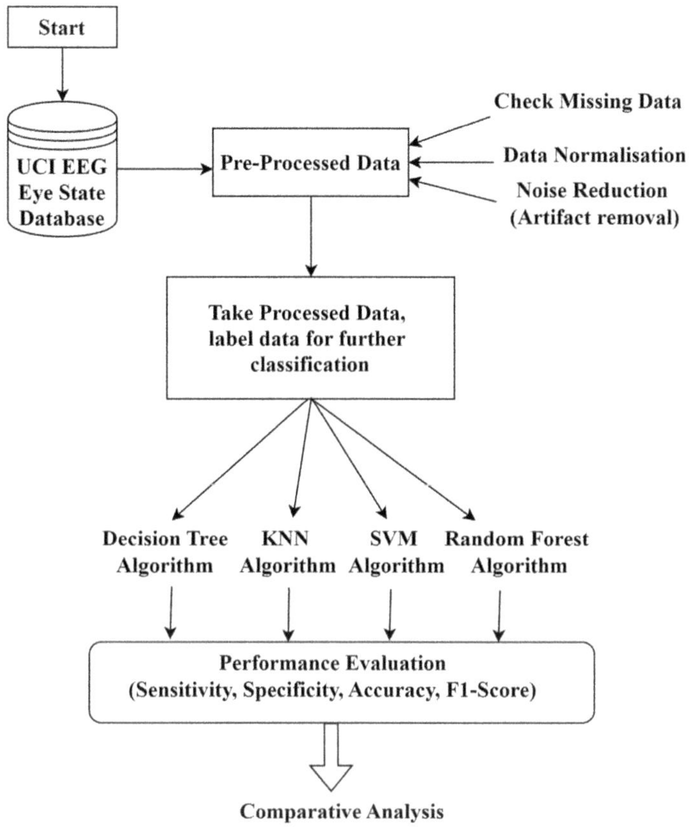

Figure 5.9. Block diagram for the proposed work.

decision tree, *k*-NN, SVM, and RF—are employed to classify the labeled data. The performance of these algorithms is evaluated using metrics such as sensitivity, specificity, accuracy, and F1-score. Finally, a comparative analysis is conducted to determine the most effective algorithm based on the evaluation metrics.

Algorithm 1: Eye state classification using RF.

Input: EEG data set with eye state labels

Output: Classification accuracy

Preprocess data:

1. Rename the column containing eye state labels to 'Eye State.'
2. Encode category labels (e.g. 'Open,' 'Closed') using numerical values (e.g. 0, 1).
3. Separate the features (EEG data) from the target variable (Eye State).

Split data:

1. Split the data into training and testing sets using a common technique such as stratified random sampling.

Train the RF model:

1. Train an RF model on the training data.
2. Tune the hyperparameters of the model (e.g. number of trees, maximum depth) using techniques such as grid search or random search (optional).

Make predictions:

1. Use the trained RF model to predict eye states in the testing data.

Evaluate model performance:

1. Calculate the classification accuracy of the model on the testing data using metrics such as accuracy, precision, recall, and F1-score.

5.7 Results

The RF algorithm predicts eye state—open or closed—from the EEG feature data, using features already extracted from the original raw data. The data set is taken from the UCI ML repository data set. The EEG signal also contains data consisting of eye movement time stamps. In this study, various algorithms were compared to select the appropriate method for classification. Here, table 5.2 shows sensitivity, specificity, F1-score, and accuracy as validation parameters. For the performance analysis and comparative discussions given here, the confusion matrix and receiver operating characteristic (ROC) curve show the performance of the RF classifier on the EEG eye state data set. The confusion matrix displays the number of true positive, true negative, false positive, and false negative predictions made by the model given in figure 5.10.

The ROC curve displays the relationship between the true positive rate and the false positive rate of the classifier. Both the confusion matrix and ROC curve are used to evaluate the accuracy and performance of a binary classifier. The area under the curve (AUC) is a measure of the model's overall performance, as shown in figure 5.11.

A perfect model would have an AUC of 1, while a model that performs no better than random guessing would have an AUC of 0.5. The ROC curve in figure 5.12 has an AUC of 0.98, which indicates that the model is performing very well at distinguishing between positive and negative cases. Figure 5.11 depicts the feature importance in a RF model classifying eyes-open and eyes-closed states based on

Table 5.2. Comparative analysis of various ANN models.

Sl. No.	Method	Sensitivity	Specificity	F1-score	Accuracy
1	SVM	35.67%	81.78%	42.23%	54.89%
2	*k*-NN	87.12%	92.56%	72.56%	93.05%
3	Decision tree [63]	84.60%	82.19%	83.04%	83.35%
4	RF	**91.70%**	**94.55%**	**93.67%**	**96.79%**

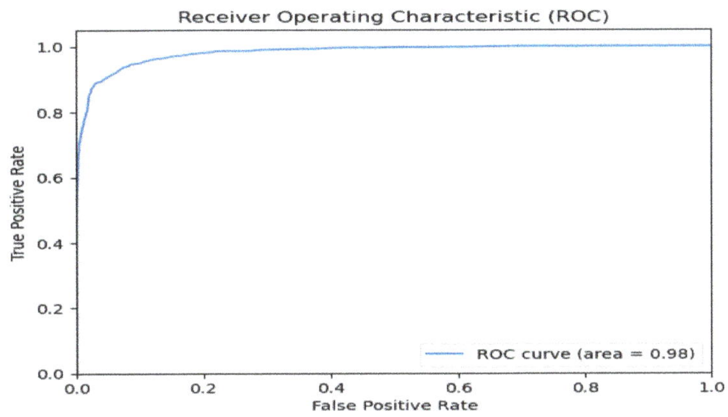

Figure 5.10. ROC matrix.

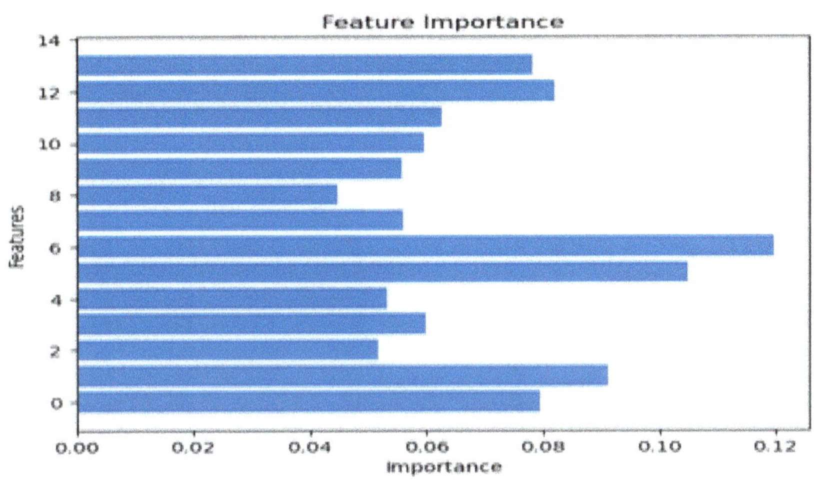

Figure 5.11. Feature importance graph.

EEG channel signals. The higher the bar on the 'importance' axis, the more a specific feature (listed on the unlabeled 'channel signals' axis) contributes to distinguishing between open and closed eyes. This helps us understand which brain activity signals captured by these features are most crucial for the model's performance. From the figure, it is clear that feature 6 and feature 7 are crucial for the classification matrix calculation.

Figure 5.12 shows a scatter plot matrix that visualizes the relationships and distributions of features used for eyes-open versus eyes-closed classification to aid in feature selection analysis. Each subplot represents a pairwise scatter plot of features, with the x-axis and y-axis corresponding to different features from the data set. The color coding distinguishes between the 'eyes-open' and 'eyes-closed' classes, typically with yellow and purple. Clear separation between colors in the subplots indicates good discriminative power, while significant overlap suggests less useful features. By

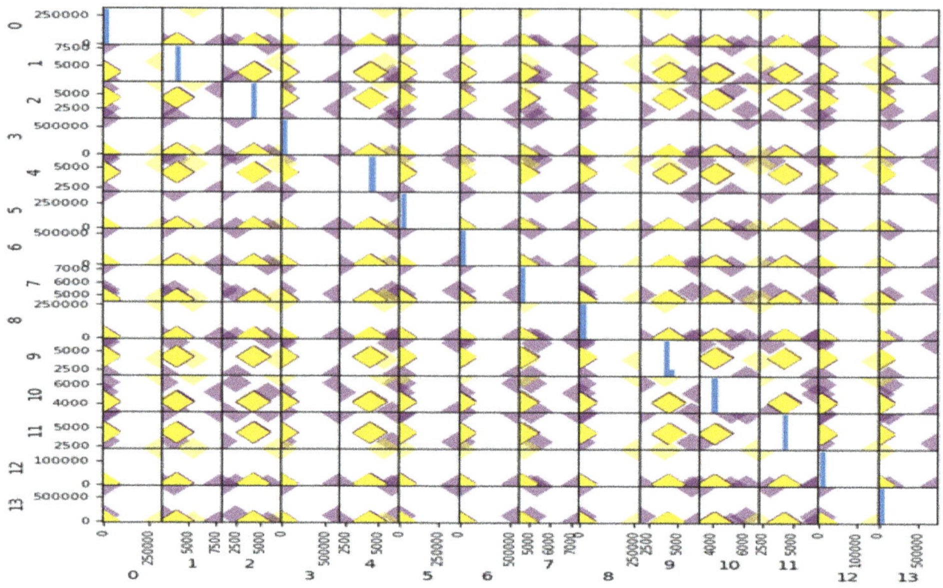

Figure 5.12. Scatter plot of features for feature selection analysis.

examining these plots, one can identify correlations, patterns, and redundancies among features, guiding the selection of the most relevant ones to improve model effectiveness and reduce complexity.

5.8 Conclusions

We conclude that an algorithm-based approach using EEG sensor input can accurately predict eye states with 96.79% accuracy, a level of accuracy that is suitable for various practical applications. The RF model developed outperforms *k*-NN, SVM, and decision tree models. Significantly, the study shows that 'P7' and 'P6' are the most critical among the 14 sensors tested. This reduces the sensor count needed compared to previous methods. The findings also suggest the potential for predicting other human gestures and activities using EEG data. In addition, this chapter discusses artifacts in EEG recordings and filtering methods, providing a comprehensive approach for eyes-open/eyes-closed classification.

References

[1] Sanei S and Chambers J A 2007 *EEG Signal Processing* (New York: Wiley)

[2] Carey J 1990 *Brain facts: a primer on the brain and nervous system* (Washington, DC: Society for Neuroscience)

[3] Siddharth T, Gajbhiye P, Tripathy R K and Pachori R B 2020 EEG-based detection of focal seizure area using FBSE–EWT rhythm and SAE-SVM network *IEEE Sens. J.* **20** 11421–8

[4] Millett D 2001 Hans Berger: from psychic energy to the EEG *Perspect. Biol. Med* **44** 522–42

[5] Li G, Lee B L and Chung W Y 2015 Smartwatch-based wearable EEG system for driver drowsiness detection *IEEE Sens. J.* **15** 7169–80

[6] Tripathy R K, Ghosh S K, Gajbhiye P and Acharya U R 2020 Development of automated sleep stage classification system using multivariate projection-based fixed boundary empirical wavelet transform and entropy features extracted from multichannel EEG signals *Entropy* **22** 1141

[7] de la O Serna J A, Paternina M R A, Zamora-Méndez A, Tripathy R K and Pachori R B 2020 EEG-Rhythm Specific Taylor–Fourier Filter Bank Implemented With O-Splines for the Detection of Epilepsy Using EEG Signals *IEEE Sens. J.* **20** 6542–51

[8] Ramirez R, Planas J, Escude N, Mercade J and Farriols C 2018 EEG-based analysis of the emotional effect of music therapy on palliative care cancer patients *Frontiers Psychol.* **9** 254

[9] Hadjileontiadis L J 2015 EEG-based tonic cold pain characterization using wavelet higher order spectral features *IEEE Trans. Biomed. Eng.* **62** 1981–91

[10] Varshney A, Ghosh S K, Padhy S, Tripathy R K and Acharya U R 2021 Automated classification of mental arithmetic tasks using recurrent neural network and entropy features obtained from multi-channel EEG signals *Electronics* **10** 1079

[11] Islam M K, Rastegarnia A and Yang Z 2016 Methods for artifact detection and removal from scalp EEG: a review *Neurophysiol. Clinique/Clin. Neurophysiol.* **46** 287–305

[12] Kurkcuoglu A, Zagyapan R and Pelin C 2010 Stereological Evaluation of Temporal Lobe/Telencephalon Volume in Temporal Lobe Epilepsy Using the Cavalieri Principle *Turk. Neurosurg.* **20** 358–63

[13] Ribas G C 2010 The cerebral sulci and gyri *Neurosurg. Focus* **28** E2

[14] Brown S and Sharpey-Schafer E A 1888 An investigation into the functions of the occipital and temporal lobes of the monkey's brain *Phil. Trans. R. Soc.* B **179** 303–27

[15] Fletcher P C and Henson R N A 2001 Frontal lobes and human memory: insights from functional neuroimaging *Brain* **124** 849–81

[16] Fogassi L and Luppino G 2005 Motor functions of the parietal lobe *Curr. Opin. Neurobiol.* **15** 626–31

[17] Engel J Jr 1996 Introduction to temporal lobe epilepsy *Epilepsy Res.* **26** 141–50

[18] Williamson P, Thadani V, Darcey T, Spencer D, Spencer S and Mattson R 1992 Occipital lobe epilepsy: clinical characteristics, seizure spread patterns, and results of surgery *Ann. Neurol.: Official J. Am. Neurol. Assoc. Child Neurol. Soc.* **31** 3–13

[19] Lagopoulos J *et al* 2009 Increased theta and alpha EEG activity during nondirective meditation *J. Alternat. Complement. Med.* **15** 1187–92

[20] Homan R W, Herman J and Purdy P 1987 Cerebral location of international 10-20 system electrode placement *Electroencephalogr. Clin. Neurophysiol.* **66** 376–82

[21] Natarajan K, Acharya R, Alias F, Tiboleng T and Puthusserypady S K 2004 Nonlinear analysis of EEG signals at different mental states *Biomed. Eng. Online* **3** 1–11

[22] Fiedler P, Pedrosa P, Griebel S, Fonseca C, Vaz F, Supriyanto E, Zanow F and Haueisen J 2015 Novel multipin electrode cap system for dry electroencephalography *Brain Topogr.* **28** 647–56

[23] Flink R, Pedersen B, Guekht A, Malmgren K, Michelucci R, Neville B, Pinto F, Stephani U and Özkara C 2002 Guidelines for the use of EEG methodology in the diagnosis of epilepsy: international league against epilepsy: commission report commission on European affairs: subcommission on European guidelines *Acta Neurol. Scand.* **106** 1–7

[24] Maheshwari D, Ghosh S, Tripathy R, Sharma M and Acharya U R 2021 Automated accurate emotion recognition system using rhythm-specific deep convolutional neural network technique with multi-channel EEG signals *Comput. Biol. Med.* **134** 104428

[25] Gilliam F, Kuzniecky R and Faught E 1999 Ambulatory EEG monitoring *J. Clin. Neurophysiol.* **16** 111–5
[26] Sawangjai P, Hompoonsup S, Leelaarporn P, Kongwudhikunakorn S and Wilaiprasitporn T 2020 Consumer grade EEG measuring sensors as research tools: a review *IEEE Sens. J.* **20** 3996–4024
[27] Seneviratne U, Mohamed A, Cook M and D'Souza W 2013 The utility of ambulatory electroencephalography in routine clinical practice: a critical review *Epilepsy Res.* **105** 1–12
[28] Gwin J T, Gramann K, Makeig S and Ferris D P 2010 Removal of movement artifact from high-density EEG recorded during walking and running *J. Neurophysiol.* **103** 3526–34
[29] Chen X, Peng H, Yu F and Wang K 2017 Independent vector analysis applied to remove muscle artifacts in EEG data *IEEE Trans. Instrum. Meas.* **66** 1770–9
[30] Chen X, Liu Q, Tao W, Li L, Lee S, Liu A, Chen Q, Cheng J, McKeown M J and Wang Z 2019 ReMAE: user-friendly toolbox for removing muscle artifacts from EEG *IEEE Trans. Instrum. Meas.* **69** 2105–19
[31] Babiloni C *et al* 2020 International Federation of Clinical Neurophysiology (IFCN)–EEG research workgroup: recommendations on frequency and topographic analysis of resting state EEG rhythms. Part 1: applications in clinical research studies *Clin. Neurophysiol.* **131** 285–307
[32] Maddirala A K 2017 Efficient subspace based techniques for processing single channel electroencephalogram signals *PhD Dissertation* Indian Institute of Technology Guwahati https://gyan.iitg.ac.in/handle/123456789/879
[33] Sazgar M and Young M G 2019 EEG artifacts *Absolute Epilepsy and EEG Rotation Review* (Berlin: Springer) pp 149–62
[34] Islam M S, El-Hajj A M, Alawieh H, Dawy Z, Abbas N and El-Imad J 2020 EEG mobility artifact removal for ambulatory epileptic seizure prediction applications *Biomed. Signal Process. Control* **55** 101638
[35] Kilicarslan A and Vidal J L C 2019 Characterization and real-time removal of motion artifacts from EEG signals *J. Neural Eng.* **16** 056027
[36] Peng H, Hu B, Shi Q, Ratcliffe M, Zhao Q, Qi Y and Gao G 2013 Removal of ocular artifacts in EEG—an improved approach combining DWT and ANC for portable applications *IEEE J. Biomed. Health Inform.* **17** 600–7
[37] McFarland D J, McCane L M, David S V and Wolpaw J R 1997 Spatial filter selection for EEG-based communication *Electroencephalogr. Clin. Neurophysiol.* **103** 386–94
[38] Krishnaveni V, Jayaraman S, Aravind S, Hariharasudhan V and Ramadoss K 2006 Automatic identification and removal of ocular artifacts from EEG using wavelet transform *Meas. Sci. Rev.* **6** 45–57 https://www.measurement.sk/2006/S2/Krishnaveni.pdf
[39] Dora C and Biswal P K 2016 Robust ECG artifact removal from EEG using continuous wavelet transformation and linear regression *2016 Int. Conf. on Signal Processing and Communications (SPCOM)* (Piscataway, NJ: IEEE) 1–5
[40] Cooper R, Osselton J W and Shaw J C 2014 *EEG Technology* 2nd edn (Oxford: Butterworth–Heinemann)
[41] Chen X, Liu A, Chiang J, Wang Z J, McKeown M J and Ward R K 2015 Removing muscle artifacts from EEG data: multichannel or single-channel techniques? *IEEE Sens. J.* **16** 1986–97
[42] Crespo-Garcia M, Atienza M and Cantero J L 2008 Muscle artifact removal from human sleep EEG by using independent component analysis *Ann. Biomed. Eng.* **36** 467–75

[43] Jiang X, Bian G B and Tian Z 2019 Removal of artifacts from EEG signals: a review *Sensors* **19** 98

[44] Sweeney K T, Ward T E and McLoone S F 2012 Artifact removal in physiological signals–practices and possibilities *IEEE Trans. Inf. Technol. Biomed.* **16** 488–500

[45] Salis C I, Malissovas A E, Bizopoulos P A, Tzallas A T, Angelidis P A and Tsalikakis D G 2013 Denoising simulated EEG signals: A comparative study of EMD, wavelet transform and Kalman filter *13th IEEE Int. Conf. on BioInformatics and BioEngineering* (Piscataway, NJ: IEEE) 1–4

[46] Chen X, Xu X, Liu A, McKeown M J and Wang Z J 2017 The use of multivariate EMD and CCA for denoising muscle artifacts from few-channel EEG recordings *IEEE Trans. Instrum. Meas.* **67** 359–70

[47] Maddirala A K and Shaik R A 2016 Removal of EOG artifacts from single channel EEG signals using combined singular spectrum analysis and adaptive noise canceler *IEEE Sens. J.* **6** 8279–87

[48] Albera L, Kachenoura A, Comon P, Karfoul A, Wendling F, Senhadji L and Merlet I 2012 ICA-based EEG denoising: a comparative analysis of fifteen methods *Bull. Polish Acad. Sci.: Tech. Sci.* **60** 407–18 Special issue on Data Mining in Bioengineering

[49] Turnip A 2014 Automatic artifacts removal of EEG signals using robust principal component analysis *2014 2nd Int. Conf. on Technology, Informatics, Management, Engineering & Environment* (Piscataway, NJ: IEEE) 331–4

[50] Xiao J, Bian G-B and Tian Z 2019 Removal of artifacts from EEG signals: a review *Sensors* **19** 987

[51] Elbert T, Lutzenberger W, Rockstroh B and Birbaumer N 1985 Removal of ocular artifacts from the EEG—a biophysical approach to the EOG *Electroencephalogr. Clin. Neurophysiol.* **60** 455–63

[52] Khatun S, Mahajan R and Morshed B I 2016 Comparative study of wavelet-based unsupervised ocular artifact removal techniques for single-channel EEG data *IEEE J. Transl. Eng. Health Med.* **4** 1–8

[53] Hsu W Y, Lin C H, Hsu H J, Chen P H and Chen I R 2012 Wavelet-based envelope features with automatic EOG artifact removal: application to single-trial EEG data *Expert Syst. Appl.* **39** 2743–9

[54] Li Y, Ma Z, Lu W and Li Y 2006 Automatic removal of the eye blink artifact from EEG using an ICA-based template matching approach *Physiol. Meas.* **27** 425

[55] Patel R, Sengottuvel S, Janawadkar M, Gireesan K, Radhakrishnan T and Mariyappa N 2016 Ocular artifact suppression from EEG using ensemble empirical mode decomposition with principal component analysis *Comput. Electr. Eng.* **54** 78–86

[56] Akhtar M T, Mitsuhashi W and James C J 2012 Employing spatially constrained ICA and wavelet denoising, for automatic removal of artifacts from multichannel EEG data *Signal Process.* **92** 401–16

[57] Klados M A, Papadelis C L and Bamidis P D 2009 REG-ICA: a new hybrid method for EOG artifact rejection *2009 9th Int. Conf. on Information Technology and Applications in Biomedicine* (Piscataway, NJ: IEEE) 1–4

[58] Yang B, Duan K, Fan C, Hu C and Wang J 2018 Automatic ocular artifacts removal in EEG using deep learning *Biomed. Signal Process. Control* **43** 148–58

[59] Xu K, Jiang X and Chen W 2019 Photoplethysmography motion artifacts removal based on signal–noise interaction modeling utilizing envelope filtering and time-delay neural network *IEEE Sens. J.* **20** 3732–44

[60] Agarwal S, Rani A, Singh V and Mittal A P 2017 EEG signal enhancement using cascaded S-Golay filter *Biomed. Signal Process. Control* **36** 194–204

[61] Gajbhiye P, Tripathy R K and Pachori R B 2019 Elimination of ocular artifacts from single channel EEG signals using FBSE–EWT based rhythms *IEEE Sens. J.* **20** 3687–96

[62] Roesler O 2013 EEG eye state UCI Machine Learning Repository https://archive.ics.uci.edu/dataset/264/eeg+eye+state

[63] Rajesh K, Sabarinathan V, Sarath Kumar V and Sugumaran V 2015 Eye state prediction using EEG signal and c4. 5 decision tree algorithm *Int. J. Appl. Eng. Res.* **10** Special issue No. 68 167–71 https://www.ripublication.com/Volume/ijaerv10n68spl.htm

Chapter 6

Hybrid reptile search algorithm–snake optimizer and rational wavelet filter banks for Alzheimer's disease detection

Digambar V Puri, Pramod H Kachare, Sandeep B Sangle and Sanjay L Nalbalwar

Alzheimer's disease (AD) is a frequently encountered type of dementia that is characterized by a slowing effect and reduced synchronization in electroencephalogram (EEG) signals. Several previously reported combinations of signal-dependent features and machine learning (ML) models exploited these characteristics for automatic AD detection. The performance of most approaches is limited by high computational time and feature redundancy. This chapter explores the use of a less complex wavelet filter bank to decompose the EEG signal. This approach uses orthogonal filters with rational coefficients to reduce complexity. A high-dimensional supervector of EEG features is input into a parallel combination of the snake optimizer (SO) and the reptile search algorithm (RSA) to select the salient feature subset. The efficiency of the proposed approach is quantitatively evaluated using two open-source AD data sets and different classifiers. Comparative analysis shows that the salient feature subset has the best performance, achieving AD detection accuracies of 97.60% and 96.95% for two-class and three-class classification, respectively. The proposed approach outperforms several earlier approaches.

6.1 Introduction

This section of this chapter has been reprinted from [39].

AD refers to the progressive decline of mental faculties, encompassing aspects such as speech, memory, and cognition. The decline of these faculties hinders daily activities [1]. Individuals aged sixty and above are particularly vulnerable to this condition. The primary early indication often involves challenges in recalling recent events [2]. The initial stage of dementia is generally called mild cognitive impairment (MCI). While MCI causes cognitive changes that can be observed by affected

doi:10.1088/978-0-7503-5964-1ch6

subjects or their caregivers, it does not significantly affect their daily activities [3]. MCI does not usually interfere with day-to-day activities because it does not fit AD detection. However, those with MCI face an elevated risk of progressing to AD or another type of dementia, and around 20%–25% of the MCI population advances to AD annually [4].

The recent approval by the Food and Drug Administration of a novel drug named Lecanemab for AD underscores the significance of early AD detection during the MCI stage. Detecting AD at this early phase can substantially slow its progression rate. Identifying AD in its initial stages allows patients to potentially benefit from upcoming therapies before the condition advances to a more critical stage [5]. The diagnostic process for MCI or AD typically encompasses a range of procedures, such as magnetic resonance imaging, blood tests, neurological examinations, positron emission tomography, mini-mental state examinations, and electroencephalography [6].

EEG is a non-invasive method for monitoring electrical fluctuations in the brain, specifically the electrical potential differences generated by numerous neurons. Electrodes positioned on the scalp detect these electrical potentials, and the spatial precision of the EEG depends on the number and placement of these electrodes [7]. Unlike neuroimaging tools, EEG recording techniques deliver outstanding temporal information and are less expensive. Various investigations have employed ML approaches for EEG analysis to identify diverse neurological conditions, such as epilepsy [8], AD, schizophrenia, and emotion recognition [9]. Moreover, the combination of EEG signals with ML has been utilized in several studies for the automated detection of MCI through resting-state or task-state paradigms. In task-state EEG, participants partake in predefined activities; for example, a study by Kulkarni focused on identifying five contrasting speech sounds on vowel continuums; subjects were tasked with recognizing sounds while their EEG data were collected from a single channel [10].

Various EEG-based methods have been reported for the classification of AD, MCI, and normal control (NC) subjects. These studies evaluate either two-way (AD: MCI, AD:NC, and MCI:NC) or three-way (MCI:AD:NC) detection [11]. Several entropy-based approaches, such as approximation entropy (ApEn) [12], auto-mutual information (AMI), sample entropy [13], spectral entropy (SpEn) [14], Tsallis entropy (TsEn), generalized multiscale entropy [15], epoch-based entropy, wavelet entropy, Shannon entropy (ShEn), sure entropy, permutation entropy (PrEn), fuzzy entropy, detrended fluctuation analysis [16], Lempel–Ziv complexity (LZC) [17], Higuchi's fractal dimension [18], distance-based LZC [19], and Kolmogorov complexity [20] have been proposed in the literature. Sharma *et al* [21] suggested a combination of spectral crest factor and power spectral density (PSD), achieving an accuracy of 95%. These quantities were employed in regard to EEG signals without considering their duration.

The existing and reported AD detection methods often use discrete wavelet transform (DWT) and fast Fourier transform-based spectral feature sets. Oltu *et al* [22] proposed DWT and coherence feature vector with support vector machine (SVM) for AD detection and obtained an accuracy of 96.50%. Fiscon *et al* [23] used Fourier and DWT-based statistical features and obtained a 92% classification rate using a decision tree. Recently, Safi *et al* [24] utilized empirical mode decomposition and DWT sub-band-based Hjorth parameters (HPs) as features to improve AD detection. The authors achieved 97.4% accuracy using linear discriminant analysis (LDA). However, the use of the leave-one-subject-out cross validation (LOSO-CV) technique reduced the classification accuracy to 86%. Similarly, Seker [25] investigated a three-class classification with eyes-closed and eyes-open EEG data sets. Logistic regression (LR) was used to examine the PrEn features in various brain regions. McBride *et al* [26] analyzed complex spectral features of NC, MCI, and AD participants to distinguish between the groups using an SVM classifier and reported 85.40% accuracy. Ruiz-Gomez *et al* [27] combined neuro-markers based on entropy, such as SpEn, sample entropy (SampEn), and AMI, with relative median frequency and power band. Using LDA, EEGs from patients with MCI and AD were classified under eyes-closed and eyes-open conditions with a diagnosis rate of 78.43%.

Recently, Miltiadous *et al* [28] reported PSD-based spectral features and performed classification using a random forest (RF) model on sleep AD EEG signals, achieving a leave-one-subject-out (LOSO) accuracy of 77.01% for AD vs. NC detection. Toural *et al* [28] used relative beta power, theta power, and entropy from wavelet-based sub-bands as features for separating AD, MCI, and NC participants. SVM was implemented at the decision stage, and the accuracy obtained was 92.60% [28]. Fouad *et al* [30] compared contrast, homogeneity, and wavelet-based features to diagnose MCI and AD. The classification was performed using various ML models, and the highest detection rate of 97.82% was obtained for AD [29]. However, they evaluated their approach using all EEG channels.

Similarly, Geng *et al* [31] investigated the effect of complexity and spectral features using the gated recurrent unit model to identify AD, reaching an accuracy of 93.46% [31]. Calub *et al* [32] combined nonlinear and linear features using principal component analysis to achieve 93.74% accuracy in distinguishing MCI and AD from normal subjects with neural networks. Ding *et al* [33] combined complexity, spectral, and functional connectivity features to differentiate MCI and AD participants with a classification rate of 72.43% [32]. Rodrigues *et al* [34] investigated lateral wavelet-based TsEn, LZC, and Higuchi's fractal dimension features for three-way (MCI vs. AD vs. NC) detection using various ML models and obtained an accuracy of 95.55% using SVM [34].

The diagnosis of AD and NC makes it difficult to identify the appropriate EEG features. Numerous algorithms have been used in attempts to solve this problem, yet determining the most effective algorithm often involves a trial-and-error process. An automated system capable of pinpointing significant features would be highly advantageous for researchers. This study seeks to create a method for investigating the most representative features. We reviewed existing methods and extracted different features of sub-bands derived from less complex orthogonal filter banks (LCOWFBs). Metaheuristic algorithms (MHAs) have recently been widely utilized to select the salient feature subset (SFS). In our study, different MHAs were employed to find effective features. The classification of AD, NC, and MCI EEGs was then performed.

The proposed MHA-based salient feature selection method supports various activities, as follows:

- Developing an automatic AD detection algorithm based on an optimal feature selection model.
- Decomposing the EEG signal utilizing recently designed LCOWFBs for effective feature investigation in wavelet-based time and frequency analysis.
- Identifying EEG sub-bands using significant features by spectral, temporal, statistical, and complexity analysis.
- Comparing the performance of the RSA, the SO, and RSA-SO-based feature selection using two publicly available and open-source AD data sets to improve three- and two-way detection and classification.
- Improving accuracy using RSA-SO-based efficient features to achieve better AD detection accuracy than previously reported and published work.

The rest of the chapter is structured as follows: section 6.2 provides details of the LCOWFBs, features, and RSA-SO feature selection utilized in our proposed method. Section 6.3 gives experimental analysis and the results obtained. The results are analyzed and discussed in section 6.4. Finally, conclusions are presented in section 6.5.

This section of this chapter has been reprinted from [39].

6.2 Methodology

The proposed automatic AD detection system, as illustrated in figure 6.1, comprises six modules, namely: signal acquisition, EEG decomposition, feature extraction, channel selection, classification, and performance metric calculation. The EEG signals of healthy subjects and participants with AD and MCI are recorded. The process begins with the preprocessing of EEG signals obtained from both data sets.

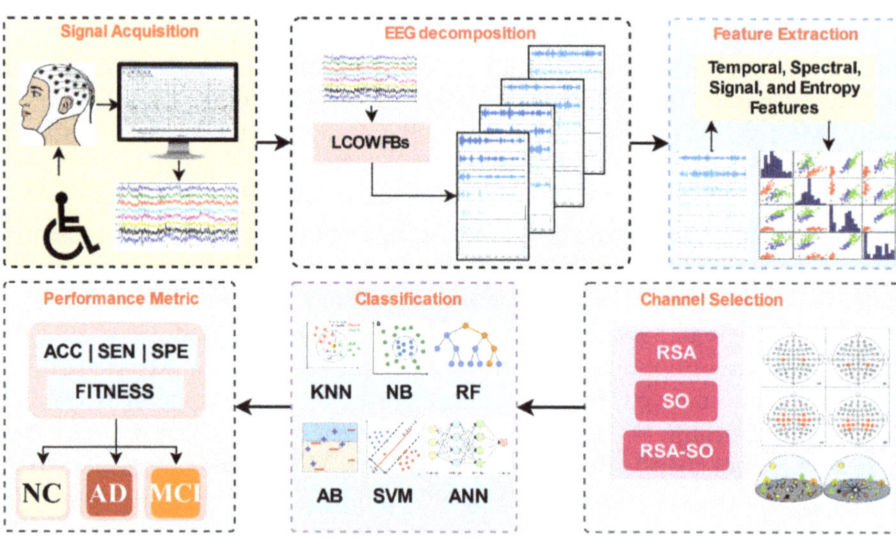

Figure 6.1. Proposed schematics for automatic AD detection.

A Butterworth bandpass filter is applied with a cutoff frequency of 100 Hz, effectively eliminating high-frequency noise and ensuring cleaner signal inputs. Subsequently, the EEG signals undergo decomposition into seven distinct sub-bands. To capture relevant information from these sub-bands, various features are extracted, providing a comprehensive representation of the underlying neurological patterns. The proposed system employs the reptile search algorithm with snake optimization (RSA-SO) method for feature selection. This method is designed to identify and prioritize salient features that are crucial for effective AD detection.

The next phase involves the utilization of diverse ML models for the training and testing stages of the classification and detection process for AD. The synergy of sophisticated feature selection and ML techniques enhances the system's ability to discern patterns indicative of AD, contributing to more accurate and reliable diagnoses. In summary, the proposed method combines signal preprocessing, sub-band decomposition, feature extraction, and a robust feature selection algorithm with ML models for efficient AD detection. This integrated approach holds promise for advancing the accuracy and effectiveness of automated AD diagnosis systems.

6.2.1 Data set details

Two data sets were used in this study. The data sets are described below.

Data set I: the subjects for EEG recording were recruited from the Alzheimer's Patients' Relatives Association of Valladolid (AFAVA) [35]. The details of this data set are presented in table 6.1. Following the removal of artifacts and the application of preprocessing, a total of 9849 epochs were included in the analysis, with 5648 stemming from the AD group and 4201 from the NC group [36]. Sample AD and NC EEG signals for five-second periods are shown in figure 6.2.

Data set II: the second data set contained three classes of EEG signals, namely AD, MCI, and NC. The subject details of this data set are presented in table 6.2. Every EEG wave was recorded with the eyes closed in a resting position. The details of data set II are available in [37]. This data set was approved by the Ethics Committee of Charles University in Prague, Czech Republic (CUPCR). The 'runICA' command in EEGLAB was used to eliminate noise.

Table 6.1. Details of data set I.

Parameters	AD patient	NC subject
Sampling frequency	256 Hz	256 Hz
No. of recordings	400	263
No. of subjects	12	11
Age (years)	72.8 ± 8	72.5 ± 6.1
Electrode placement system	10–20	10–20
Signal duration (seconds)	5	5
Number of electrodes	16	16
EEG samples per electrode	1280	1280

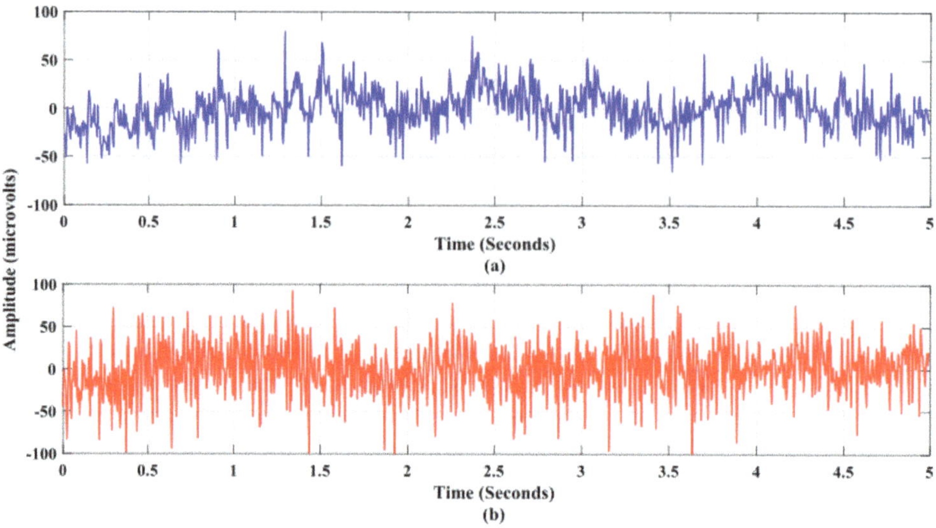

Figure 6.2. Sample EEGs showing (a) an AD subject and (b) an NC.

Table 6.2. Details of data set II.

Parameters	AD patient	MCI patient	NC subject
Sampling frequency (fs)	256 Hz	256 Hz	256 Hz
No. of recordings	305	56	110
No. of subjects	59 (29 M + 31 F)	70 (30 M + 40 F)	102 (43 M + 59 F)
Age (years)	70.5 ± 4.9	67 ± 7.6	72 ± 5.3
Electrode placement system	10–20	10–20	10–20
Signal duration (seconds)	7.8	7.8	7.8
Number of electrodes	19	19	19
EEG samples per electrode	1000	1000	1000

6.2.2 Low-complexity orthogonal wavelet filter banks

Rational and dyadic LCOWFBs with vanishing moments were varied to obtain the desired frequency response [37]. This type of filter bank is efficient in terms of implementation. It takes a smaller number of adders and shifters to implement the filter coefficients on a digital signal processing (DSP) processor. It has been proven that this filter bank performs well in detecting AD. The LCOWFB is available for different vanishing moments, such as $v = 2$, 4, and 6. Our study utilized $v = 6$ to decompose the EEG signals whose filter coefficients were obtained from the following equation:

$$F(z) = F_1(z) + F_2(z) \tag{6.1}$$

where

$$F_1(z) = \sum_{p=0}^{5}(c(p,\, 0)a(0) + c(p,\, 1)a(1) + \cdots + c(p,\, p)a(p))z^{-p}$$

and

$$F_2(z) = \sum_{p=0}^{5}(c(p,\, p)a(0) + c(p,\, p - 1)a(1) + \cdots + c(p,\, 0)a(p))z^{-p+6}$$

where $a(0)$ to $a(5)$ are constants determined by the iterative process mentioned in [37]. The impulse response of the low-pass analysis filter in LCOWFB coefficients is as follows:

$$f(n) = [\quad 2,\ 10,\ 1,\quad 66,\quad 58,\ 208,\quad 272,\quad 472,\ 660,\ 1572,\ 1036,\ 232]/2048 \tag{6.2}$$

6.2.3 Feature extraction

Feature extraction is a crucial aspect of pattern recognition and ML, as it reduces computation costs and improves classification performance. To extract features from sub-bands, three categories are used here: the time–frequency domain, non-linear complexity characteristics, and other features. A total of 21 features are used. This feature list is presented in table 6.3. These features are then input into RSA, SO, and RSA-SO MHAs for optimal feature selection. This produces the highest AD and MCI detection rate by reducing the number of features input to the classifiers, thus reducing the computation time. MHAs are discussed briefly in the following section.

Table 6.3. Features used in this study.

Time domain	Frequency domain	Complexity features
Band power	Average band power	Approximate entropy
Root mean square	Relative power of β	Higuchi's fractal dimension
Zero crossing	Log energy entropy	Karl's fractal dimension
Interquartile range	Petrosian fractal dimension (PFD)	Sample entropy
Skewness	Shannon entropy	Conditional entropy
Kurtosis	Log-root sum of sequential variations (LRSSV)	Tsallis entropy
Mobility	Kraskov entropy (KE)	Petrosian fractal dimension (PFD)

6.2.4 Feature selection

Because it reduces computational costs and enhances classification performance, the feature selection process is essential to ML and pattern recognition. One of the biggest challenges in ML and data mining is finding a suitable data representation that incorporates all attributes. The SFS that improves accuracy while requiring the fewest features is investigated using two of the most well-known metaheuristic algorithms: the SO and the RSA.

- RSA

  The RSA is a nature-inspired metaheuristic method that draws inspiration from the hunting and circling behaviors of crocodiles. The computation of the *j*th feature $X_{i,\,j}$,s, *i*th candidate solution is obtained using the expression

$$X_{i,j} = (Ub_j - Lb_j) \times r + Lb_j \quad i, j \in 1, 2, 3, \ldots, N \tag{6.3}$$

  where Ub_j and Lb_j are the boundaries of the *j*th feature dimension, $r \in [0, 1]$, N is the number of search crocodiles, and M is the degree of features. The encircling of the region starts with a search which is computed as shown below:

$$X_{i,j} = \begin{cases} [-\eta_{i,\,j}(g)\ \gamma\ B_j(g)] - [rR_{i,\,j}(g)] & g \leqslant \dfrac{G}{2}, \\ ES(g)B_j(g)x & g \leqslant \dfrac{G}{2} \text{ and } g \geqslant \dfrac{G}{4} \end{cases} \tag{6.4}$$

  where $B_j(g)$ is the best solution for the *j*th features, $\eta_{i,j}$ is the hunting operator, $\gamma = 0.1$, $R_{i,j}$ is the reduction function, and ES is the sense of evolution. Details of the RSA and the fitness function used in this study are provided in [38].

- SO

  An optimization technique called the SO algorithm was motivated by the group behavior of snake swarms. The SO uses the following ratio to split the swarm equally between male and female groups:

$$N_{\text{male}} \approx \frac{N}{2} \tag{6.5}$$

$$N_f = N - N_{\text{male}} \tag{6.6}$$

  where N is the total number of individuals, N_{male} is the number of male individuals, and N_f is the number of female individuals. For each iteration, the first male (f_{bm}) with a female f_{bf} candidate is found by evaluating every group. The food quality (Q_f) is expressed as:

$$Q_f = c_1 \exp\left(\frac{\tilde{g} - I}{I}\right) \tag{6.7}$$

$$T1 = \exp\left(\frac{\tilde{g}}{I}\right) \tag{6.8}$$

where $c = 1$, g is the current iteration, and I is the number of total iterations. When < 0.5, the snake moves randomly in search of food, updating its position every time. The following expression can be used to calculate the nature of female and male snakes:

$$x_{i,j}(1+g) = x(g) \pm c_2 \exp\left[\frac{-f_{r,\text{male}}}{f_{i,\text{male}}}((Ub_j - Lb_j) \times r + Lb_j)\right] \tag{6.9}$$

where $x_{i,j}$ is the snake position, $x(g)$ is the random position of a male, and $f_{r,\text{male}}$ is a value computed previously. Details of the SO are provided in [38].

- **Hybrid RSA-SO Approach**

  An overview of the steps involved in the fusion of the RSA and SO is presented in figure 6.3. Initially, RSA, SO, and shared hyperparameters are initialized. A random number generator initializes N solutions for M features. The candidate solutions are divided equally between the RSA and SO. For the kth iteration, the candidate solutions $x_i(k)$,$1 \leqslant i \leqslant N$ are divided into two parts, where one half is passed to the RSA and the other to SO, as follows,

$$x_i^{\text{RSA}-\text{SO}} = \begin{cases} x_i^{\text{RSA}}, \ 1 \leqslant i \leqslant N/2 \\ x_i^{\text{SO}}, \ N/2 < i \leqslant N \end{cases}. \tag{6.10}$$

The solutions derived from equation (6.9) are arranged in ascending order with fitness values. Candidates with lower fitness values are chosen from the population. The top N/2 solutions are carried forward to both algorithms for the next iteration. Subsequently, the candidate solutions are updated using the following method:

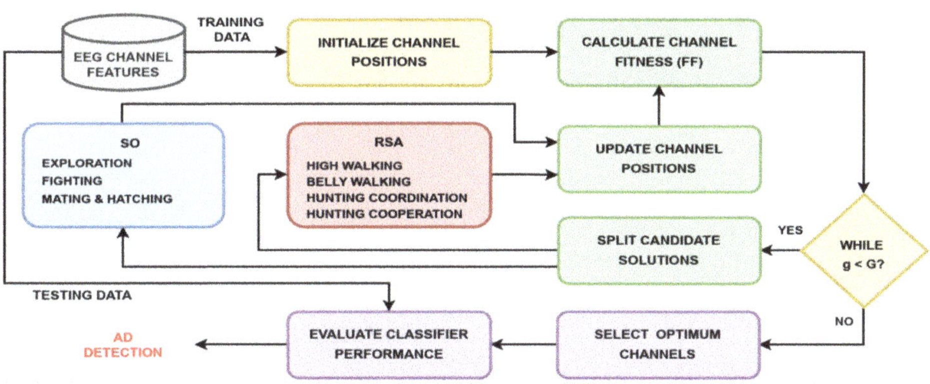

Figure 6.3. RSA-SO flowchart.

$$x_i^{\mathrm{RSA}}(g+1) = x_i^{\mathrm{SO}}(g+1) = \widehat{x}_i(g) \tag{6.11}$$

where $\widehat{x}_i(g) = x_{\arg\min(f(g))}(g)$. Hence, the solution with the fewer features and best accuracy has the smallest fitness f_i, which is given by

$$f_i = \alpha \times \gamma + \beta \times \frac{SF_i}{M} \tag{6.12}$$

where α, β are the weight parameters such that $\alpha + \beta = 1$, γ is the error rate, and SF_i is the number of features in SFS.

6.2.5 Classification models

The various features are computed from the EEG sub-bands of data sets I and II. The selected features from RSA, SO, and RSA-SO are used to train the multiple ML classifiers, namely SVM [39], neural network (NN), naive Bayes (NB) [40], AdaBoost (AB) [41], and RF [42], and the tenfold cross validation (CV), random sampling, and LOSO-CV methods are used to reduce overfitting issues. Tenfold CV breaks the total feature set into ten mutually exclusive subsets. Of these, nine are used to train the model, and the rest are utilized for testing [43]. A fivefold nested loop is adopted to obtain the optimal hyperparameters [6]. It cannot be predetermined which classifier will perform better on the AD, MCI, and NC EEG data sets. Hence, we select the classifier with the highest classification performance. The hyperparameters are tuned to enhance the performance of the classifiers. The performance parameters are obtained by considering confusion matrices and are presented in figures 6.4 and 6.5.

	AD	NC	MCI
AD	True AD (TA)	False AD_2 (FA-2)	False AD_1 (FA-1)
NC	False NC (FC-1)	True NC (TC)	False NC (FC-2)
MCI	False MCI (FM-1)	False MCI (FM-2)	True MCI (TM)

Figure 6.4. Schematic of the confusion matrix for three classes (AD vs. MCI vs. NC).

AD +MCI	TA + FA-1 + TM + FM-1	FA_2 + FM-2
NC	FC-1 + FC-2	TC

(a)

AD	TA	FA-1
MCI	FM-1	TM

(b)

AD	TA	FA-2
NC	FC-1	TC

(c)

Figure 6.5. Table used to convert the confusion matrix from three to two classes (a) NC vs. (AD + MCI), (b) AD vs. MCI, and (c) AD vs. NC.

6.3 Results

A computer running Linux with an Nvidia P100 GPU, a 1.32 GHz clock speed, 16 GB of RAM, and a Windows 10 operating system was used for this experimental work. The convolutional neural network (CNN) architecture was implemented in Python. Other libraries, such as NumPy, Pandas, Seaborn, and Matplotlib, were also used for data processing, evaluation, and reporting tasks. The performance of the RSA, SO, and proposed RSA-SO approach for the LCOWFBs method are listed in table 6.4 in terms of the number of salient features, fitness values, and computational time. The RSA, SO, and RSA-SO algorithms were compiled ten times and used for 100 iterations for each MHA to obtain statistically reliable evaluation metrics. The fitness metric gives an indication of how well the models perform based on the fitness criterion. The fitness value of the RSA-SO approach was 0.019 68, which was less than the fitness values of the RSA and SO. The SO had a higher fitness value. These fitness values were evaluated using the number of features in SFS. The RSA-SO selected only 214 features while achieving the highest performance and requiring the lowest computational time. The RSA took longer then the RSA-SO approach to obtain good performance. The optimal features common to both the RSA and SO that provided the optimal performance were selected by RSA-SO. Feature selection maps for both data sets indicating a particular sub-band and corresponding selected features are depicted in figure 6.6(a).

The performances of the various ML models were evaluated using features selected by RSA-SO and all features. Figure 6.7 shows the accuracies obtained from five ML models using LCOWFBs with RSA-SO features for data set I. The performance was obtained using a random sampling method (RSM) (80%–20%), LOSO-CV, and tenfold CV. SVM and k-nearest neighbors (k-NN) tended to

Table 6.4. Performance parameters obtained for data sets I and II.

		Data set I (AD vs. NC)			Data set II (AD vs. MCI vs. NC)		
Parameter	Value	RSA	SO	RSA-SO	RSA	SO	RSA-SO
Fitness	Min	0.0599	0.0820	0.019 683	0.1401	0.1432	0.078 043
	Max	0.0510	0.1122	0.046 042	0.1462	0.1487	0.103 255
	Mean	0.0170	0.0997	0.015 583	0.1438	0.1460	0.091 132
	Std. dev.	0.0123	0.0106	0.018 373	0.0023	0.0017	0.007 668
Computational time (sec)	Min	1908.38	3737.09	1775.890	2116.16	1495.60	982.08
	Max	2152.94	4038.98	1977.947	2634.85	1506.00	7652.993
	Mean	1998.53	3830.08	913.6399	2221.41	1499.53	1716.745
	Std. dev.	98.97	125.32	968.1814	154.5	3.39	2086.314
Optimal features	Min	115	2361	22	1723	1817	5
	Max	547	3369	214	1962	2019	15
	Mean	325	2657	103	1749	1951	6.4
	Std. dev.	156	326	73.9713	75	54	3.864

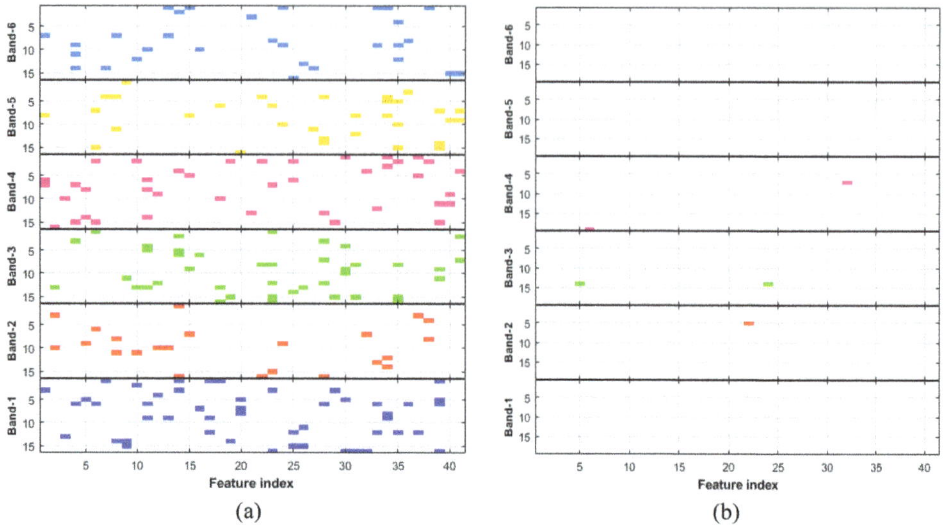

Figure 6.6. LCOWFB feature selection using RSA-SO for (a) data set I and (b) data set II.

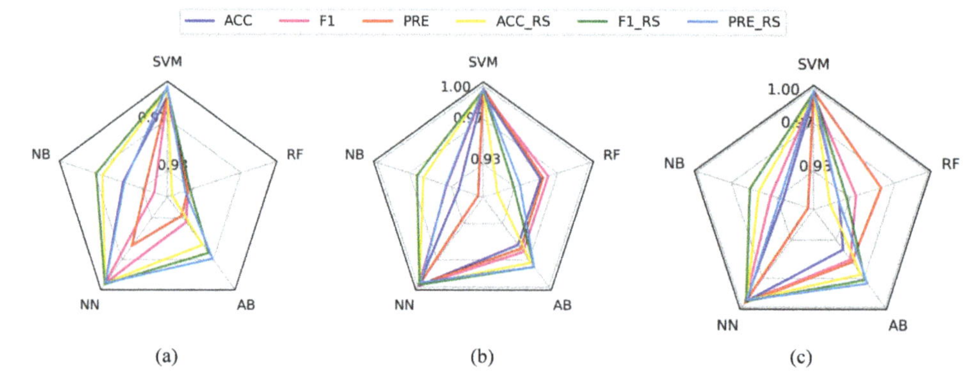

Figure 6.7. Comparison of accuracy of LCOWFBs and RSA-SO for data set I utilizing (a) RSM, (b) LOSO, and (c) 10-fold CV.

perform well across various validation techniques. LCOWFB with RSA-SO often outperformed LCOWFB without feature selection, especially in the SVM and AB models. Tenfold CV generally resulted in higher accuracy than RSM and LOSO-CV. The highest accuracy obtained from the SVM was 97.90%. The lowest accuracy was 91.55%, which was obtained from the NB classifier. The RF, NB, and AB algorithms performed poorly, whereas SVM and *k*-NN performed better for two-class data using LCOWFBs and RSA-SO.

The performances of the RSA, SO, and proposed RSA-SO approaches with the LCOWFB method using data set II are presented in table 6.4 in terms of the number of salient features, fitness values, and computational time. As for data set I, all MHAs were compiled ten times and used for 100 iterations to obtain statistically reliable results. The fitness metric gives an indication of how well the models performed based on the fitness criterion. The fitness value of RSA-SO was 0.078 043, which was smaller than those of the RSA and SO. The fitness values were evaluated using the number of optimal features selected. The RSA-SO selected only five features, while achieving the highest performance and lowest computational time. However, the RSA took a little more time than RSA-SO to obtain good performance. The salient features common to the RSA and SO that provided optimal performance were selected by RSA-SO. Figure 6.6(b) depicts the sub-band and corresponding selected features.

The performances of the various ML models were evaluated using selected features from RSA-SO and all features. Table 6.5 shows the accuracies obtained from five ML models using LCOWFBs with RSO-SO features for data set II. The performances were obtained using RSM (80%-20%), LOSO-CV, and tenfold CV. As in the case of data set I, SVM and *k*-NN performed well across various models and validation techniques. LCOWFBs with RSA-SO often outperformed LCOWFBs, especially in the SVM and AB models. Tenfold CV generally resulted in higher

Table 6.5. Accuracy comparison of LCOWFBs with and without RSA-SO for data sets I and II.

Data set	Method	Model	RSM	LOSO CV	Tenfold CV
Data set I (AD vs. NC)	LCOWFBs	SVM	94.64	92.40	96.90
		NB	91.55	93.00	93.60
		NN	92.30	94.30	94.10
		AB	93.21	94.27	93.80
		RF	89.63	92.91	92.40
		k-NN	92.26	93.56	95.24
	LCOWFBs with RSA-SO	SVM	96.60	96.40	**97.90**
		NB	95.80	94.00	95.60
		NN	96.20	95.30	96.10
		AB	93.70	96.27	96.80
		RF	94.27	93.91	93.40
		k-NN	96.56	94.52	95.45
Data set II (AD vs. MCI vs. NC)	LCOWFBs	SVM	89.64	91.40	95.90
		NB	90.55	91.00	92.60
		NN	91.30	91.30	94.10
		AB	91.21	92.27	93.80
		RF	90.63	90.91	90.40
		k-NN	91.56	90.80	92.47
	LCOWFBs with RSA-SO	SVM	96.55	93.40	**96.95**
		NB	94.80	92.00	95.60
		NN	95.20	95.30	96.10
		AB	92.70	95.27	95.80
		RF	93.27	94.91	95.40
		k-NN	95.33	95.87	95.78

Bold indicates maximum accuracy.

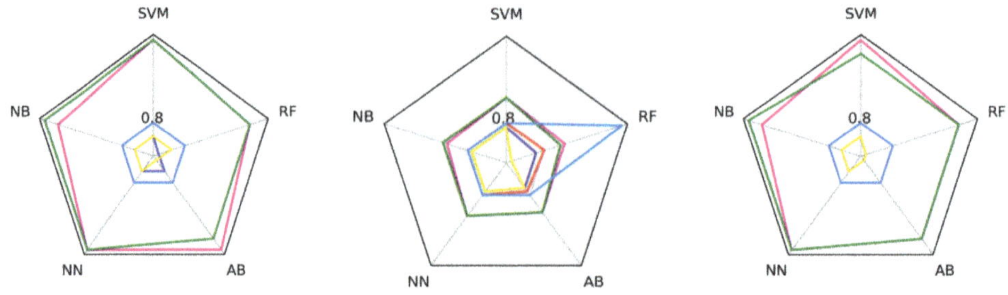

(a) (b) (c)

Figure 6.8. Two-class (AD + MCI vs. NC) ML model accuracies of LCOWFB and RSA-SO for data set II using (a) RSM, (b) LOSO, and (c) tenfold CV.

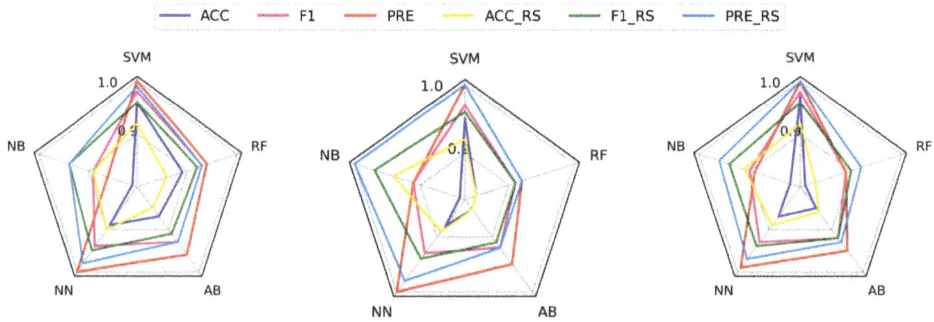

(a) (b) (c)

Figure 6.9. Two-class (AD vs. MCI) ML model accuracies of LCOWFB and RSA-SO for data set II using (a) RSM, (b) LOSO, and (c) tenfold CV.

accuracy than random sampling and LOSO-CV. The highest accuracy obtained from the SVM was 96.95%. The lowest accuracy was 90.40%, which obtained using the NB classifier. The RF, NB, and AB algorithms performed poorly, whereas SVM and *k*-NN performed better for two-class data using LCOWFBs and RSA-SO. Moreover, binary classification (AD + MCI vs. NC, MCI vs. NC, and AD vs. MCI) was performed for different split methods (RSM, LOSO, and tenfold CV) using data set II. The corresponding performances are shown in figures 6.8–6.10.

6.4 Discussion

Various methods for the detection of AD and MCI using NC EEG signals have been reported in the research literature. A comparative analysis of the proposed method and existing methods is presented in table 6.6. Abasolo *et al* [14–18] reported the use of various complexity-based features to distinguish AD EEG signals from normal signals, such as MSEn, fuzzy entropy, quadratic sample entropy (QSE), ApEn, LZC, and AMI. However, these methods were able to achieve only 92.90% accuracy. Abasolo *et al* also reported that the complexity of the AD EEG signals is less than that of NC signals.

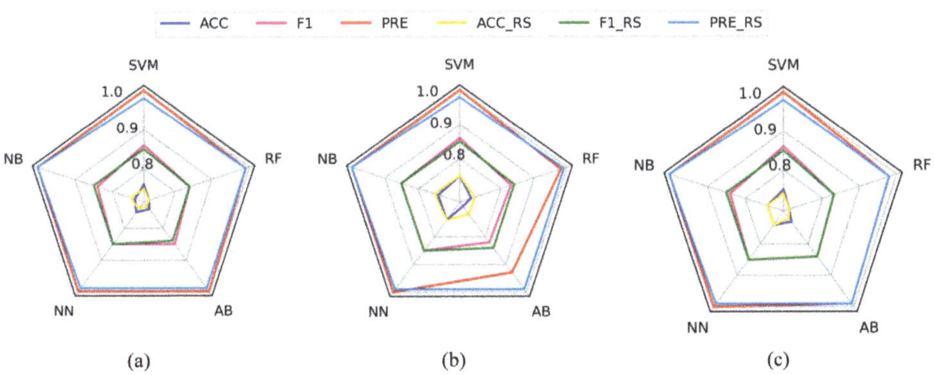

Figure 6.10. Two-class (AD vs. NC) ML model accuracies of LCOWFB and RSA-SO for data set II using (a) RSM, (b) LOSO, and (c) tenfold CV.

Table 6.6. Comparative analysis of state-of-the-art-methods.

Reference	Year	data set (subjects)	Method	Classifier	Validation strategy	ACC (%)	SEN (%)	SPE (%)
[15]	2006	AD:12 NC:11	Generalized MSEn	SM	—	74.73	83.82	72.73
[14]	2006	AD:12 NC:11	SpEn and ShEn	SM	—	77.27	90.91	63.64
[12]	2008	AD:11 NC:11	ApEn and AMI	SM	—	90.91	95.56	81.82
[16]	2015	AD:11 NC:11	QSE	SM	—	77.27	—	—
[13]	2018	AD:11 NC:11	Fuzzy entropy	SM	—	81.82	90.91	86.36
[19]	2018	AD:12 NC:11	Distance-based LZC	SM	—	72.74	81.82	77.28
[18]	2021	AD:12 NC:11	Kolmogorov Complexity (KMC) and SpEn	ML	10-fold	92.9	92.8	93
Proposed		AD:12 NC:11	RSA-SO hybrid approach and LCOWFB-based feature selection	SVM	10-fold	**97.50**	96.05	96.83

[a]SM—statistical method, KMC—Kolmogorov complexity, ML—machine learning models.
Bold indicates maximum accuracy.

Moreover, the AD EEG signals are more regular. The slowing effect was also observed in the AD EEG signals. All features are considered in the existing methods to increase performance. However, this leads to increased complexity and time consumption and poor performance. The proposed method performs well compared to other methods that only use selected features. This increases the efficiency of the AD detection method. The RSA-SO feature selection methods also reduce the time complexity. On the other hand, the more dominant channels in the AD can be easily detected from the selected features. This allows the brain area that AD may be affecting to be identified. This helps in treating the patient and observing their symptoms.

The proposed method was employed on two publicly available AD EEG data sets. These data sets have pretty small populations. In the current work, just seven MHAs were employed. Nonetheless, a hybrid feature selection model can be created by combining MHAs with nature-inspired models. Our automatic AD detection algorithm could be used in the future with private data sets that have EEG recordings of large populations. In this instance, we combined four decomposition techniques with seven MHAs, allowing a comparative analysis of different filter banks to be performed.

6.5 Conclusions

The rate of prevalence of AD is increasing exponentially. The performance of most approaches is limited by long computational times and feature redundancy. This study explored the use of LCOWFBs to decompose EEG signals into sub-bands. It used orthogonal filters with rational coefficients to reduce the complexity. A super-vector of EEG features was generated by extracting ten spectral features for each sub-band. A hybrid metaheuristic optimizer, a parallel combination of the RSA and SO, was used to select an SFS. The efficiencies of LCOWFBs and RSA-SO were compared using different ML models. Two open-source AD data sets were used to evaluate the proposed approach quantitatively. The results showed that RSA-SO effectively reduced the supervector feature dimension, thereby improving AD detection. A comparative analysis of the previously reported approaches showed that the SFS has the highest performance in AD detection, achieving accuracies of 97.90% and 96.95% for two-class and three-class classification, respectively. The LCOWFBs and hybrid RSA-SO provided the highest classification performance compared to several previously reported literature approaches, while reducing feature dimensions and computational cost. The proposed approach can be used to detect other neurodegenerative diseases.

Acknowledgments

The authors would like to thank AFAVA and CUPCR for making the AD and NC EEG data sets open source and thus usable by other researchers.

References

[1] Vicchietti M L, Ramos F M, Betting L E and Campanharo A S 2023 Computational methods of EEG signals analysis for Alzheimer's disease classification *Sci. Rep.* **13** 8184

[2] Alvi A M, Siuly S and Wang H 2022 A long short-term memory based framework for early detection of mild cognitive impairment from EEG signals *IEEE Trans. Emerg. Top. Comput. Intell.* **7** 375–88
[3] Jeong J, Gore J C and Peterson B S 2001 Mutual information analysis of the EEG in patients with Alzheimer's disease *Clin. Neurophysiol.* **112** 827–35
[4] Al-Jumeily D, Iram S, Vialatte F B, Fergus P and Hussain A 2015 A novel method of early diagnosis of Alzheimer's disease based on EEG signals *Sci. World J.* **2015** 931387
[5] Khare S K and Acharya U R 2023 Adazd-Net: automated adaptive and explainable Alzheimer's disease detection system using EEG signals *Knowledge-Based Syst.* **278** 110858
[6] Khare S K, Bajaj V, Gaikwad N B and Sinha G R 2023 Ensemble wavelet decomposition-based detection of mental states using electroencephalography signals *Sensors* **23** 7860
[7] Puri D V, Nalbalwar S, Nandgaonkar A and Wagh A 2022 Alzheimer's disease detection from optimal electroencephalogram channels and tunable Q-wavelet transform *Indones. J. Electr. Eng. Comput. Sci.* **25** 1420–8
[8] Puri D, Chudiwal R and Kachare P 2022 Detection of epilepsy using wavelet packet sub-bands from EEG signals *Int. Conf. on Computing in Engineering and Technology* (Singapore: Springer Nature) pp 302–10
[9] Khare S K, Blanes-Vidal V, Nadimi E S and Acharya U R 2023 Emotion recognition and artificial intelligence: a systematic review (2014–2023) and research recommendations *Inf. Fusion.* **102** 102019
[10] Kulkarni N 2018 Use of complexity based features in diagnosis of mild Alzheimer disease using EEG signals *Int. J. Inf. Technol.* **10** 59–64
[11] Puri D V, Nalbalwar S L and Ingle P P 2023 EEG-based systematic explainable Alzheimer's disease and mild cognitive impairment identification using novel rational dyadic biorthogonal wavelet filter banks *Circ. Syst. Signal Process.* **43** 1792–822
[12] Abásolo D, Escudero J, Hornero R, Gómez C and Espino P 2008 Approximate entropy and auto mutual information analysis of the electroencephalogram in Alzheimer's disease patients *Med. Biol. Eng. Comput.* **46** 1019–28
[13] Simons S, Espino P and Abásolo D 2018 Fuzzy entropy analysis of the electroencephalogram in patients with Alzheimer's disease: is the method superior to sample entropy? *Entropy* **20** 21
[14] Abásolo D, Hornero R, Espino P, Alvarez D and Poza J 2006 Entropy analysis of the EEG background activity in Alzheimer's disease patients *Physiol. Meas.* **27** 241
[15] Azami H, Abásolo D, Simons S and Escudero J 2017 Univariate and multivariate generalised multiscale entropy to characterize EEG signals in Alzheimer's disease *Entropy* **19** 31
[16] Abásolo D, Hornero R, Escudero J and Espino P 2008 A study on the possible usefulness of detrended fluctuation analysis of the electroencephalogram background activity in Alzheimer's disease *IEEE Trans. Biomed. Eng.* **55** 2171–9
[17] Abásolo D, Hornero R, Gómez C, García M and López M 2006 Analysis of EEG background activity in Alzheimer's disease patients with Lempel–Ziv complexity and central tendency measure *Med. Eng. Phys.* **28** 315–22
[18] Puri D V, Gawande J P, Rajput J L and Nalbalwar S L 2023 A novel optimal wavelet filter banks for automated diagnosis of Alzheimer's disease and mild cognitive impairment using Electroencephalogram signals *Decis. Anal. J.* **9** 100336
[19] Simons S and Abásolo D 2017 Distance-based Lempel–Ziv complexity for the analysis of electroencephalograms in patients with alzheimer's disease *Entropy* **19** 129

[20] Puri D, Nalbalwar S, Nandgaonkar A and Wagh A 2022 EEG-based diagnosis of Alzheimer's disease using Kolmogorov complexity *Applied Information Processing Systems: Proc. ICCET 2021* (Singapore: Springer) pp 157–65

[21] Sharma N, Kolekar M H and Jha K 2020 Iterative filtering decomposition based early dementia diagnosis using EEG with cognitive tests *IEEE Trans. Neural Syst. Rehabil. Eng.* **28** 1890–8

[22] Oltu B, Akşahin M F and Kibaroğlu S 2021 A novel electroencephalography based approach for Alzheimer's disease and mild cognitive impairment detection *Biomed. Signal Process. Control* **63** 102223

[23] Fiscon G, Weitschek E, De Cola M C, Felici G and Bertolazzi P 2018 An integrated approach based on EEG signals processing combined with supervised methods to classify Alzheimer's disease patients *2018 IEEE Int. Conf. on Bioinformatics and Biomedicine (BIBM)* (Piscataway, NJ: IEEE) pp 2750–2

[24] Safi M S and Safi S M M 2021 Early detection of Alzheimer's disease from EEG signals using Hjorth parameters *Biomed. Signal Process. Control* **65** 102338

[25] Şeker M, Özbek Y, Yener G and Özerdem M S 2021 Complexity of EEG dynamics for early diagnosis of Alzheimer's disease using permutation entropy neuromarker *Comput. Methods Programs Biomed.* **206** 106116

[26] McBride J C, Zhao X, Munro N B, Smith C D, Jicha G A, Hively L, Broster L S, Schmitt F A, Kryscio R J and Jiang Y 2014 Spectral and complexity analysis of scalp EEG characteristics for mild cognitive impairment and early Alzheimer's disease *Comput. Methods Programs Biomed.* **114** 153–63

[27] Ruiz-Gómez S J, Gómez C, Poza J, Gutiérrez-Tobal G C, Tola-Arribas M A, Cano M and Hornero R 2018 Automated multiclass classification of spontaneous EEG activity in Alzheimer's disease and mild cognitive impairment *Entropy* **20** 35

[28] Miltiadous A, Tzimourta K D, Afrantou T, Ioannidis P, Grigoriadis N, Tsalikakis D G and Tzallas A T 2023 A dataset of scalp EEG recordings of Alzheimer's disease, frontotemporal dementia and healthy subjects from routine EEG *Data* **8** 95

[29] Toural J E, Montoya Pedrón A and Marañón Reyes E J 2021 Classification among healthy, mild cognitive impairment and Alzheimer's disease subjects based on wavelet entropy and relative beta and theta power *Pattern Anal. Appl.* **24** 413–22

[30] Fouad I A and Labib F E Z M 2023 Identification of Alzheimer's disease from central lobe EEG signals utilising machine learning and residual neural network *Biomed. Signal Process. Control* **86** 105266

[31] Geng D, Wang C, Fu Z, Zhang Y, Yang K and An H 2022 Sleep EEG-based approach to detect mild cognitive impairment *Front. Aging Neurosci.* **14** 865558

[32] Calub G I A, Elefante E N, Galisanao J C A, Iguid S L B G, Salise J C and Prado S V 2023 EEG-based classification of stages of alzheimer's disease (AD) and mild cognitive impairment (MCI) *2023 5th Int. Conf. on Bio-engineering for Smart Technologies (BioSMART)* (Piscataway, NJ: IEEE) pp 1–6

[33] Ding Y, Chu Y, Liu M, Ling Z, Wang S, Li X and Li Y 2022 Fully automated discrimination of Alzheimer's disease using resting-state electroencephalography signals *Quant. Imaging Med. Surg.* **12** 1063

[34] Rodrigues P M, Bispo B C, Garrett C, Alves D, Teixeira J P and Freitas D 2021 Lacsogram: a new EEG tool to diagnose Alzheimer's disease *IEEE J. Biomed. Health Inform.* **25** 3384–95

[35] Puri D, Nalbalwar S, Nandgaonkar A, Rajput J and Wagh A 2023 Identification of Alzheimer's disease using novel dual decomposition technique and machine learning algorithms from EEG signals *Int. J. Adv. Sci. Eng. Inf. Technol.* **13** 658–65

[36] Puri D, Nalbalwar S, Nandgaonkar A, Kachare P, Rajput J and Wagh A 2022 Alzheimer's disease detection using empirical mode decomposition and Hjorth parameters of EEG signal *2022 Int. Conf. on Decision Aid Sciences and Applications (DASA)* (Piscataway, NJ: IEEE) pp 23–8

[37] Puri D V, Nalbalwar S L, Nandgaonkar A B, Gawande J P and Wagh A 2023 Automatic detection of Alzheimer's disease from EEG signals using low-complexity orthogonal wavelet filter banks *Biomed. Signal Process. Control* **81** 104439

[38] Al-Shourbaji I, Kachare P H, Alshathri S, Duraibi S, Elnaim B and Abd Elaziz M 2022 An efficient parallel reptile search algorithm and snake optimizer approach for feature selection *Mathematics* **10** 2351

[39] Puri D V, Kachare P H and Nalbalwar S L 2024 Metaheuristic optimized time–frequency features for enhancing Alzheimer's disease identification *Biomed. Signal Process. Control* **94** 106244

[40] Kamble K and Sengupta J 2023 A comprehensive survey on emotion recognition based on electroencephalograph (EEG) signals *Multimed. Tools Appl.* **82** 27269–304

[41] Khare S K and Acharya U R 2023 An explainable and interpretable model for attention deficit hyperactivity disorder in children using EEG signals *Comput. Biol. Med.* **155** 106676

[42] Puri D, Chudiwal R, Rajput J, Nalbalwar S, Nandgaonkar A and Wagh A 2021 Detection of Alcoholism from EEG signals using Spectral and Tsallis Entropy with SVM *2021 Int. Conf. on Communication Information and Computing Technology (ICCICT)* (Piscataway, NJ: IEEE) pp 1–5

[43] Kehri V, Puri D and Awale R N 2020 Entropy-based facial movements recognition using CPVM *Applied Computer Vision and Image Processing: Proc. ICCET 2020* (Singapore: Springer Singapore) pp 17–27

Chapter 7

Mother tree optimization for early detection of focal seizure using entropy-based features

Hesam Akbari and Wael Korani

A seizure is an electrical disturbance in the human brain that affects its normal functions. There are different kinds of seizures that have different origins in the brain: focal, generalized, or unknown onset. After a patient experiences a seizure, a physician identifies where the seizure starts in the brain. The accurate classification of seizures helps professional healthcare providers to diagnose and treat epilepsy patients. The focal seizure (hemisphere) happens on one side of the brain, and it affects 60% of people with epilepsy. Patients with focal seizures who are unresponsive to standard medical therapy might have the option of a surgical operation. In surgery, surgeons carefully remove some parts of the brain that cause the seizure. Focal seizure patients have abnormal signals in one or more brain places. An electroencephalogram (EEG) is one of the most successful ways to distinguish between focal seizure areas and non-focal seizure areas. However, EEGs are time-consuming and prone to errors when surgeons manually evaluate them to detect focal seizure areas. Therefore, automated computer-based systems are beneficial and efficient at differentiating between focal and non-focal EEGs. This chapter introduces a novel automated system called EEG-focal to classify EEGs in focal and non-focal groups. Our proposed system separates the EEGs into 32 sub-bands in the fixed empirical wavelet transform domain. Then, three entropy-based features, Stein's unbiased risk estimation, log energy, and threshold entropy are computed from each sub-band, totaling 96 features. Finally, a novel feature selection technique built on the Mother Tree Optimization (MTO) algorithm is used to select the best features fed to the feed-forward neural network classifier. Our experiments use a ten-fold cross validation strategy to avoid bias in the results. The results show that the EEG-focal system achieves a classification accuracy of 93%, which outperforms other previous related work. The proposed EEG-focal system is robust and reliable enough to be used as a supportive tool for physicians in surgery rooms.

doi:10.1088/978-0-7503-5964-1ch7

7.1 Introduction

Epilepsy is a chaotic situation in the brain in which the central nervous system is affected [1–3]. Epilepsy is a disorder of the nervous system that can lead to seizures, unusual sensations, and even loss of awareness [4]. These symptoms characterize epilepsy. Epileptic individuals experience periodic seizures due to increased cerebral nerve impulses, which disrupt synaptic connectivity in the brain. Even though the symptoms of a seizure may manifest in any region of the body, the primary cause of the underlying electrical abnormalities is in the brain. Understanding epilepsy symptoms and how the condition affects the brain is one of the most challenging problems to solve in the field of neuroscience. Determining which type of seizure, where it is located within the brain, how it spreads across the brain, how much of the brain is involved, and how long it lasts are all critical factors. Epilepsy affects around fifty million people worldwide, the vast majority of whom live in countries that are still developing [5]. Epilepsy is often broken down into three distinct subtypes by neurologists: partial or focal epilepsy, generalized, and unknown epilepsy. When seizures are confined to certain regions of the brain, this condition is known as focal epilepsy, while seizures that affect the whole brain are referred to as generalized epilepsy. Figure 7.1 is an illustration of focal epilepsy and generalized epilepsy.

Epilepsy can affect anyone at any stage of life, but the condition is often treatable with antiepileptic drugs. Even though the outcomes of anti-epileptic medications are encouraging, roughly 25% of patients do not react well to medication [6]. Anti-epileptic medicines are ineffective for around 20% of people who have generalized epilepsy and 60% of those who have focal epilepsy. When a patient with focal epilepsy does not react effectively to anti-epileptic medications as a treatment option, surgery becomes an alternative that should be considered. In such cases, the parts of the patient's brain that are responsible for epilepsy attacks are removed during surgery by physicians. Before surgery, it is essential to accurately identify these specific regions of the brain. Despite the fact that positron emission tomography (PET) scans [7], single-photon emission computed

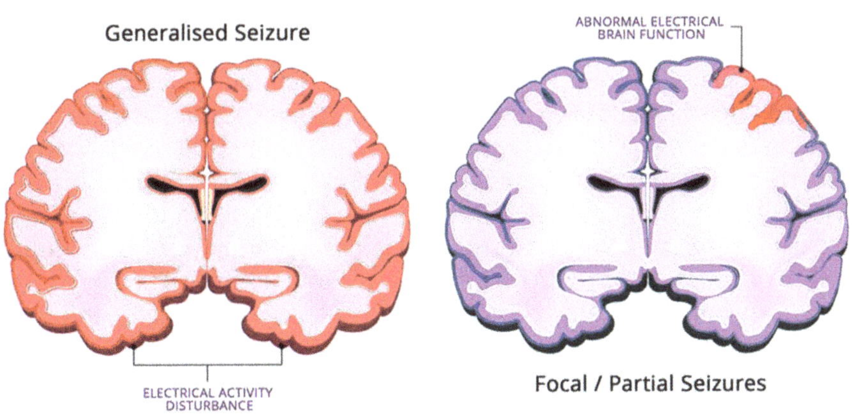

Figure 7.1. A comparison between focal and generalized seizure.

tomography (SPECT) scans [8], and magnetic resonance imaging (MRI) scans [9] may reveal focal regions in the brain, the most significant obstacle is that there is a limited number of such medical imaging instruments in most of the undeveloped and developing countries. EEG signals have been used by physicians to identify brain illnesses and monitor brain functions [10]. EEG readings represent the synaptic electrical activity of the brain. Doctors can identify specific brain areas by visually analyzing EEG data. In patients diagnosed with focal epilepsy, EEG signals captured from the regions of the brain experiencing the condition display unique patterns known as focal EEG signals while non-focal signals are those captured from different brain areas. Visually inspecting several EEG channels requires much time and is prone to mistakes. This is done to distinguish focal signals from non-focal signals during surgery. For this reason, creating a computer diagnostic system (CAD) is necessary if reliable identification of focused signals is to be accomplished [11]. Any CAD system has four steps, including processing, feature extraction, feature selection, and classification. Here, we review previous investigations that have been suggested for the identification of focal EEG signals using these specific procedures.

As the processing step, several time-frequency methods have been utilized to decompose the focal and non-focal EEG signals into subbands (SBs) including empirical mode decomposition (EMD) [12–14], s-transform [15], discrete wavelet transform (DWT) [16–18], EMD-DWT [6], empirical wavelet transform (EWT) [19–21], flexible analytic wavelet transform (FAWT) [22, 23], Fourier–Bessel series expansion domain empirical wavelet transform filter bank [24], Fourier–Bessel series expansion-based flexible time-frequency coverage wavelet transform [25], sliding mode-singular spectrum analysis (SM-SSA) [26], variational mode decomposition (VMD) [27, 28], and VMD-DWT [29]. Although time-frequency methods have been proposed for focal detection, the performance of classification in some of them is not impressive.

As a feature extraction step, several linear features like statistical-based features and nonlin- ear features like chaotic-based features have been applied to EEG signals to classify focal and non-focal groups. Statistical features, such as mean, standard deviation (std), and variance, offer significant insights into the central tendency and spread of EEG signals, but these features cannot be significant features to decode the hidden information of EEG signals [30]. On the other hand, chaotic-based features like fractal dimension, large Lyapunov exponent, and entropies offer a detailed understanding of the complex function and dynamics of signals [31]. However, the problem is that chaotic-based features involve complicated computational steps, which is not desirable for a real-time CAD system to detect focal EEG signals during surgery. In the literature, entropy-based features, including sample entropy [12, 13], Shannon entropy [6, 13, 16], and Renyi's entropy [6, 13, 16], approximate entropy [13], phase entropies [13, 16], log energy (LE) entropy [6, 14, 23, 32, 33], Stein's unbiased risk estimate (SURE) entropy [14, 21, 22], Tsallis wavelet entropy [16], fuzzy entropy [23, 29], and permutation entropy [16] have been utilized as discriminating features in the identification of focal and non-focal EEG signals.

In the feature selection step, once the features have been extracted, it is necessary to select the most important features and input them into classifiers. Feature selection is a crucial component in the development of machine learning applications. When the classifier is provided with many features, the system's complexity is heightened. On the other hand, if the number of features is restricted, the system's accuracy declines and the machine cannot make reliable decisions. The majority of previous machine learning methods suggested employing the p-value as a feature selection technique [6, 13, 14, 16, 19, 20, 22, 23, 29, 34–39] for classifying EEG signals into focal and non-focal groups so that the features with p-values below 0.05 were deemed suitable to feed the classification algorithms [40]. While the traditional technique can identify essential features in most applications, it is ineffective where all extracted features have a p-value lower than 0.05.

As a classification step, most of the previous works used support vector machine (SVM) and K-nearest neighbor (KNN) classifiers which are popular classification algorithms [41, 42]. Nevertheless, checking the classification accuracies for other classification methods is essential when applying focal and non-focal EEG signal detection.

To address the mentioned weakness in the literature, we propose a new framework that is based on decomposing the EEG signals by Fixed EWT and extracting three entropy-based features that have straightforward computation, selecting the best features with a new feature selection algorithm called mother tree optimization (MTO), and checking the performance of nine various classifiers.

It has been suggested to use the EWT to analyze non-stationary, nonlinear, and oscillation signals like EEG signals [43]. Although focal detection using EWT has been done before, the reported results needed to be significantly more accurate [19]. In order to decompose focal and non-focal EEG signals, this study employs EWT as a processing method. In fact, in EWT, the input signal's spectrum is separated by considering its frequency components in such a way that the Fourier transform (FT) computes the frequency spectrum, and then the bandwidths of EWT filter banks are made based on the maximum frequency components on the spectrum, and finally, the signal is decomposed by designed filters in the EWT domain. The EWT filters are changed for input signals, an adaptive signal processing tool. However, for focal EEG signal detection applications, the adaptive characteristic of EWT cannot be helpful because the nature of EWT can introduce variability in the signal decomposition, potentially leading to unreliable results. Therefore, to address this issue, we used a modified version of EWT called Fixed EWT, designed explicitly for focal EEG signal detection by fixing the bandwidths of the filter bank. We aim to provide more consistent and reliable results for focal detection tasks. Fixed EWT retains its ability to effectively decompose EEG signals while mitigating the adaptability issues that could hinder its utility in this context.

Following the SB decomposition of the EEG signal by Fixed EWT, three entropy-based features with straightforward computation, named log energy (LE) entropy, SURE entropy, and threshold (TH) entropy are computed for all SBs to classify EEG signals into focal and non-focal groups. To choose the best features for classification, search heuristic methods can be used as a feature selection technique.

Therefore, optimization techniques can be used to minimize the number of feature vector arrays and, at the same time, try to increase the classification performance. In this work, a new feature selection technique based on MTO is proposed to select the best entropy-based features. Finally, the ability of nine various classifiers is evaluated by applying focal EEG signal detection.

The contribution of the current study can be listed as follows:

- A new automated method is developed to classify focal and non-focal EEG signals.
- A new version of EWT is designed for focal EEG signal detection called Fixed EWT.
- A new feature selection technique called MTO is developed and applied on focal EEG signal detection application.
- The performance of the framework is tested using ten-fold cross-validation (CV) to avoid bias in results that makes the framework robust and reliable.
- Improved classification performance compared to the previous studies reported in the literature.
- Design of a low-cost time framework.

The chapter is organized as follows: section 7.2 gives a thorough overview of the database used for this study; section 7.3 describes the suggested framework and includes details on the Fixed EWT, entropy-based features, MTO, and classification algorithms; section 7.4 shows the results; section 7.5 discusses them; and finally, the chapter concludes in section 7.6.

7.2 Used database

This study used the Bern–Barcelona EEG dataset, which includes EEG data for more than 41.6 h, to assess the proposed framework [44]. The Bern–Barcelona dataset contains EEG signals obtained from five surgical candidates with focal epilepsy. The format of the database is text. There are 3750 files for the focal group and 3750 files for the non-focal group. Each file has two EEG signals, named '*X*' and '*Y*'. '*X*' and '*Y*' are EEG signals from neighboring channels. Each of the '*X*' and '*Y*' signals has 10 240 samples since they were sampled at 512 hertz (HZ) for 20 s. In previous works, it has been emphasized that using '*X*–*Y*' can result in better performance [38], so in the current study, we use '*X*–*Y*' as the input EEG signal. Figure 7.2 shows a sample of focal and non-focal EEG signals.

7.3 Proposed framework

The difference between the EEG signals is computed in the first stage of the suggested framework. Following this, fixed EWT is utilized in order to divide the EEG signals into a total of 32 SBs. The next step involves computing three entropies from each SB, which results in a total of $32 \times 3 = 96$ features for each single EEG signal. MTO is utilized to choose the best features. Finally, the classifiers feed using the selected features by MTO. This section describes the step-by-step implementation of the proposed framework. The suggested approach is tested using the

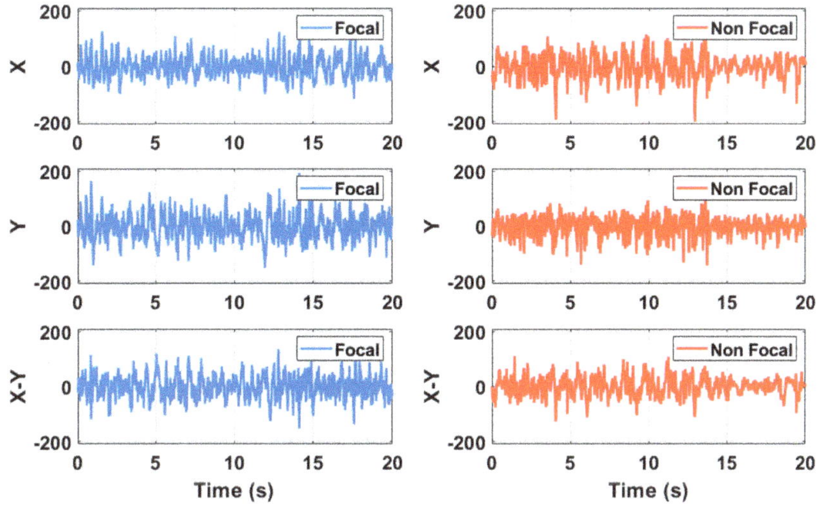

Figure 7.2. An example of '*X*', '*Y*', and '*X–Y*' for focal and non-focal EEG signals.

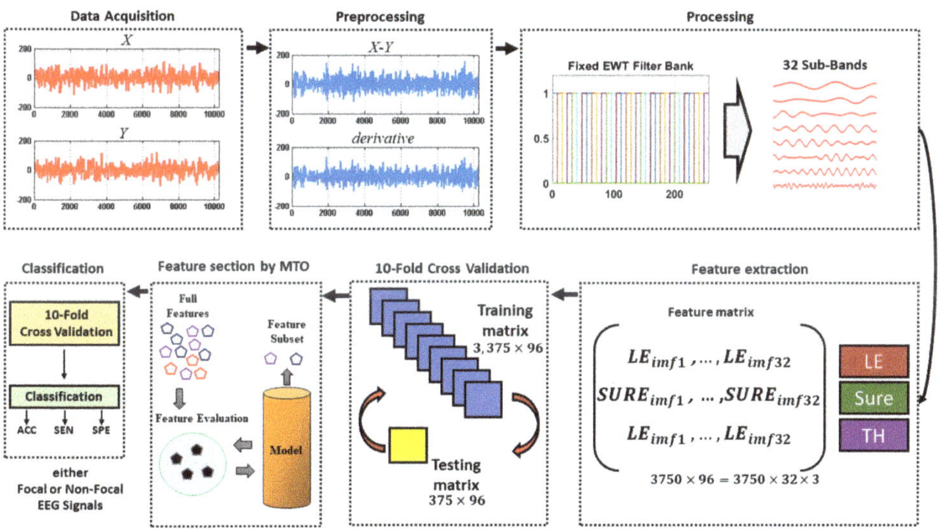

Figure 7.3. The block diagram of the proposed framework for focal and non-focal EEG signals classification.

MATLAB 2023a software on a PC with an i7-4790 CPU operating at 3.60 GHz and 16 GB of RAM. A diagrammatic representation of the proposed framework is shown in figure 7.3.

7.3.1 Derivative operator

The derivative operator is a mathematical operator applied to bio-signals to show their variations. Here, the derivative of EEG signals is computed before decomposing by Fixed EWT. let us assume $x(n) = [s_1, s_2, \ldots, s_n]$ represents a signal with n samples, the derivative operator can be formulated as follows:

$$x'(n) = [s_2 - s_1, s_3 - s_2, \ldots, s_n - s_{n-1}] \tag{7.1}$$

where $x'(n)$ is the derivative of x with the length of $n - 1$ samples.

7.3.2 Fixed EWT

The EWT is an adaptive signal processing technique used in signal processing and data analysis. In the current work, EWT is utilized for analyzing EEG signals as a nonlinear and non-stationary time sequence. The EWT has been developed to solve the issue of mode mixing that occurs in the EMD technique.

Whereas the DWT extracts specific frequency bandwidths for input signals, the EWT employs filters with variable bandwidths that adjust to the input signal spectrum for adaptive decomposition. In the EWT procedure, it is necessary to ascertain the number of SBs. To produce m SBs, the frequency spectrum of the signal is calculated using the FFT technique, and then $m - 1$ maximums are identified as the primary frequency components and are denoted as $L = L_1, L_2, \ldots, L_{m-1}$ [43]. Next, the midpoints between the local maximums are identified and denoted as $B = B_1, B_2, \ldots, B_{m-1}$. The assumption is that the initial midpoint is within the range of 0 and L1. The bounds of the EWT are ultimately defined as follows:

$$\omega = \{[0B_1], [B_1B_2], \ldots, [B_{M-1}\, F_s/2]\} \tag{7.2}$$

where the B is the midpoint between the local maximums, m is the number of SBs, F_s is the sampling frequency. After frequency differentiation, the EWT filter bank is constructed using Littlewood–Paley and Meyer wavelets. The scaling filter (φ) and wavelet filters (ψ) for EWT are formulated as follows:

$$\varphi(\omega) = \begin{cases} 1, & \text{if } |\omega| \leqslant (1 - \eta)\omega_1 \\ \cos\left(\dfrac{\pi\beta(\eta, \omega_1)}{2}\right), & \text{if } (1 - \eta)\omega_1 \leqslant |\omega| \leqslant (1 + \eta)\omega_1 \\ 0, & \text{otherwise} \end{cases} \tag{7.3}$$

$$\psi_{i=2,\ldots,m}(\omega) = \begin{cases} 1, & \text{if } (1 + \eta)\omega_i \leqslant |\omega| \leqslant (1 - \eta)\omega_{i+1}. \\ \cos\left(\dfrac{\pi\Gamma(\eta, \omega_{i+1})}{2}\right), & \text{if } (1 - \eta)\omega_{i+1} \leqslant |\omega| \leqslant (1 + \eta)\omega_{i+1} \\ \sin\left(\dfrac{\pi\Gamma(\eta, \omega_i)}{2}\right), & \text{if } (1 - \eta)\omega_i \leqslant |\omega| \leqslant (1 + \eta)\omega_i. \\ 0, & \text{otherwise.} \end{cases} \tag{7.4}$$

where

$$\Gamma(\eta, \omega_i) = \Gamma(\frac{|\omega| - (1 - \eta)\omega_i}{2\eta\omega_i}) \tag{7.5}$$

where η is a parameter to provide the tight window of the empirical scaling filter and empirical wavelet filter in $L^2(R)$. The condition of a tight window can be satisfied by $<\min(\frac{\omega_{i+1} - \omega_i}{\omega_{i+1} + \omega_i})$, and $\Gamma(y)$ is an arbitrary function as follows:

$$\Gamma(y) = \begin{cases} 0 & \text{if } y \leqslant 0 \\ \Gamma(y) + \Gamma(1 - y) = 1 \,\forall\, y \in [0, 1] & \\ 1 & \text{if } y \geqslant 1 \end{cases} \tag{7.6}$$

The parameter η has a vital role in determining the structure of the filter bank, as it influences the degree of overlap between adjacent filters' bandwidths, particularly in the lower and higher frequency ranges. Including the factor Γ in the EWT filter bank design results in the generation of negligible stop-band ripples, effectively addressing the issue of mode-mixing. The computation of the inner product between the input signal and the scaling filter yields SB_1, whereas the inner product with the wavelet filter produces SB_2, SB_3,…, SB_m, correspondingly.

In the current work, instead of using the adaptive nature of EWT to separate the spectrum of input signals based on local maximums, the Fixed EWT is used by separating the spectrum of EEG signals into 32 equal parts with an 8 Hz duration, which means each input EEG signal is decomposed into 32 SBs. In other words, the boundaries of the scaling and wavelet filters in the EWT domain are fixed to decompose the EEG signals with 32 filters with equal lengths of 8 Hz from 0 to 256 Hz (i.e. $F_s/2$). Figure 7.4 shows the designed Fixed EWT to separate the EEG signal into 32 SBs.

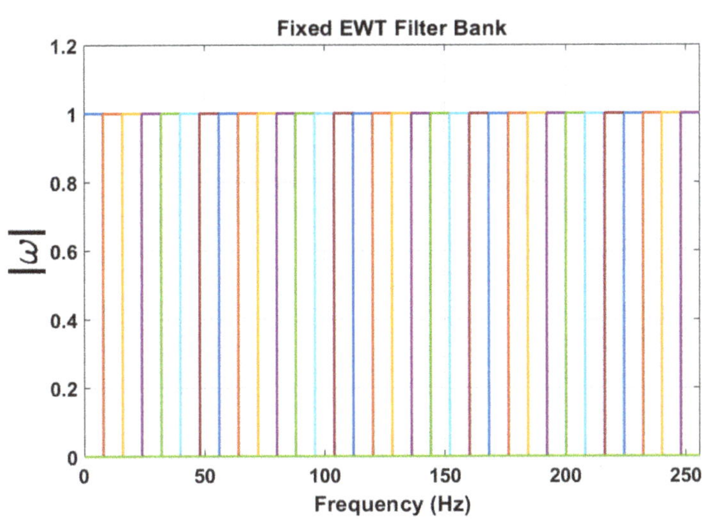

Figure 7.4. The designed fixed EWT filter bank.

7.3.3 Feature extraction

In advanced digital signal processing, entropy is a common technique. In telecommunications, entropy is used to determine the value of missing information; in physics, it is used to quantify the stability of disorder. The complexity of a nonlinear system, such as the brain, can be quantified using entropy. This research used three types of entropy to separate focal and non-focal groups. These included log energy (LE) entropy, Stein's unbiased risk estimation (SURE) entropy, and threshold (TH) entropy.

Let us say that a SB of Fixed EWT is represented by the time series $V(m) = [v_1, v_2, \ldots, v_m]$; then the following definitions for the LE [6, 14], SURE [14, 45], and TH [14] entropies can be defined as follows:

$$\mathrm{LE} = \sum_{i=1}^{m} \log_2 (v_i^2) \tag{7.7}$$

$$\mathrm{SURE} = m - \#\{i \text{ such that } |v_i| \leqslant \gamma\} + \sum_{i=1}^{m} \min(v_i^2, \gamma^2) \tag{7.8}$$

$$\mathrm{TH}(v_i) = \begin{cases} 1 & |v_i| > \gamma \\ 0 & \text{elsewhere} \end{cases} \tag{7.9}$$

So,

$$\mathrm{TH} = \#\{i \text{ such that } |v_i| > \gamma\} \tag{7.10}$$

Where, v_i and γ are ith sample of the input signal and the threshold with positive value, respectively. Here, the value of γ in both SURE and TH entropies is set to 0.5. The '*wentropy*' function is used to compute the LE, SURE, and TH entropies on Matlab.

7.3.4 Mother tree optimization for feature selection (MTO-FS)

The MTO method is a computational technique that draws inspiration from the symbiotic relationship between Douglas fir trees and mycorrhizal fungal networks [46]. Within MTO, candidate solutions operate in accordance with a proposed topology known as fixed-offspring (FO). The algorithm categorizes agents into three main groups based on this topology: top mother tree (TMT), partially connected trees (PCTs), and fully connected trees (FCTs).

7.3.4.1 Top mother tree

The TMT's primary food source actively explores solutions across two distinct tiers: root and mycorrhizal levels. At the fundamental level, it aims to find enhanced solutions by exploring randomly with a step size α. The updated position can be calculated in the following manner:

$$\beta_1(x_{k+1}) = \beta_1(x_k) + \alpha E(d) \tag{7.11}$$

Where $E(d) = \frac{E}{\sqrt{E \cdot E^{T}}}$, is a step size, $E(d)$ is a random vector, $E = 2$ (round (rand $(d, 1)) - 1)$ and d is the dimension of the problem. In the mycorrhizal level, the TMT's position is updated as follows:

$$\beta_1(x_{k+1}) = \beta_1(x_k) + \Delta E(d) \tag{7.12}$$

where Δ is a smaller step size.

7.3.4.2 Partially connected trees

PCTs are situated at both ends of the population: the first-PCTs and last-PCTs. Agents belonging to the first-PCTs group are within the range $[2: \frac{N_T}{2} - 1]$, and their active positions for food sources are adjusted using the following procedure:

$$\beta_n(x_{k+1}) = \beta_n(x_k) + \sum_{i=1}^{n-1} \frac{1}{n - i + 1}(\beta_i(x_k) - \beta_n(x_k)) \tag{7.13}$$

where the population size is N_T, the updated position of agent n is $\beta_n(x_{k+1})$, the current positions of agent n and i are $\beta_n(x_k)$ and $\beta_i(x_k)$, respectively. So, in the event that any individual inside this group employs the defensive mechanism, the position is subsequently updated by utilizing:

$$\beta_n(x_{k+1}) = \beta_n(x_k) + \phi E(d) \tag{7.14}$$

where ϕ represents a little deviation from the current position. Agents of last-PCTs group are in the range $[\frac{N_T}{2} + 3: N_T]$, and the update of the active food source positions for them is modified as follows:

$$\beta_n(x_{k+1}) = \beta_n(x_k) + \sum_{i=n-N_{os}}^{N_T - N_{os}} \frac{1}{n - i + 1}(\beta_i(x_k) - \beta_n(x_k)) \tag{7.15}$$

7.3.4.3 Fully connected trees

The members of the FCTs group are within the range of $[\frac{N_T}{2}: \frac{N_T}{2} + 2]$, and the positions of these agents are modified using the following procedure:

$$\beta_n(x_{k+1}) = \beta_n(x_k) + \sum_{i=n-N_{os}}^{n-1} \frac{1}{n - i + 1}(\beta_i(x_k) - \beta_n(x_k)) \tag{7.16}$$

In [47], a modification of MTO known as DMTO was introduced to address the traveling salesman problem through a swap concept operation. The paper presents a distinct variant of MTO named binary-MTO (BMTO) designed for solving feature selection problems.

7.3.5 Evaluation of method and classification

The current work presents the outcomes of classifiers using a ten-fold CV technique [34]. In the ten-fold CV, the database is partitioned into ten subsets in a way that all subsets have equal size. Subsequently, one subset is utilized for each iteration as data for testing the classifier, while the other nine subsets are employed as data for training the classifier. Here, the EEG signals are utilized nine times to train and once to test the classifier. The label of test data can be either focal or non-focal. There are four scenarios for each testing data after classification based on its labels and the label assigned by the classifier, which are described in the following:

- True positive (TP): this occurs when a focal signal is accurately classified as focal by the trained model.
- True negative (TN): this occurs when a non-focal signal is accurately classified as non-focal by the trained model.
- False positive (FP): this occurs when a non-focal signal is incorrectly classified as focal by the trained model.
- False positive (FN): this occurs when a focal signal is incorrectly classified as non-focal by the trained model.

The equations shown below have been used to assess the accuracy (ACC), sensitivity (SEN), and specificity (SPE) of the classifier [20].

$$\mathrm{ACC}=\frac{T_{\mathrm{TP}}+T_{\mathrm{TN}}}{T_{\mathrm{TP}}+T_{\mathrm{TN}}+T_{\mathrm{FP}}+T_{\mathrm{FN}}}\times 100 \tag{7.17}$$

$$\mathrm{SEN}=\frac{T_{\mathrm{TP}}}{T_{\mathrm{TP}}+T_{\mathrm{FN}}}\times 100 \tag{7.18}$$

$$\mathrm{SPE}=\frac{T_{\mathrm{TN}}}{T_{\mathrm{TN}}+T_{\mathrm{FP}}}\times 100 \tag{7.19}$$

where T_{TP}, T_{TN}, T_{FP} and T_{FN} represent the sum of TP, TN, FP, and FN after ten rounds of testing the classifier by ten-fold CV technique.

Nine algorithms are analyzed and compared for their ability to classify EEG signals as either focal or non-focal. The decision trees (DT); random forest (RF); artificial neural network (ANN) such as multi-layer perceptron neural network (MLPNN), recurrent neural network (RNN), feed-forward neural network (FFNN), probability neural network (PNN), cascade forward neural net-work (CFNN), neural network (NN), generalized regression neural network (GRNN); naive Bayes (NB) with four probability distribution assumptions including Gaussian, kernel, multinomial, multivariate multinomial; support vector machine (SVM) with three kernel functions including linear, polynomial with degree 3 and radial basis function (RBF) with a sigma of 1; K-nearest neighbors (KNN) with eight distance metrices including City-block, Minkowski, Cosine, Spearman, Euclidean, Hamming, Chebyshev and Mahalanobis; Discriminate analysis (DA) with five assumptions such as linear, diagonal-linear, diagonal-quadratic, pseudo-linear, pseudo-quadratic; and ensemble tree (ET) algorithms are eval- uated to classify the extracted features in focal and nonfocal groups. The parameter configurations for the employed classification algorithms can be seen in table 7.1.

Table 7.1. The parameters of the classifiers.

Method	Parameter	Value
DT	Number of splits	50
RF	Number of trees	20
MLPNN, RNN, FFNN, PNN, CFNN, NN	Hidden layer size	10
	Maximum epochs allowed	50
GRNN	Spread of radial basis functions	1
NB	Probability distribution assumption	Multivariate multinomial Multinomial Kernel Gaussian
SVM	Kernel Function	Linear RBF Polynomial
KNN	Distance metric	City-block Minkowski Cosine Spearman Euclidean Hamming Chebyshev Mahalanobis
	Number of nearest neighbors	5
DA	Data distribution assumption	Pseudo-quadratic Pseudo-linear Diagonal-quadratic Diagonal-linear Linear
ET	Number of branches	50

7.4 Result and discussion

The present study uses EEG data from the Bern–Barcelona benchmark dataset to evaluate the proposed framework. Figure 7.2 shows an example of EEG signal for focal and non-focal groups from the Bern–Barcelona benchmark database. Figure 7.3 illustrates the proposed framework steps. As preprocessing, the '*X*–*Y*' is calculated by the difference between two neighboring channels of '*X*' and '*Y*' to reduce the effect of noise [20], and then the first derivative operator is applied to the

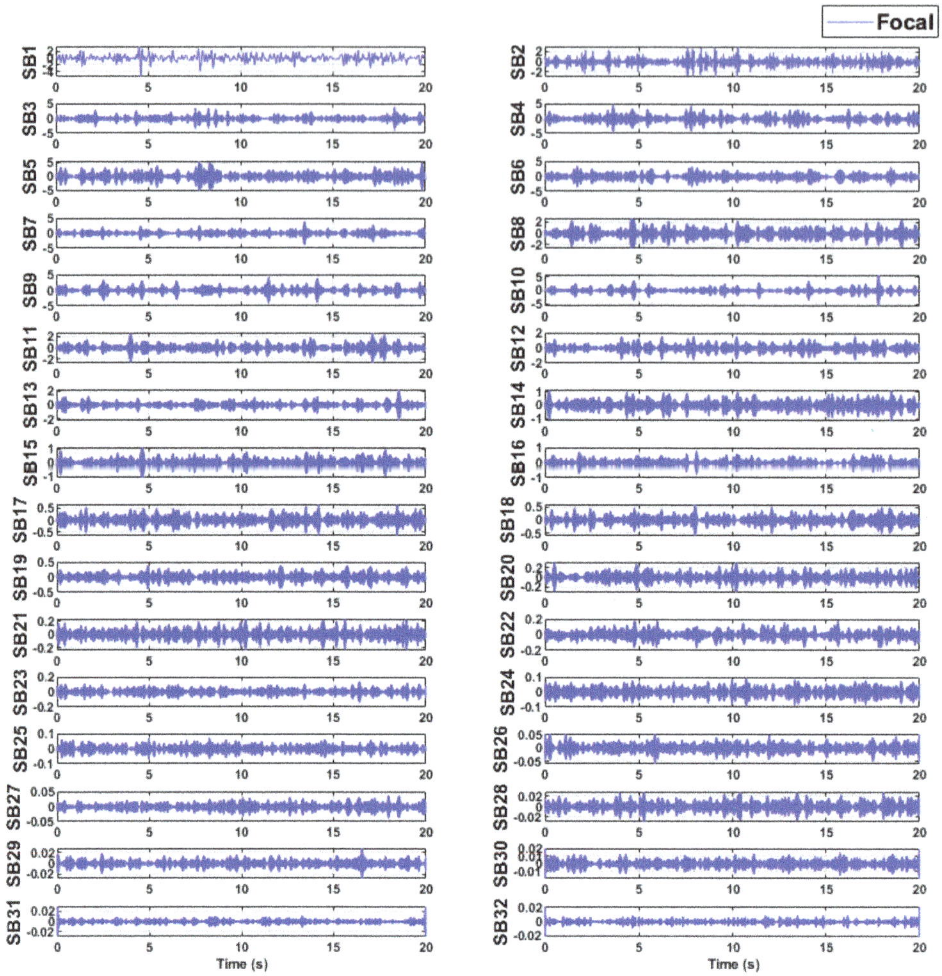

Figure 7.5. A sample of focal EEG signals.

'*X*–*Y*' signal, which has been proven in previous studies to increase the efficiency of CAD systems in recognizing focal and non-focal EEG signals.

The EEG signals are decomposed into 32 SBs in the processing step by Fixed EWT. Figure 7.4 shows the bandwidth of the filter bank in the Fourier domain. Figures 7.5 and 7.6 show the separated 32 SBs of EEG signals in focal and non-focal groups, respectively.

After the decomposition of the EEGs into 32 SBs, in the feature extraction phase, three entropies, including SURE, THE, and LE, are extracted from the SBs. Each SB is quantized with three features, which makes $32 \times 3 = 96$ features in total. The mean, std, and p-value of the features for SBs are written in tables 7.2 and 7.3. The focal group has a lower mean and std than the non-focal group. The focal EEGs are collected from the points of the brain that are the source of the seizure attack, and one possible explanation for the lower entropy of the focal data is the synchronous

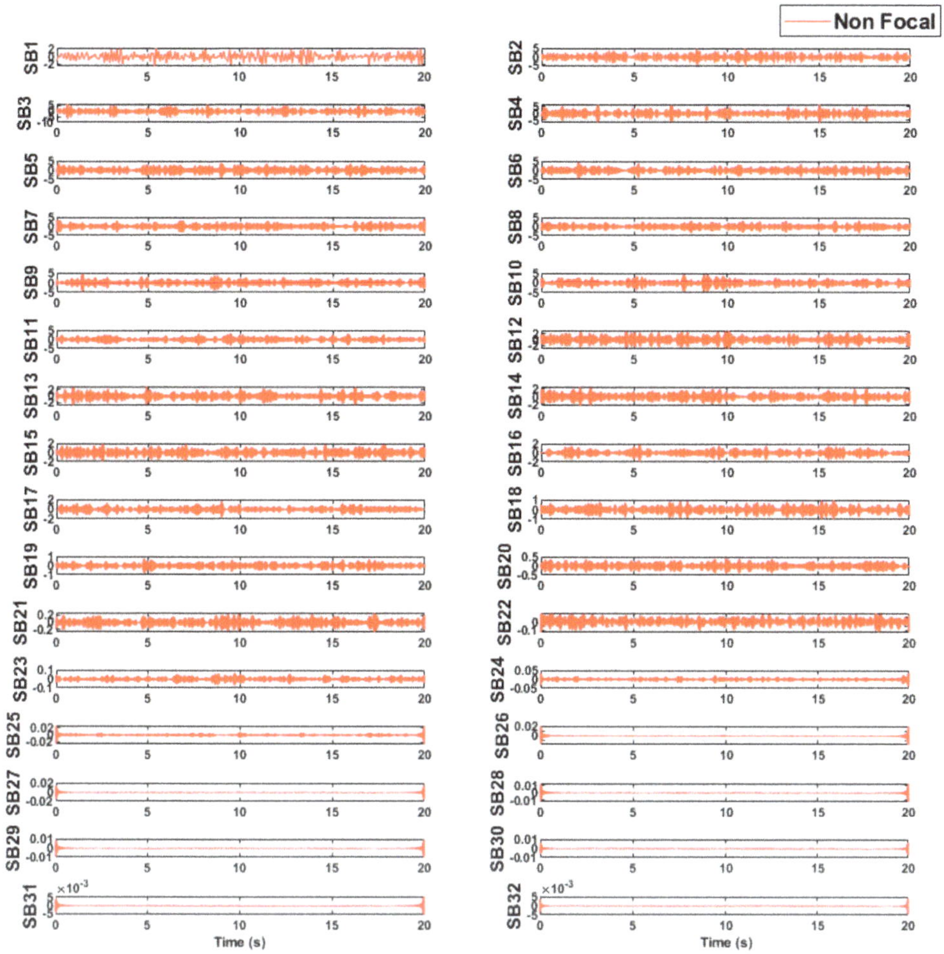

Figure 7.6. A sample of non-focal EEG signals.

activation of neurons inside the epileptogenic region. Since the entropy measures and quantifies the irregularity of the systems, the lower entropy values of focal EEGs indicate a lower connection between the synapses in the focal areas. In [20], the SODP of EEGs and in [19], the PSR of EEGs have been plotted on a two-dimensional space for focal and non-focal groups and it was reported that the 2D shape of the focal EEGs has a simpler and more predictable shape than non-focal EEG signals; Here, the same concept can be concluded by lower entropy values for focal EEGs than non-focal.

Another observation in table 7.3 is that all 96 SBs have a *p*-value below 0.05. Statistically speaking, there is a proper difference between the features of two groups (i.e., the focal and non-focal groups) when the p-value is lower than 0.05. All the extracted features can be used in classifiers if the traditional statistical-based methods are used to select the best features that show their inability. In order to

Table 7.2. The mean and std of features in focal and non-focal groups.

	LE				SURE				TH			
	Focal		Non-focal		Focal		Non-focal		Focal		Non-focal	
SB	Mean	Std	Mean	Std	Mean	Std	Mean	Std	Mean	Std	Mean	Std
1	−11 517	13 526	−15 126	17 123	5472	3721	4329	5338	7480	1800	6931	2573
2	−11 959	14 228	−9167	17 750	5256	4049	5584	5289	7376	1958	7538	2553
3	−12 456	13 935	−10 684	18 358	5228	4013	5215	5579	7362	1940	7360	2692
4	−13 328	13 863	−13 102	18 789	5070	4059	4642	5871	7286	1961	7084	2831
5	−14 056	13 895	−14 917	19 318	4897	4141	4211	6083	7203	1999	6876	2931
6	−15 320	13 669	−15 821	19 536	4595	4167	3986	6173	7057	2012	6768	2974
7	−15 570	13 270	−13 610	16 983	4546	4044	4683	5386	7032	1955	7100	2601
8	−17 363	13 820	−17 560	19 942	3975	4300	3559	6287	6756	2077	6562	3026
9	−18 360	14 238	−18 499	19 933	3610	4416	3324	6313	6579	2133	6449	3038
10	−20 053	13 999	−19 587	19 740	3116	4474	3051	6321	6340	2160	6317	3041
11	−22 545	13 104	−20 910	19 429	2437	4483	2706	6321	6011	2164	6150	3041
12	−25 043	12 336	−22 697	19 059	1669	4485	2250	6308	5640	2164	5930	3034
13	−27 378	11 824	−24 478	18 074	875	4487	1735	6203	5256	2164	5680	2984
14	−29 807	11 500	−27 177	17 775	−24	4496	1006	6162	4822	2167	5329	2961
15	−32 516	11 156	−29 908	16 917	−1075	4464	170	5994	4315	2150	4925	2879
16	−35 589	10 870	−33 040	16 066	−2296	4377	−853	5745	3727	2105	4432	2757
17	−39 284	10 464	−36 810	15 318	−3778	4129	−2145	5376	3014	1982	3809	2575
18	−43 860	9988	−41 511	14 696	−5521	3641	−3800	4814	2179	1741	3014	2299
19	−49 509	9335	−46 145	13 516	−7386	2761	−5576	4091	1291	1311	2162	1948
20	−57 044	8783	−54 847	14 641	−9074	1469	−7734	2859	499	685	1138	1346
21	−65 925	8953	−63 800	15 744	−9923	515	−9120	1700	116	231	490	787
22	−76 401	10 722	−74 359	17 935	−10 143	231	−9834	789	30	103	164	353
23	−88 479	14 392	−86 610	21 576	−10 201	139	−10 125	339	11	62	37	150

(*Continued*)

Table 7.2. (*Continued*)

	LE				SURE				TH			
	Focal		Non-focal		Focal		Non-focal		Focal		Non-focal	
SB	Mean	Std	Mean	Std	Mean	Std	Mean	Std	Mean	Std	Mean	Std
24	−102 456	20 053	−100 804	26 917	−10 220	107	−10 202	220	5	49	8	102
25	−118 743	28 035	−117 315	34 368	−10 227	86	−10 219	176	4	40	5	82
26	−135 223	36 924	−133 972	42 943	−10 231	70	−10 227	128	3	32	3	59
27	−144 980	41 216	−144 406	47 762	−10 233	53	−10 231	73	2	25	2	33
28	−148 886	39 970	−148 694	46 687	−10 234	41	−10 234	41	2	19	2	19
29	−152 018	37 719	−151 912	44 269	−10 235	32	−10 235	27	1	15	1	12
30	−154 963	35 612	−154 978	41 936	−10 236	27	−10 236	19	1	12	1	9
31	−157 557	33 899	−157 696	39 950	−10 236	23	−10 236	15	1	11	1	7
32	−159 496	32 904	−159 662	38 718	−10 236	18	−10 236	12	1	8	1	6

Table 7.3. The p-value of features.

Sub-band	LE	SURE	TH
1	4.66×10^{-06}	9.91×10^{-09}	9.89×10^{-08}
2	2.81×10^{-08}	1.02×10^{-00}	1.04×10^{-00}
3	6.16×10^{-01}	1.61×10^{-53}	1.66×10^{-06}
4	2.25×10^{-02}	2.93×10^{-09}	3.00×10^{-00}
5	4.78×10^{-07}	2.55×10^{-05}	2.62×10^{-06}
6	3.90×10^{-16}	1.55×10^{-21}	1.62×10^{-21}
7	8.25×10^{-02}	9.49×10^{-43}	1.03×10^{-00}
8	5.37×10^{-03}	1.16×10^{-23}	1.18×10^{-23}
9	2.14×10^{-01}	1.05×10^{-00}	1.07×10^{-00}
10	1.79×10^{-07}	3.59×10^{-05}	3.61×10^{-06}
11	9.70×10^{-07}	4.05×10^{-00}	4.06×10^{-00}
12	1.24×10^{-02}	3.60×10^{-06}	3.52×10^{-05}
13	1.90×10^{-09}	2.67×10^{-06}	2.74×10^{-07}
14	7.40×10^{-04}	5.15×10^{-01}	5.09×10^{-00}
15	5.13×10^{-01}	1.37×10^{-03}	1.29×10^{-02}
16	4.56×10^{-05}	4.39×10^{-03}	3.71×10^{-07}
17	1.01×10^{-00}	2.44×10^{-04}	1.66×10^{-06}
18	3.57×10^{-05}	3.70×10^{-07}	6.58×10^{-05}
19	1.14×10^{-01}	2.94×10^{-09}	4.24×10^{-02}
20	1.47×10^{-04}	1.62×10^{-06}	8.88×10^{-08}
21	9.58×10^{-05}	3.92×10^{-09}	1.68×10^{-06}
22	4.12×10^{-0}	7.32×10^{-0}	2.43×10^{-04}
23	4.37×10^{-0}	7.98×10^{-0}	1.11×10^{-01}
24	1.14×10^{-0}	3.41×10^{-0}	1.25×10^{-02}
25	8.17×10^{-0}	6.60×10^{-0}	1.11×10^{-0}
26	6.12×10^{-0}	1.88×10^{-0}	1.40×10^{-0}
27	4.03×10^{-0}	6.79×10^{-0}	6.91×10^{-0}
28	2.34×10^{-0}	4.60×10^{-06}	2.19×10^{-0}
29	2.00×10^{-0}	3.51×10^{-05}	5.19×10^{-0}
30	2.73×10^{-0}	1.30×10^{-03}	6.28×10^{-0}
31	4.36×10^{-0}	2.39×10^{-03}	9.77×10^{-0}
32	2.16×10^{-0}	3.82×10^{-08}	8.20×10^{-0}

overcome the inefficiency of traditional methods, the MTO is used to select the best features before feeding the classifiers. After feature selection, 49 out of all 96 features were selected. The MTO selected 23 lE entropy from 1, 2, 4, 5, 6, 7, 8, 11, 12, 13, 16, 17, 18, 19, 20, 23, 24, 25, 27, 29, 30, 31, and 32 SBs; 15 SURE entropy from 4, 5, 8, 9, 10, 11, 12, 16, 17, 22, 25, 27, 28, 29, and 32 SBs; and 11 TH entropy from 1, 2, 7, 8, 9, 12, 14, 15, 20, 21, and 32.

The resulting classifications of ACC, SEN, and SPE before and after using feature selection are listed in table 7.4. Although the ACC has become slightly lower after

Table 7.4. Performance of classification algorithms before and after feature selection.

	Performance of all features			Performance of MTO features		
Classification method	ACC	SEN	SPE	ACC	SEN	SPE
DT	80.12	86.93	73.31	79.84	87.33	72.35
RF	90.69	93.12	88.27	90.51	93.01	88.00
MLPNN	87.19	88.00	86.37	87.69	87.97	87.41
RNN	92.71	93.73	91.68	91.81	92.13	91.49
CFNN	92.44	92.61	92.27	92.27	92.27	92.27
PNN	72.22	71.36	76.59	71.92	72.13	71.59
FFNN	92.76	93.71	91.81	93.00	93.52	92.48
NN	87.55	87.89	87.20	86.52	87.20	85.84
GRNN	87.56	88.69	86.43	86.43	87.23	85.63
NB Gaussian	68.12	76.29	59.95	68.13	74.24	62.03
NB Kernel	66.81	84.99	53.00	66.81	82.59	51.04
NB multinomial	73.25	74.50	75.75	73.81	74.12	75.69
NB multivariate multinomial	73.33	75.42	76.89	73.66	74.25	76.51
SVM linear	73.95	74.63	76.18	73.42	74.77	76.05
SVM polynomial	73.58	74.94	76.37	73.79	74.12	76.62
SVM rbf	80.12	86.93	73.31	79.33	80.14	81.69
KNN City-Block	90.69	93.12	88.27	86.47	88.69	84.24
KNN Minkowski	87.19	88.00	86.37	87.03	89.39	84.67
KNN Cosine	92.71	93.73	91.68	86.92	89.33	84.51
KNN Spearman	92.44	92.61	92.27	86.76	89.39	84.13
KNN Euclidean	72.22	71.36	76.59	86.81	89.07	84.56
KNN Hamming	92.76	93.71	91.81	87.05	89.25	84.85
KNN Chebyshev	87.55	87.89	87.20	86.92	89.44	84.40
KNN Mahalanobis	87.56	88.69	86.43	86.95	89.28	84.61
DA linear	68.12	76.29	59.95	82.59	85.81	79.36
DA diagonal-linear	66.81	84.99	53.00	60.99	69.36	52.61
DA diagonal-quadratic	73.25	74.50	75.75	66.71	82.45	50.96
DA pseudo-linear	73.33	75.42	76.89	82.68	85.97	79.39
DA pseudo-quadratic	73.95	74.63	76.18	75.81	93.76	57.87
ET	73.58	74.94	76.37	83.36	92.13	74.59

using the best features in most of the classifiers, the point is that instead of 96 features, 49 features are used, which means that the feature vector has become 45.12% smaller, which makes the system fast, which is desired in CAD systems. Another observation that is obvious in table 7.4 is that the classification ACCs for RF, RNN, CFNN, and FFNN are higher than 90% before and after selecting the significant features, which indicates the efficacy of these classifications in recognizing focal and non-focal EEGs. Similarly, the classification ACCs for MLPNN, NN, GRNN, and KNNs are higher than 85%, which is acceptable in a CAD system.

In table 7.5, The effectiveness of the proposed framework is studied with previous methods. The Bern–Barcelona database has been utilized in all the mentioned

Table 7.5. Comparison of the performance of the proposed framework with the previous works on the Bern–Barcelona database.

Refercences	Method	Pairs of EEG signals	CV	ACC (%)
[6]	DWT + EMD, entropies, Knn	3750	Not used	89.40
[48]	Delay permutation entropy, SVM	750	Not used	75
[12]	EMD, sample entropy, LS-SVM	50	Ten-fold	85
[13]	Seven entropies in the EMD domain, LS-SVM	50	Ten-fold	87
[14]	Four nonlinear features in the EEMD domain, SVM	50	Ten-fold	89
[15]	Time-frequency entropy of spectrum, S-transform, SVM	50	Not used	86
[16]	DWT, entropies, LS-SVM	50	Ten-fold	84
[17]	Nine linear features, DWT, SVM	3750	Not used	83.07
[36]	Mean frequency and root mean square of rhythms in Fourier domain, LS-SVM	3750	Ten-fold	89.52
[19]	Central tendency measure of PSR of rhythms in the EWT domain, LS-SVM	750	Ten-fold	82.53
[34]	Twenty-three nonlinear features, LS-SVM	3750	Not used	87.93
[49]	Linear and nonlinear features, SVM	3750	Not used	92.15
[35]	Multifractal detrended fluctuation analysis, KNN	50	Ten-fold	92.18
[37]	Multi-scale entropy, TQWT, LS-SVM	3750	Ten-fold	84.67
[33]	Differential operator, nonlinear features, SVM	3750	Not used	88.14
[21]	Nonlinear features of rhythm in EWT domain, KNN	50	Ten-fold	93
[38]	KNN-En, CC, FzEn, TQWT, LS-SVM	3750	Ten-fold	95
[27]	VMD, clustering	750	Ten-fold	96
[29]	VMD-DWT, entropies, SVM	3750	Not used	95.2
[23]	Flexible analytic wavelet transform (36 levels), SVM	3750	Ten-fold	94.8
[50]	TQWT (27 levels), entropies, GRNN	3750	Ten-fold	97.68
Ours	Fixed EWT, entropies, MTO, FFNN	3750	Ten-fold	93

methods in table 7.5. It can be seen that the classification ACC of 93% is higher than all previous works instead of [23, 27, 29, 38, 50]. In [38], the reported classification ACC of 95% is 2% higher than ours. However, the LE, TH, and SURE entropies in our proposed framework have simple and straightforward computation, while the KNN entropy estimator (KNN-En), centered correntropy (CC), and fuzzy entropy (FzEn), which have been extracted as features in [38] have complex and heavy calculations, which makes their work not suitable for applications that operate in real time. Although the classification ACC of 96% in [27] is 3% higher than ours, in their work to assess the efficiency of methods, 750 pairs of EEGs have been utilized, while the resulting classification ACC of 93% for our framework has resulted from 3750 pairs of EEGs, which makes our proposed framework more reliable than theirs.

In [29], the classification ACC is 95.2%, which is 2.2% higher than ours, but the main weakness of their method is that it needs to use two time-frequency methods, including VMD and DWT, back-to-back to extract the SBs, which means in the processing step it is more complex than our use of just Fixed EWT. In [23], the resulted classification ACC is 1.8% higher than ours, but the decomposition level in their method is 36 levels while ours is 32, which means their work is less complicated than ours. The reported ACC of 97.68% by [50] is 4.68% higher than ours. The TQWT has been utilized in the processing step to distinguish the EEGs into 27 SBs. The TQWT has three parameters that have to be set by the operator to get the best results. In fact, by changing the sampling frequency, their method cannot be used, while our proposed framework is not sensitive to the sampling frequency, and it can be used even after changing the sampling frequency; in another work, our proposed framework is not sensitive to changing the sampling frequency while their method is.

The suggested framework exhibits some advantages in comparison to previous investigations, which are listed below:

- This is the first time that the application of MTO as a feature selection algorithm has been defined and used in a focal EEG detection application.
- This is the first study to compare how well various classification algorithms can classify EEGs, either in focal or non-focal groups.
- To assess the efficacy of the present study, the entire Bern–Barcelona dataset consisting of 7500 pairs of EEG signals for each group (i.e 3750 focal and 3750 non-focal) was used while in [12–16, 21, 35], only 100 EEG signals (i.e. 50 focal and 50 non-focal) were utilized to evaluate the methods.
- In this study, we used a total of three entropies to distinguish EEGs either in focal or non-focal groups. However, previous research [13, 16–18, 34, 49] used various features, making our framework simpler than theirs by using just three entropies, which have straightforward computational costs.
- We report our results in a ten-fold CV approach to avoid the bias effect, while in [6, 15, 17, 29, 33, 34, 48, 49] the results have been reported without using the CV technique.
- The proposed framework requires a processing time of 0.0.3 s for classifying an input EEGs which indicates that there is significant processing time for real-time applications.
- The proposed framework offers cost-effective and user-friendly implementation via the use of a computer and EEG recording equipment, hence enabling hospitals to employ it extensively in pre-surgical procedures.

- The proposed methodology effectively identifies focal EEG patterns without human error.
- The recommended technique needed 0.03 s for preprocessing, processing, and feature extraction for any '*X*' and '*Y*' pair of EEG signals. Furthermore, classifying any test signal took less than 0.002 s with FFNN, confirming the speed and efficacy of the suggested framework.

The limitation of the present framework is the number of patients in the database. Additionally, the number of SBs should be selected manually in the Fixed EWT; it would be better to choose it automatically. In the future, the performance of the proposed framework will be tested using another database with more patients. Moreover, an automatic variant of Fixed EWT will be introduced.

7.5 Conclusion

Before surgery, doctors may locate the brain's surface by visually examining EEG signals. Physicians have to visually recognize the focal and non-focal EEGs for a very long duration, which is quite confusing, time-consuming, and potentially susceptible to human errors. In order to effectively differentiate between focal and non-focal EEGs, a computer-based procedure needs to be developed. In the current work, we propose a technique using features based on entropy taken from Fixed EWT SBs. The Fixed EWT and MTO algorithms were implemented as an effective signal decomposition technique and feature selection method, respectively, and aligned with multiple classification models to classify more than 41.6 h of EEGs in the benchmark Bern–Barcelona dataset, either in focal or non-focal groups. With distinct entropy-based features chosen using the MTO approach extracted from the Fixed EWT domain and classified using the FFNN, our framework resulted in an ACC of 93% in a ten-fold CV situation. In the future, the performance of MTO as a reliable feature selection algorithm in mental disorder applications such as the detection of depression, stress, Parkinson's disease, Alzheimer's disease, autism, and attention deficit hyperactivity disorder (ADHD) will be tested.

List of abbreviations

CV	Cross validation	**VMD**	Variational mode decomposition	**TP**	True positive
EEG	Electroencephalogram	T_{TP}	Total number of TPin cv	**TN**	True negative
FO	Fixed offspring	T_{TN}	Total number of TN in cv	**FP**	False positive
CC	Centered correntropy	T_{FP}	Total number of FP in cv	**FN**	False positive
N_T	Population size	T_{FN}	Total number of FN in cv	**NB**	Naive Bayes
Δ	Smaller step size	**BMTO**	Binary-MTO	**NN**	Neural network
SB	Sub-band	**MTO**	Mother tree optimization	**ET**	Ensemble Tree

(Continued)

FzEn	Fuzzy entropy	**DWT**	Discrete wavelet transform	**TMT**	Top Mother Tree
FT	Fourier transform	**EMD**	Empirical mode decomposition	**ACC**	Accuracy
LE	Log energy entropy	$\boldsymbol{\Gamma(y)}$	An arbitrary function	**SEN**	Sensitivity
TH	Threshold entropy	**PET**	Positron emission tomography	**SPE**	Specificity
HZ	Hertz	**MRI**	Magnetic resonance imaging	**DT**	Decision Trees
$\boldsymbol{x(n)}$	Signal with n samples	**CAD**	Computer diagnostic system	**RF**	Random Forest
s	Samples of input signal	**EWT**	Empirical wavelet transform	φ	Scaling filter
$\boldsymbol{x'(n)}$	Derivative of signal x	**SVM**	Support vector machine	ψ	Wavelet filter
$\boldsymbol{m}$	Number of subbands	**RBF**	Radial basis function	$\boldsymbol{L^2(R)}$	Two norm space
ω	Frequency bandwidth	**KNN**	K-nearest neighbors	γ	Threshold
$\boldsymbol{F_s}$	Sampling frequency	**DA**	Discriminate analysis	**V**	A time series
α	Step size in MTO	**ANN**	Artificial Neural Network	$\boldsymbol{E(d)}$	A random vector

FFNN	Feed-forward neural network	**SPECT**	Single-photon emission computed tomography
PNN	Probability Neural Network	**GRNN**	Generalized regression neural network
CFNN	Cascade forward neural network	$\boldsymbol{\beta_n(x_{k+1})}$	The position of the agent at $k + 1$ iteration
TQWT	Tunable Q wavelet transform	**L**	Number of local maximums in EWT
ϕ	Deviation from the current position	**B**	Midpoint within two local maximums
PCTs	Partially Connected Trees	**FAWT**	Flexible analytic wavelet transform
FCTs	Fully connected trees	**SURE**	Stein's unbiased risk estimate entropy
SODP	Second order difference plot	**MLPNN**	Multi-layer Perceptron Neural Network
PSR	Phase space reconstruction	**KNNEn**	KNN entropy estimator
ADHD	Attention deficit hyperactivity disorder	η	Parameter to determine the structure of EWT filter bank

References

[1] Khare S K and Bajaj V 2020 Constrained based tunable Q wavelet transform for efficient decomposition of EEG signals *Appl. Acoust.* **163** 107234

[2] Akbari H and Esmaili S 2020 A novel geometrical method for discrimination of normal, interictal and ictal EEG signals *Trait. Signal* **37** 59–68

[3] Akbari H, Sadiq M T and Rehman A U 2021 Classification of normal and depressed EEG signals based on centered correntropy of rhythms in empirical wavelet transform domain *Health Inf. Sci. Syst.* **9** 1–15

[4] Hussain W, Sadiq M T, Siuly S and Rehman A U 2021 Epileptic seizure detection using 1D-convolutional long short-term memory neural networks *Appl. Acoust.* **177** 107941

[5] de la O Serna J A, Paternina M R A, Zamora-Méndez A, Tripathy R K and Pachori R B 2020 EEG-rhythm specific Taylor–Fourier filter bank implemented with o-splines for the detection of epilepsy using EEG signals *IEEE Sens. J.* **20** 6542–51

[6] Das A B and Bhuiyan M I H 2016 Discrimination and classification of focal and non-focal EEG signals using entropy-based features in the EMD-DWT domain *Biomed. Signal Process. Control* **29** 11–21

[7] Savic I, Thorell J O and Roland P 1995 [11C] flumazenil positron emission tomography visualizes frontal epileptogenic regions *Epilepsia* **36** 1225–32

[8] Newton M R, Berkovic S F, Austin M C, Rowe C C, McKay W J and Bladin P F 1995 SPECT in the localisation of extratemporal and temporal seizure foci *J. Neurol. Neurosurg. Psychiatry* **59** 26–30

[9] Woermann F G and Vollmar C 2009 Clinical MRI in children and adults with focal epilepsy: a critical review *Epilepsy Behav.* **15** 40–9

[10] Khare S K, Bajaj V and Acharya U R 2023 SchizoNet: a robust and accurate Margenau–Hill time-frequency distribution based deep neural network model for schizophrenia detection using EEG signals *Physiol. Meas.* **44** 035005

[11] Khare S K, Blanes-Vidal V, Nadimi E S and Acharya U R 2023 Emotion recognition and artificial intelligence: a systematic review (2014–2023) and research recommendations *Inf. Fusion.* **102** 102019

[12] Sharma R, Pachori R B and Gautam S 2014 Empirical mode decomposition based classification of focal and non-focal EEG signals *2014 Int. Conf. on Medical Biometrics* (Piscataway, NJ: IEEE) pp 135–40

[13] Sharma R, Pachori R B and Acharya U R 2014 Application of entropy measures on intrinsic mode functions for the automated identification of focal electroencephalogram signals *Entropy* **17** 669–91

[14] Ghofrani S and Akbari H 2019 Comparing nonlinear features extracted in EEMD for discriminating focal and non-focal EEG signals *Proc. 10th Int. Conf. Signal Process. Syst.* (Bellingham, WA: SPIE) vol 11071 pp 25–9

[15] Krishnan P T and Balasubramanian P 2016 Automated EEG seizure detection based on S-transform *2016 IEEE Int. Conf. on Computational Intelligence and Computing Research (ICCIC)* (Piscataway, NJ: IEEE) pp 1–5

[16] Sharma R, Pachori R B and Acharya U R 2015 An integrated index for the identification of focal electroencephalogram signals using discrete wavelet transform and entropy measures *Entropy* **17** 5218–40

[17] Chen D, Wan S and Bao F S 2016 Epileptic focus localization using discrete wavelet transform based on interictal intracranial EEG *IEEE Trans. Neural Syst. Rehabil. Eng.* **25** 413–25

[18] Madhavan S, Tripathy R K and Pachori R B 2019 Time-frequency domain deep convolutional neural network for the classification of focal and non-focal EEG signals *IEEE Sens. J.* **20** 3078–86

[19] Sharma R and Pachori R B 2015 Classification of epileptic seizures in EEG signals based on phase space representation of intrinsic mode functions *Expert Syst. Appl.* **42** 1106–17

[20] Akbari H, Ghofrani S and Ghofrani S 2019 Fast and accurate classification F and NF EEG by using SODP and EWT *Int. J. Image Graph. Signal Process.* **11** 29–35

[21] Akbari H and Sadiq M T 2021 Detection of focal and non-focal EEG signals using non-linear features derived from empirical wavelet transform rhythms *Phys. Eng. Sci. Med.* **44** 157–71

[22] Gupta V, Priya T, Yadav A K, Pachori R B and Acharya U R 2017 Automated detection of focal EEG signals using features extracted from flexible analytic wavelet transform *Pattern Recognit. Lett.* **94** 180–8

[23] You Y, Chen W, Li M, Zhang T, Jiang Y and Zheng X 2020 Automatic focal and non-focal EEG detection using entropy-based features from flexible analytic wavelet transform *Biomed. Signal Process. Control* **57** 101761

[24] Siddharth T, Gajbhiye P, Tripathy R K and Pachori R B 2020 EEG-based detection of focal seizure area using FBSE-EWT rhythm and SAE-SVM network *IEEE Sens. J.* **20** 11421–8

[25] Gupta V and Pachori R B 2020 Classification of focal EEG signals using FBSE based flexible time-frequency coverage wavelet transform *Biomed. Signal Process. Control* **62** 102124

[26] Siddharth T, Tripathy R K and Pachori R B 2019 Discrimination of focal and non-focal seizures from EEG signals using sliding mode singular spectrum analysis *IEEE Sens. J.* **19** 12286–96

[27] Taran S and Bajaj V 2018 Clustering variational mode decomposition for identification of focal EEG signals *IEEE Sens. Lett.* **2** 1–4

[28] Khare S K, Gaikwad N B and Bajaj V 2022 VHERs: a novel variational mode decomposition and Hilbert transform-based EEG rhythm separation for automatic ADHD detection *IEEE Trans. Instrum. Meas.* **71** 1–10

[29] Rahman M M, Bhuiyan M I H and Das A B 2019 Classification of focal and non-focal EEG signals in VMD-DWT domain using ensemble stacking *Biomed. Signal Process. Control* **50** 72–82

[30] Khare S K, Gadre V M and Acharya R 2023 ECGPsychnet: an optimized hybrid ensemble model for automatic detection of psychiatric disorders using ECG signals *Physiol. Meas.* **44** 115004

[31] Khare S K and Acharya U R 2023 ADAZD-Net: Automated adaptive and explainable Alzheimer's disease detection system using EEG signals *Knowl. Based Syst.* **278** 110858

[32] Akbari H, Sadiq M T, Rehman A U, Ghazvini M, Naqvi R A, Payan M, Bagheri H and Bagheri H 2021 Depression recognition based on the reconstruction of phase space of EEG signals and geometrical features *Appl. Acoust.* **179** 108078

[33] Fasil O, Rajesh R and Thasleema T 2017 Influence of differential features in focal and non-focal EEG signal classification *Proc. IEEE Region 10 Humanitarian Technol. Conf. (R10-HTC) (IEEE)* (Piscataway, NJ: IEEE) pp 646–9

[34] Acharya U R, Hagiwara Y, Deshpande S N, Suren S, Koh J E W, Oh S L, Arunkumar N, Ciaccio E J and Lim C M 2019 Characterization of focal EEG signals: a review *Future Gener. Comput. Syst.* **91** 290–9

[35] Chatterjee S, Pratiher S and Bose R 2017 Multifractal detrended fluctuation analysis based novel feature extraction technique for automated detection of focal and non-focal electroencephalogram signals *IET Sci. Meas. Technol.* **11** 1014–21

[36] Singh P and Pachori R B 2017 Classification of focal and nonfocal EEG signals using features derived from Fourier-based rhythms *J. Mech. Med. Biol.* **17** 1–22

[37] Bhattacharyya A, Pachori R B, Upadhyay A and Acharya U R 2017 Tunable-q wavelet transform based multiscale entropy measure for automated classification of epileptic EEG signals *Appl. Sci.* **7** 385

[38] Sharma R, Kumar M, Pachori R B and Acharya U R 2017 Decision support system for focal EEG signals using tunable-q wavelet transform *J. Comput. Sci.* **20** 52–60

[39] Sharma M, Achuth P, Deb D, Puthankattil S D and Acharya U R 2018 An automated diagnosis of depression using three channel bandwidth-duration localized wavelet filter bank with EEG signals *Cogn. Syst. Res.* **52** 508–20

[40] Khare S K, Bajaj V and Sinha G 2020 Automatic drowsiness detection based on variational non-linear chirp mode decomposition using electroencephalogram signals *Modelling and Analysis of Active Biopotential Signals in Healthcare* **vol 1** (Bristol: IOP Publishing) pp 5-1–25

[41] Sharma R, Khare S K, Bajaj V and Ansari I A 2021 Improving the separability of drowsiness and alert EEG signals using analytic form of wavelet transform *Appl. Acoust.* **181** 108164

[42] Khare S K, March S, Barua P D, Gadre V M and Acharya U R 2033 Application of data fusion for automated detection of children with developmental and mental disorders: a systematic review of the last decade *Inform. Fusion* **99** 101898

[43] Gilles J 2013 Empirical wavelet transform *IEEE Trans. Signal Process.* **61** 3999–4010

[44] Andrzejak R G, Schindler K and Rummel C 2012 Nonrandomness, nonlinear dependence, and nonstationarity of electroencephalographic recordings from epilepsy patients *Phys. Rev.* E **86** 046206

[45] Li T, Dong H and Sun J 2019 Binary differential evolution based on individual entropy for feature subset optimization *IEEE Access* **7** 24109–21

[46] Korani W, Mouhoub M and Spiteri R J 2019 Mother tree optimization *IEEE Intl Conf. on Systems, Man and Cybernetics (SMC)* pp 2206–13

[47] Korani W and Mouhoub M 2020 Discrete mother tree optimization for the traveling salesman problem *Neural Information Processing: 27th Int. Conf. ICONIP* vol 27 pp 25–37

[48] Zhu G, Li Y, Wen P P, Wang S and Xi M 2013 Epileptogenic focus detection in intracranial eeg based on delay permutation entropy *AIP Conf. Proc.* **1559** 31–6

[49] Sriraam N and Raghu S 2017 Classification of focal and non focal epileptic seizures using multi-features and SVM classifier *J. Med. Syst.* **41** 160

[50] Sadiq M T, Yu X and Yuan Z 2021 Exploiting dimensionality reduction and neural network techniques for the development of expert brain–computer interfaces *Expert Syst. Appl.* **164** 114031

Chapter 8

Automatic detection of seizure activity using EEG signals

Hesam Akbari and Wael Korani

The use nonstationary electroencephalography to identify seizure activity is a challenge in the field of brain disorders. In addition, the manual evaluation of EEG signals for different brain disorders, including seizures, is error-prone, imprecise, and time-consuming. In recent decades, many efforts have been made to provide automatic computer-based systems to help neurophysiologists detect seizure activity. In this chapter, the linear and nonlinear features of electroencephalogram (EEG) signal rhythms are utilized to develop an efficient automatic computer-based system called EEG-seizure that recognizes epileptic attacks. To evaluate the performance of the proposed system, extensive experiments are conducted by performing four different classifications: normal versus seizure, normal versus seizure-free, seizure versus seizure-free, and normal versus seizure versus seizure-free. The proposed EEG-seizure system is evaluated using a database from Bonn, Germany, and an Indian seizure database. In the study described here, a tenfold cross validation strategy is utilized to avoid bias in the results. It is essential to use a feature selection (FS) preprocessing stage to decrease computational costs; however, choosing the best FS technique for a specific classification task is challenging. In addition, selecting the best classification technique to tackle a particular task is another challenge that influences the efficiency of the model. In this regard, we evaluated the performance of eight classifiers and 14 FS techniques to choose the best techniques for the proposed EEG-seizure system. The results show that the cascade forward neural network (CFNN) classifier outperforms other classifiers for all classification tasks, as mentioned earlier. However, the best FS technique depends on the classification task, and the results show that the best FS techniques for EEG seizure systems are the whale optimization algorithm (WOA), the equilibrium optimizer, the dragonfly algorithm, and grey wolf optimization (GWO). The accuracy levels of all classification tasks, as mentioned earlier, are 100% when the CFNN classifier is combined with the best FS technique.

doi:10.1088/978-0-7503-5964-1ch8

8.1 Introduction

Epilepsy is a persistent neurological disorder that is the result of conflict due to abnormal brain activity. Epilepsy affects around 50 million individuals worldwide, the vast majority of whom are located in underdeveloped nations [1]. Finding epilepsy patients before they have a seizure may be beneficial to their treatment. The majority of epilepsy patients do not exhibit any clear clinical indications before experiencing a seizure [2]. Electroencephalographic data is often used to identify various brain illnesses and activities [3, 4]. Seizures caused by epilepsy in humans typically appear as spikes in EEG readings, which may be visually studied by specialists [5, 6]. Activity that involves the laborious and time-consuming task of visually inspecting lengthy EEG recordings in order to identify the presence of epileptic seizures may be challenging [7, 8]. As a result, it is preferable to develop an automatic computer-based system to categorize EEG signals as seizure-free (SF), indicative of seizure (S), or normal (N).

The automatic computer-based systems proposed to classify S, SF, and N EEG signals have four main components: signal decomposition, feature extraction, FS, and classification. In the signal decomposition stage, time–frequency techniques have been employed to decompose the input EEG into its sub-bands to show and analyze the behavior of EEG signals in narrow frequency bandwidths. These techniques include dual-tree complex wavelet transform (DT-CWT) [9], tunable-Q wavelet transform (TQWT) [10], localized orthogonal wavelets [11], flexible analytic wavelet transform (FAWT) [12], and variational mode decomposition (VMD) [13, 14]. In the feature extraction stage, various techniques have been proposed, such as calculating permutation entropy [15], constructing horizontal visibility graphs (HVGs) [16], performing clustering analysis [17], measuring linear prediction error energy [18], computing fractional linear prediction (FLP) error [19], generating second-order difference plots (SODPs) [20], and reconstructing phase space [21]. These techniques have been proposed to recognize seizures in EEG signals, which means that the majority of the approaches created to date are based on measuring the linear and nonlinear features of EEG signals.

Most of the previous approaches proposed for the detection of S vs. SF conditions in EEG signals have used traditional FS methods based on the p-values of the features. Features that have p-values less than or equal to 0.05 are considered significant and are included as inputs for subsequent processing stages [13, 20–22]. The main weakness of the p-value method is that it cannot determine the best features when all extracted features have p-values of less than 0.05. To overcome this problem, optimization algorithms such as the genetic algorithm (GA) [23] and particle swarm optimization (PSO) [2] have been proposed, since they not only reduce the number of features used but also improve classification performance. The use of a suitable classification algorithm has a direct effect on the performance of automatic computer-based systems. In the research literature, several classification algorithms, such as support vector machine (SVM) [16, 20, 24], k-nearest neighbors (k-NN) [19, 25, 26], and neural networks (NN) [27–29], have been reported for the categorization of EEG data.

The fundamental problem of the previous techniques based on time–frequency methods, as shown by the literature review, is the lack of a clear justification for choosing the number of decomposition levels [2, 5, 7, 10–12]. In addition, although several methods have been proposed based on the linearity and nonlinearity of EEG data, a comprehensive list of these features is still lacking [15, 18, 20, 21, 23, 26]. Furthermore, the EEG signal classification field needs more solid work to evaluate the effectiveness of different optimization methods for FS algorithms [4, 29, 40–43]. Finally, a lack of evaluation of the efficacy of different classification algorithms in EEG signal classification is another problem that still needs to be solved [44–50].

In this chapter, we propose a new framework based on EEG rhythms. In this approach, both linear and nonlinear features are extracted to decode the nonlinear and nonstationary nature of EEG signals. In the final stage, we assess the effectiveness of combining multiple FS techniques with classification algorithms to achieve optimal performance.

The contributions of the current chapter are as follows:

- By extracting the five principal brain rhythms, including delta, theta, alpha, beta, and gamma, instead of decomposing the EEGs into several sub-bands, we address the lack of rationale for the number of decomposition levels. The frequency ranges of these five rhythms can reveal the signs of mental disorders better than other frequency ranges. Empirical wavelet transform (EWT) is used to separate the EEG signals into five rhythms.
- Seventeen features to be extracted from the EEG signals are listed and introduced. This constitutes a comprehensive list of features for the EEG data classification field.
- The performances of fourteen optimization algorithm techniques are checked to evaluate their effectiveness in EEG data classification.
- The efficacy of eight classification algorithms is checked to evaluate their effectiveness in EEG data classification.

The structure of this chapter is as follows: section 8.2 describes the suggested methodology, outlining the utilization of the database, the process of rhythm separation by EWT, feature extraction, FS, and the classification model. The findings and analysis are outlined in section 8.3, while conclusions are drawn in the final section.

8.2 Resources and method

8.2.1 Databases used

The Bonn database, a benchmark database, and an Indian database recently recorded at the Neurology and Sleep Clinic in India were used to evaluate the EEG-seizure framework. These two databases are briefly described in this section.

The Bonn database is freely accessible for download from Bonn University's official website. The Bonn database includes five distinct folders named *A*, *B*, *C*, *D*, and *E* [30]. Every folder contains 100 EEGs in .text format recorded at a rate of 173.61 hertz (Hz). Each EEG signal has a length of 23.6 s, corresponding to a total of 4096 samples per signal. Folders *A* and *B* contain samples taken from five normal subjects. The EEGs in folder *A* were collected while the subjects had their eyes open, whereas those from folder *B* were collected when the subjects had closed eyes. Folders *C* and *D* were obtained from five patients who had fully recovered from seizure episodes after surgery. Folder *E* comprises EEG signals that display epileptic seizure activity detected inside the epileptogenic zone. In this study, EEGs in folders *A* and *B* are considered the N group, EEGs in folders *C* and *D* are considered the SF group, and EEGs in folder *E* are considered the S group. Figure 8.1 illustrates examples of EEG readings from the N, S, and SF classes.

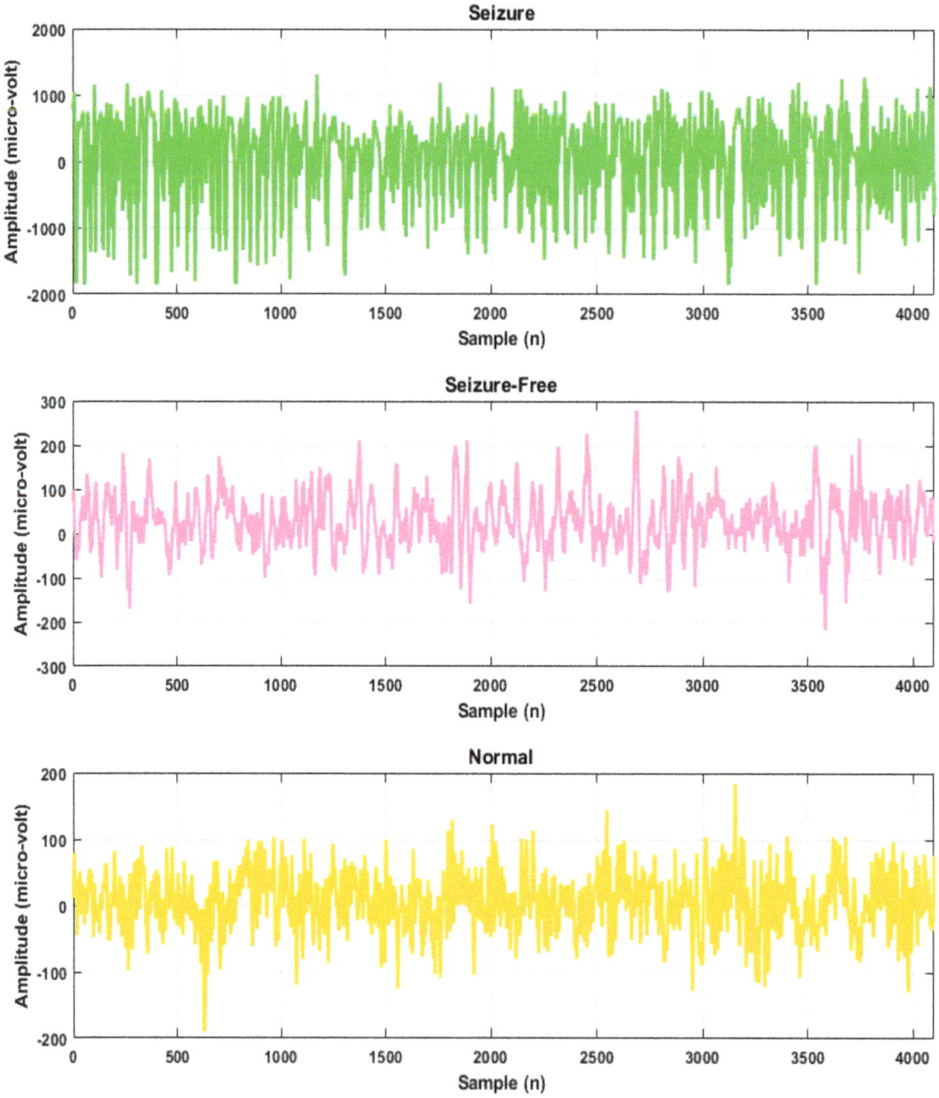

Figure 8.1. A sample of S, SF, and N EEG signals.

The Indian database was recently recorded at the Neurology and Sleep Centre, Hauz Khas, New Delhi [31–33]. This database has three folders, and each folder has 50 files in .mat format. The normal, interictal, and ictal folders in the Indian database have EEG signals from the N, SF, and S groups, respectively. Each .mat file has one EEG signal with a length of 1024 samples. The signals in the Indian database were recorded for a total of 2.56 s at a sampling rate of 400 Hz. The EEG signals in the Bonn and Indian databases were recorded using a 10–20 system with gold-plated electrodes, an international standard.

8.2.2 Setting up empirical wavelet transform to separate EEG rhythms

Gilles [34] proposed EWT as a technique for separating the input data into several modes using an adaptive filter bank. Figure 8.2 illustrates the steps required to decompose an input signal using EWT. We assume that M, the total number of modes, remains constant in the EWT process [35]. Subsequently, we apply a fast Fourier transform to the signal to compute the spectrum. The frequency point is selected by identifying two local maximum points, which are sorted according to equation (8.1):

$$L_{\text{max}} = \{\text{max}_1, \text{max}_2, \ldots, \text{max}_{M-1}\}. \tag{8.1}$$

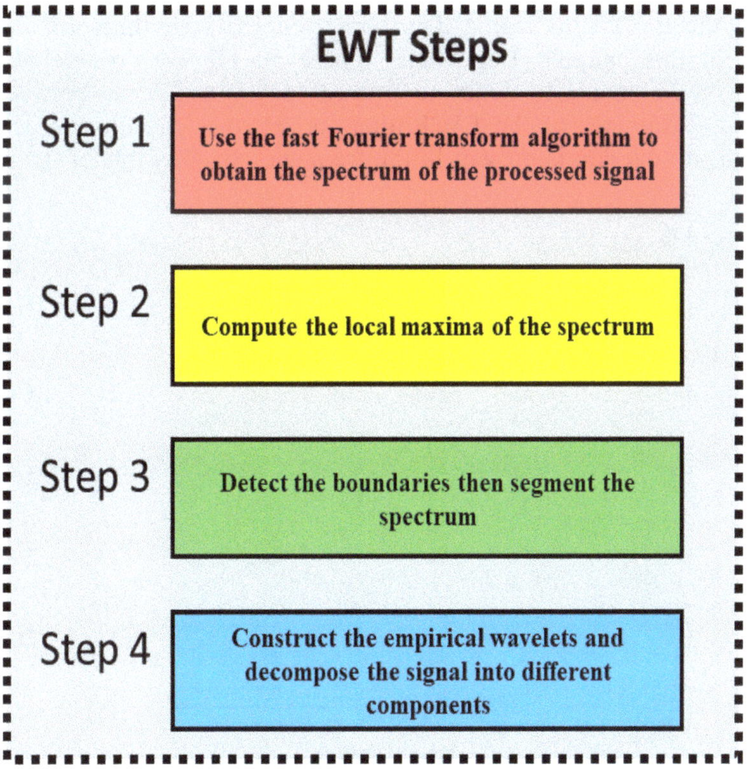

Figure 8.2. The EWT process used to decompose the input signal.

The number of M bandwidths that can be established between the cutoff frequencies is presented in equation (8.2):

$$f_{\text{out}} = \{f_1, f_2, \ldots, f_n\}. \tag{8.2}$$

Finally, the M bandwidths can be defined as follows:

$$\omega_{i=1,\,2\ldots,\,m} = \{[0, f_1], [f_1, f_2], \ldots, [f_{m-1}, f_m], [f_m, f_s/2]\}. \tag{8.3}$$

This chapter describes the use of EWT as an operator for rhythm separation. The selection of bandwidths for the EWT filter bank determines the bandwidths of the EEG rhythms. Consequently, the selection of frequency bandwidths is used to extract brain rhythms, with delta in the range of 0–4 Hz, theta in the range of 4–8 Hz, alpha in the range of 8–13 Hz, beta in the range of 13–30 Hz, and gamma in the range of 30–60 Hz. The EWT filter bank designed to determine the brain rhythms is shown in figure 8.3.

In the filter settings, it can be observed that the transition band has a particularly small size. Similarly, the band-pass filters demonstrate minimal ripples in the pass-band and stop-band regions [36]. The separated rhythms reduce aliasing, giving the measurement increased accuracy (ACC). The filters used for scaling and wavelet functions in the Fourier domain are constructed using the Littlewood–Paley and Meyer wavelet principles [37]. The filtering of EEG signals to separate the rhythms is done using the EWT filter bank. The separated EEG rhythms are illustrated in figure 8.4. In this chapter, frequencies above 60 Hz are considered noise and consequently eliminated. In order to prevent any interference between the sub-bands, the λ parameter of the EWT filters is set to a constant value of 0.1825, ensuring that no overlap is present in the frequency bandwidths of the rhythms.

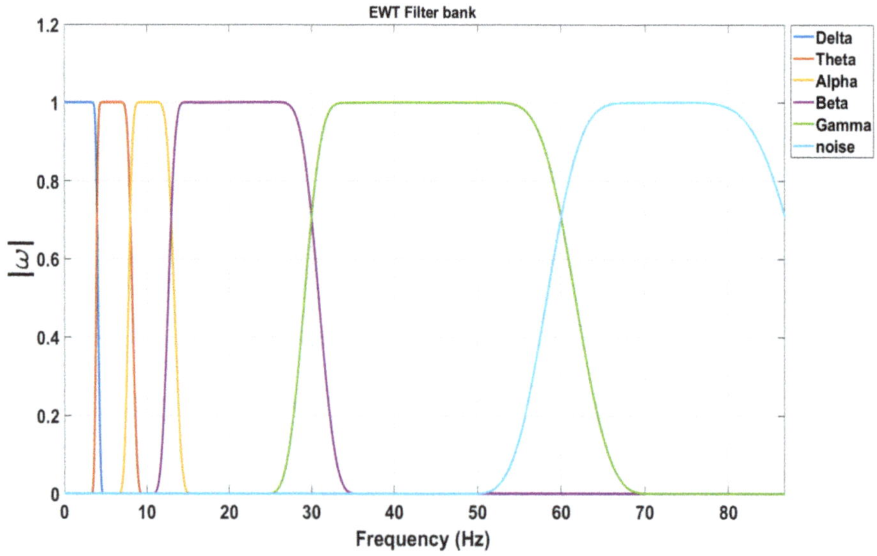

Figure 8.3. The designed EWT filter bank.

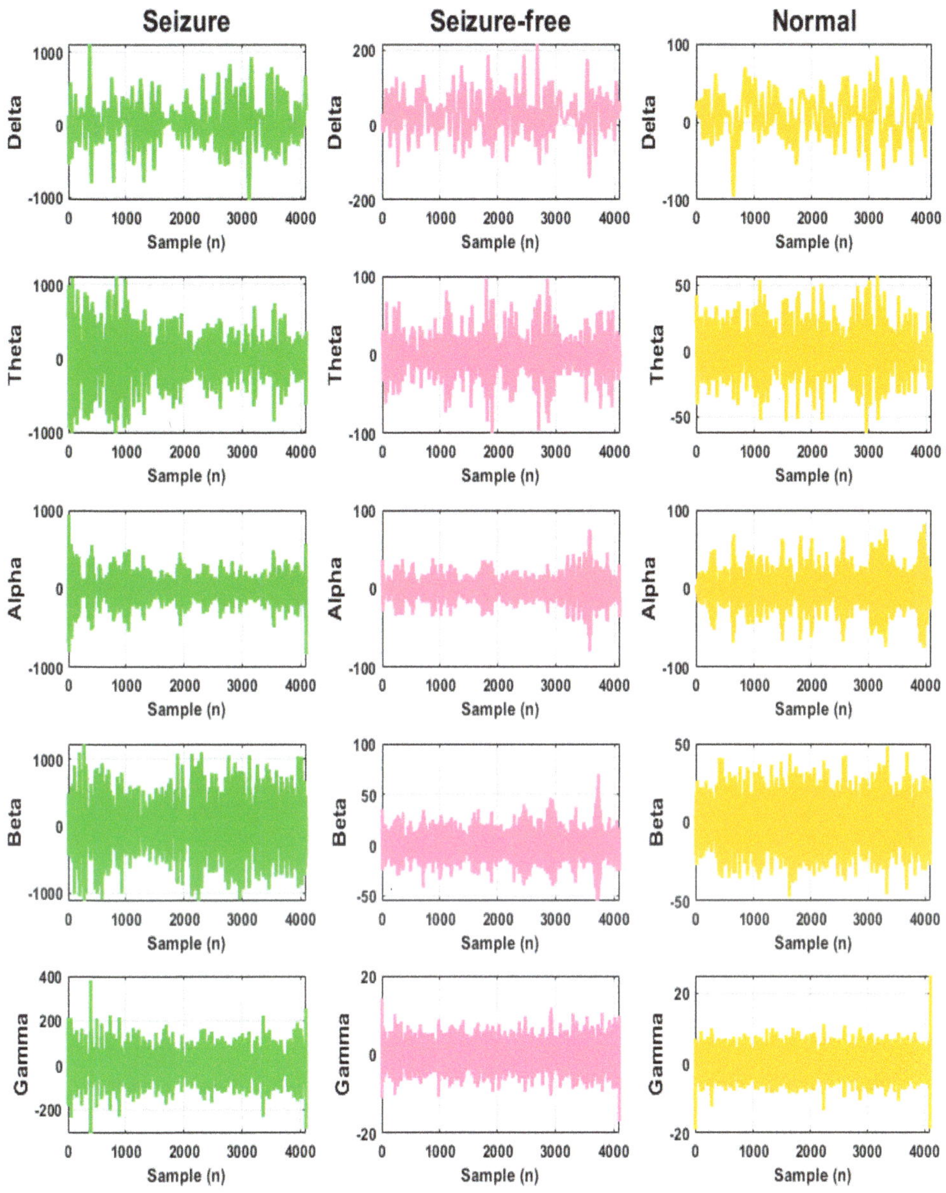

Figure 8.4. The EEG signal rhythms extracted by EWT.

8.2.3 Feature extraction

The computation of pertinent features enhances the efficacy of models in effectively recognizing EEGs. To unravel the intricate operations of the brain, prior research has established many characteristics that are used to delineate EEG signals. In our study, a total of 17 linear and nonlinear features are utilized to classify EEG signals.

Table 8.1. Description of linear and nonlinear features.

Feature name	Feature equation
Mean (μ) [22]	$F_1 = \frac{\sum_{i=1}^{n} x_i}{n}$
Standard deviation (σ) [14]	$F_2 = \sqrt{\frac{\sum_{i=1}^{n}(x_i-\mu)^2}{(n-1)}}$
Variance [8]	$F_3 = \frac{\sum_{i=1}^{n}(x_i-\mu)^2}{(n-1)}$
Skewness [29]	$F_4 = \frac{\sum_{i=1}^{n}(x_i-\mu)^3}{(n\cdot\sigma^3)}$
Kurtosis [6]	$F_5 = \frac{\sum_{i=1}^{n}(x_i-\mu)^4}{(n\cdot\sigma^4)}$
Maximum (max) [7]	$F_6 = \max(x)$
Minimum (min) [38]	$F_7 = \min(x)$
Range [38]	$F_8 = \max(x) - \min(x)$
Median (Med)	$F_9 = \text{Med}(x)$
Interquartile range [20]	$F_{10} = Q3 - Q1$
Correlation coefficient [28]	$F_{11} = \frac{\sum_{i=1}^{n}(x_i-\mu_x)(y_i-\mu_y)}{\sqrt{\sum_{i=1}^{n}(x_i-\mu_x)^2\sum_{i=1}^{n}(y_i-\mu_y)^2}}$
Sum of power spectral density [7]	$F_{12} = \sum\frac{1}{N}\sum_{i=1}^{N}\lvert \gamma_i(f)\rvert^2$
Shannon entropy [10]	$F_{13} = -\sum x_i \ \log_2 x_i$
Log energy entropy [38]	$F_{14} = -\sum \log_2 x_i$
Threshold entropy [4]	$F_{15} = \sum_{i=1}^{n}\mathbf{1}_{\{\forall\ x_i>\varepsilon\}}$
Sure entropy [39]	$F_{16} = n - \sum_{i=1}^{n}\mathbf{1}_{\{\forall\ x_i<\varepsilon\}} + \sum\min(x_i^2, \varepsilon^2)$
Norm entropy [32]	$F_{17} = -\frac{1}{\log(n)}\sum_{i=1}^{n} x_i \log x_i$

Let us define $x = [x_1, x_2, \dots, x_n]$ as a time series with length n. These features can then be defined as listed in table 8.1.

Here, x_i and y_i are the ith sample of the time series with length n and its difference, respectively, Q 3 and Q 1 are the 75th and 25th percentile of the time series, N is the number of windows, $\gamma_i(f)$ is the Fourier transform of the ith window of the signal, f is the frequency, and ε is the threshold.

8.2.4 Feature selection

To assess the efficacy of using a prominent metaheuristic algorithm for FS, we experimented to evaluate the efficacy of thirteen techniques in the context of EEG signal recognition. This section describes the algorithms and their corresponding parameters.

Recently, the use of the FS technique has been widely employed in the domains of machine learning and data mining. The principal aim of the FS technique is to minimize the total number of features as well as the model's error rate. Typically, a data set may have many features obtained during the feature extraction step. In some cases, an overlarge number of features can have a detrimental impact on the efficacy of the classifier [40]. Therefore, the use of an FS approach becomes imperative in the context of handling a data set of such substantial magnitude [38].

Generally, an FS method aims to identify and choose a subset of highly discriminating features from all extracted features. Wrapper techniques are strongly prevalent among FS algorithms, primarily because of their exceptional performance in addressing this intricate challenge [41]. The wrapper approach involves representing the features using a vector of size Φ, where Φ corresponds to the total number of extracted features [42]. The wrapper strategies primarily generate a set of randomized solutions. During the feature subset assessment phase, a learning algorithm is used as a metric to evaluate the solution's efficacy. The wrapper methods undergo iterative processes to refine the obtained solutions until the specified end condition is reached [43]. Ultimately, the optimum feature subset, i.e. the subset that represents the best solution, is recognized.

In this study, we employ a selection of 14 recent FS methods, namely ant colony optimization (ACO), differential evolution (DE), the binary dragonfly algorithm (BDA), the binary equilibrium optimizer (BEO), the GA, GWO, Harris's hawk optimization (HHO), Henry gas solubility optimization (HGSO), PSO, atom search optimization (ASO), the salp swarm algorithm (SSA), the tree growth algorithm (TGA), the WOA, and the sine cosine algorithm (SCA). In order to provide an equitable comparison, our study employs identical parameters for each approach, namely a population size of ten and a maximum iteration limit of 100. The validation strategy involves the use of a classifier to quantify error rates. In addition, the tenfold CV method is used throughout the validation phase. Table 8.2 presents the parameter settings of the techniques used.

8.2.5 Classification

In the study reported here, we evaluated the effectiveness of eight different classification techniques for recognizing seizures in EEG signals. These algorithms were: decision tree (DT); random forest (RF); artificial intelligence, including a NN, a multilayer neural network (MNN), a feed-forward neural network (FFNN), a CFNN, a recurrent neural network (RNN), a generalized regression neural network (GRNN); the naive Bayes (NB) classifer, which makes use of kernel and normal probability distribution assumptions; k-NN, which uses eight distance metrics, including city block, Minkowski, cosine, Spearman, Euclidean, Hamming, Chebyshev, and Mahalanobis; and discriminant analysis (DA) with three assumptions, namely diagonal–linear, pseudo-linear, and pseudo-quadratic. The specific parameter configurations for these classifiers are detailed in table 8.3. The 'Neural

Table 8.2. Parameter settings of the FS techniques used.

Method	Parameter	Value
All	Population size	10
	Maximum iterations	100
	K-fold CV	10
ACO	Number of ants	10
	Coefficient control, tau	1
	Coefficient control, eta	0.1
	Initial tau	1
	Initial eta	1
	Pheromone	0.2
ASO	Number of atoms	10
	Depth weight	50
	Multiplier weight	0.2
Binary differential evolution (BDE)	Number of solutions	10
	Crossover rate	0.9
BDA	Number of dragonflies	10
BEO	Number of particles	10
	First constant parameter	2
	Second constant parameter	1
	Generation rate control parameter	0.5
GA	Number of chromosomes	10
	Crossover rate	0.8
	Mutation rates	0.3
GWO	Number of wolves	10
HHO	Number of hawks	10
HGSO	Number of gases	10
	Number of gas types	2
	Constant parameter K	1
	Influence of other gases	1
	Constant parameter beta	1
	First initial parameter	0.005
	Second initial parameter	100
	Second initial parameter	0.01
PSO	Number of particles	10
	Cognitive factor	2
	Social factor	2
	Inertia weight	1
SSA	Number of salps	10

SCA	Number of solutions	10
	Constant parameter alpha	2
TGA	Number of trees	10
	Number of trees in the first group	3
	Number of trees in the second group	5
	Number of trees in the fourth group	3
	Tree reduction rate	0.8
	Parameter controls nearest tree	0.5
WOA	Number of whales	10
	Constant parameter	1

Table 8.3. Parameter settings for the classification algorithms.

Method	Parameter	Value
DT	Number of splits	50
RF	Number of trees	20
NN, MNN, FFNN, CFNN, and RNN	Hidden layer size	10
	Maximum epochs allowed	50
GRNN	Spread of radial basis functions	1
NB	Probability distribution assumption	Kernel Normal
k-NN	Distance metric	City-block Minkowski Cosine Spearman Euclidean Hamming Chebyshev Mahalanobis
	Number of nearest neighbors (*k*-value)	5
DA	Data distribution assumption	Diagonal–linear Pseudo-quadratic
Ensemble tree (ET)	Data distribution assumption	Pseudo-linear Pseudo-quadratic
	Number of branches	50

Network Toolbox' is utilized here, with its default parameter settings (see https://github.com/JingweiToo/Neural-Network-Toolbox).

8.3 Results and discussion

In the study described in this chapter, we utilized two distinct databases, namely the Bonn database and the Indian database, to assess the EEG-seizure framework. The Bonn database results were used to identify the most effective FS and classification algorithms. Subsequently, the selected algorithms were applied to the Indian database. Figure 8.5 shows a block diagram of the EEG-seizure framework. Four distinct classification tasks are defined: S vs. SF, S vs. N, SF vs. N, and S vs. SF vs. N. Figure 8.1 displays examples of S, SF, and N EEG signals. We filtered the five brain rhythms, namely delta (0.5–4 Hz), theta (4–8 Hz), alpha (8–13 Hz), beta (13–30 Hz), and gamma (30–60 Hz and above) using an EWT filter bank that was specifically created for this purpose.

Figure 8.3 shows the filter bank designed to filter EEG signals using EWT, and figure 8.4 shows the five brain rhythms following filtering through the filter bank. After extracting the brain rhythms, we extracted 17 different features from each rhythm to represent the complexity of the EEG signals. This totals 85 features, i.e. the result of extracting 17 features from five rhythms (i.e. $17 \times 5 = 85$). All 85 features were found to have a p-value of less than 0.05, indicating their statistical significance and thus their suitability for feeding classifiers. It is essential to choose the best features before classification because this improves model performance and at the same time simplifies the model. There are 3.86×1025 ways to set up the feature vector with 85 features. At this point, it is clear that it is not easy to check the results for all of these cases, and it can even be challenging to do on a computer.

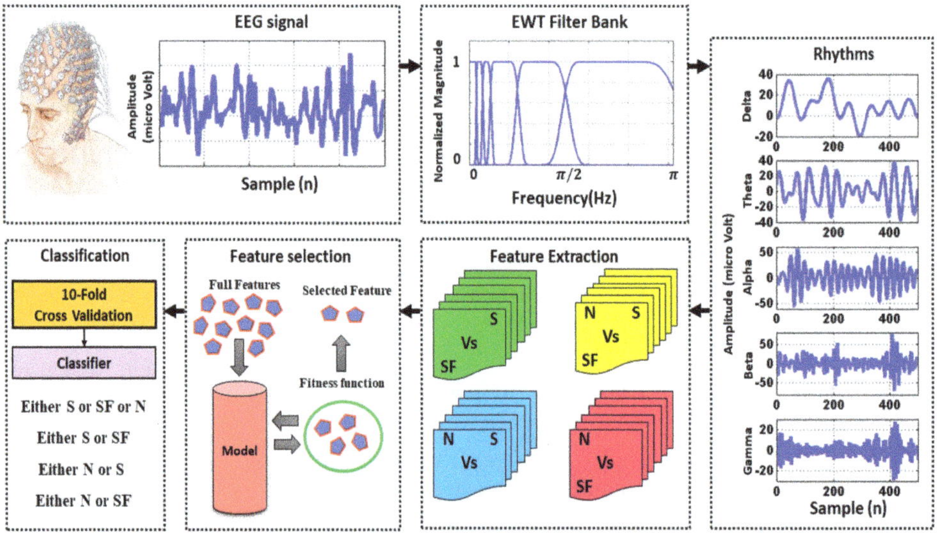

Figure 8.5. The EEG-seizure framework steps.

Because of this, scientists often use optimization algorithms to pick out the best features based on the goal of checking fewer trials.

A reliable classifier can significantly improve the ACC by identifying the hidden pattern inside the data. An effective classifier can learn from the feature space and, as a result, it can decide about new input test data. A classifier with a significant structure can decode the nonlinearity and complex links between features, which is important when processing a high-dimensional feature vector. Understanding the complex relationships inside the feature vector space allows the classifier to make a better decision, thereby improving the overall model ACC. In addition, the use of a perfect classification algorithm plays a key role in achieving higher ACC because it maximizes the use of valuable features inside the feature vector and effectively learns from the data, which also leads to a perfect and reliable prediction. For these reasons, we tested eight classifiers and 14 FS techniques to determine the best performers.

Table 8.4 reports the ACCs of different classifiers for defined classification tasks. The CFNN classifier achieved an average classification ACC of 99.75%, outperforming the other classifiers. This confirmed the CFNN classifier's strong ability to recognize EEGs. So, the CFNN classifier was chosen as the best classifier for the

Table 8.4. ACC results for the various classifiers.

Classifier	N vs. S	N vs. SF	S vs. SF	N vs. SF vs. N	Average
CFNN	100	99.5	100	99.5	99.75
DT	99	99.65	97	97.23	97.43
k-NN-Chebyshev	99.33	91	95.33	90.13	93.95
k-NN-Hamming	99.33	89.75	95.67	90.89	93.91
MNN	100	98	98.67	98.99	98.91
RF	99.33	98	97.33	97.97	98.16
DA-diagonal–linear	92.67	89	93	86.93	90.4
ET	99	98	98	98.74	98.43
k-NN-city-block	99.33	89.5	94.67	90.56	93.52
k-NN-Mahalanobis	99.33	90.25	95.33	91.39	94.08
NB-kernel	96.67	90.5	96.67	91.69	93.88
RNN	100	99.25	100	98	99.31
DA-pseudo-linear	100	98.5	98	98.5	98.75
FFNN	100	98.25	99.67	99	99.23
k-NN-cosine	99.33	90.75	95.33	90.38	93.95
k-NN-Minkowski	99.33	90.25	95	90.38	93.74
NB-normal	99.33	94.75	96.33	94.43	96.21
DA-pseudo-quadratic	99.67	97.5	97	97.7	97.97
GRNN	99.67	91.5	96.67	91.39	94.81
k-NN-Euclidean	99.33	91	95.33	90.89	94.14
k-NN-Spearman	99.33	90.5	95.33	91.39	94.14
NN	100	99.5	99.33	99.25	99.52

Table 8.5. ACC results for the various FS algorithms.

	ACC (%)/number of features used						
Task	ACO	ASO	BDA	BDE	BEO	GA	GWO
N vs. S	100/700	100/49	100/47	100/47	100/74	100/74	100/74
N vs. SF	100/56	100/47	100/55	100/72	100/28	100/46	100/55
S vs. SF	100/77	100/45	100/39	100/44	100/47	100/42	100/42
N vs. SF vs. N	99.8/81	99.6/45	99.8/51	99.8/77	99.8/33	99.6/42	100/55
Task	HGSO	HHO	PSO	SCA	SSA	TGA	WOA
N vs. S	100/47	100/47	100/47	100/47	100/47	100/47	100/44
N vs. SF	100/61	100/57	100/45	100/32	99.7/43	100/53	99.7/63
S vs. SF	100/45	100/48	100/42	100/50	100/47	100/42	100/44
N vs. SF vs. N	99.6/48	99.8/64	99.8/53	99.4/27	99.6/38	99.8/63	99.6/81

EEG recognition task. The resulting classification ACCs for the FS techniques are listed in table 8.5. In the classification task of N vs. S, all FS techniques demonstrated an outstanding classification ACC of 100%. Notably, the WOA score was achieved using 44 features, which was the lowest number of features, indicating its superior performance in this classification task. For the N vs. SF classification task, once again, all FS techniques except the WOA and SSA achieved an excellent classification ACC of 100%. However, the BEO achieved this ACC using only 28 features, which shows its effectiveness for this specific task. In the S vs. SF classification task, all FS techniques achieved a perfect classification ACC of 100%. Among them, the BDA achieved this ACC with 39 features, confirming its effectiveness for this classification. For the task of N vs. SF vs. N, where the classification involves three classes, all methods attained a remarkably high classification ACC of nearly 100%. GWO achieved 100% ACC using 55 features. This indicates the strength of GWO as a feature selector for this multiclassification task. The features selected by the best FS technique are listed for each classification task in table 8.6.

After the best classification and FS methods were selected for each classification task, the same structure was used for the Indian database. We achieved a perfect classification ACC of 100% for the N vs. S, N vs. SF, S vs. SF, and N vs. SF vs. S tasks by feeding selected features from the WOA, the BEO, the BDA, and GWO into the CFNN classifier. Table 8.7 lists previous studies that performed seizure classification using the Bonn and Indian databases. The performance of our proposed approach is higher than those of previous studies.

The most important results of this research are:

- We introduced EEG-seizure, an efficient technique for classifying epileptic seizures. This is the first comprehensive analysis of FS and classification

Table 8.6. Features of each rhythm selected for classification tasks.

Rhythm	N vs. S	N vs. SF	S vs. SF	N vs. SF vs. S
Delta	2, 4, 7, 8, 10, 11, 12, 14	2, 5, 7, 9, 10, 17	1, 2, 5, 10, 11, 15, 16	1, 4, 5, 6, 8, 9, 10, 12, 13, 14, 15, 17
Theta	1, 3, 7, 8, 9, 10, 11, 12, 15, 16	4, 6, 7, 8, 14, 16	2, 3, 4, 7, 11, 12, 13	2, 3, 5, 6, 9, 10, 12, 13, 14, 16
Alpha	4, 5, 7, 10, 11, 12, 13, 15, 16	1, 3, 5, 7, 11, 13	2, 3, 4, 5, 6, 7, 8, 9, 15, 16	1, 3, 5, 7, 8, 10, 11, 13, 14, 16
Beta	1, 3, 4, 5, 6, 7, 8, 9, 10, 14	1, 5, 7, 8	2, 7, 8, 10, 11, 13, 17	1, 3, 4, 6, 7, 9, 11, 12, 14, 15, 16, 17
Gamma	1, 2, 3, 6, 10, 11, 12	5, 8, 11, 14, 15, 16	2, 3, 4, 9, 11, 14, 16	1, 2, 3, 7, 9, 10, 11, 12, 14, 15, 16

techniques for identifying seizures in EEGs. According to our findings, for the N vs. S, N vs. SF, S vs. SF, and N vs. SF vs. S classification tasks, the WOA, BEO, BDA, and GWO algorithms outperform the others, respectively. In addition, the CFNN exhibits superior performance across all classification tasks.

- In contrast to earlier studies that used discrete wavelet transform (DWT), which requires multiple decomposition levels to separate EEG signal rhythms, EWT separated the EEG signal rhythms in a single step.
- Our EEG-seizure system demonstrates the significance of focusing on the five primary brain rhythms instead of filtering the EEGs into multiple sub-bands.
- The suggested approach achieves a perfect 100% ACC in its classifications.

Although the classification performance of the proposed framework was perfect in the defined classification tasks, the main limitation of the current study is the number of subjects in the database. Another point is that the performance of the proposed framework was not tested by adding noise to the EEG signals, whereas in [39], the performance of the method was evaluated by adding noise to the EEG signals. In addition, we decomposed the EEG signal using brain rhythms, which means that the adaptivity property of EWT was ignored. In contrast, [6] preserved the adaptivity property of the TQWT method while simultaneously optimizing the number of decomposition levels. In the future, we will work to optimize the number of sub-bands in EWT instead of using it to extract brain rhythms.

- Unlike most previous research, which only used a single database (i.e. the Bonn database), we evaluated our system utilizing two different databases.
- We simplified the procedure by filtering out frequencies over 60 Hz, while previous methods often needed a preprocessing step to eliminate noise from EEG data. To achieve this, we used EEG signal analysis inside the EWT domain.

Table 8.7. A brief overview of previous studies compared with the EEG-seizure framework.

Reference	Database	Task	ACC
[12]	Bonn	N vs. SF	92.50
Ours	Bonn	N vs. SF	100
Ours	Indian	N vs. SF	100
[15]	Bonn	N vs. S	88.83
[16]	Bonn	N vs. S	98
[17]	Bonn	N vs. S	97.69
[12]	Bonn	N vs. S	100
[9]	Bonn	N vs. S	99.18
[5]	Bonn	N vs. S	99.33
[5]	Indian	N vs. S	96.33
Ours	Bonn	N vs. S	100
Ours	Indian	N vs. S	100
[15]	Bonn	SF vs. S	83.13
[16]	Bonn	SF vs. S	93
[17]	Bonn	SF vs. S	93.91
[18]	Bonn	SF vs. S	94
[19]	Bonn	SF vs. S	95.33
[44]	Bonn	SF vs. S	97
[20]	Bonn	SF vs. S	97.75
[21]	Bonn	SF vs. S	98.67
[39]	Bonn	SF vs. S	99.13
[12]	Bonn	SF vs. S	98.67
[45]	Bonn	SF vs. S	97
[9]	Bonn	SF vs. S	95.15
[23]	Bonn	SF vs. S	98.33
[25]	Bonn	SF vs. S	99
[5]	Bonn	SF vs. S	98.33
[5]	Indian	SF vs. S	99.20
Ours	Bonn	SF vs. S	100
Ours	Indian	SF vs. S	100
[12]	Bonn	N vs. SF vs. S	99.20
[46]	Bonn	N vs. SF vs. S	97.73
[47]	Bonn	N vs. SF vs. S	97.77
[48]	Bonn	N vs. SF vs. S	96.60
[31]	Bonn	N vs. SF vs. S	95.44
[15]	Bonn	N vs. SF vs. S	86.10
[49]	Bonn	N vs. SF vs. S	98.10
[50]	Bonn	N vs. SF vs. S	99.15
[9]	Bonn	N vs. SF vs. S	95.24
Ours	Bonn	N vs. SF vs. S	100
Ours	Indian	N vs. SF vs. S	100

8.4 Conclusions

The detection of epilepsy seizures by monitoring EEG recordings for a long time is one of the oldest challenges for physicians and has always been prone to human error. In this chapter, we proposed the EEG-seizure framework, an automatic computer-based system that uses the linear and nonlinear features of rhythms in EEG signals to categorize them in a seizure detection application. In the initial step of the EEG-seizure framework, the EEGs were decomposed into rhythms by an EWT filter bank. We then computed 17 features from five rhythms and made a feature vector with 85 arrays. After that, we selected the best features to improve the efficiency of the system. Finally, we fed the most relevant selected features into the classifier. We defined four different classification tasks for the EEG-seizure system, namely S vs. SF, S vs. N, SF vs. N, and S vs. SF vs. N. The EEG-seizure framework was assessed using the Bonn database and the Indian seizure database, utilizing tenfold CV to avoid the bias effect in reporting the results. We tested fourteen FS and eight classification algorithms to design the most effective framework. In all classification tests, the CFNN classifier performed best. We showed that for N vs. S, N vs. SF, S vs. SF, and N vs. SF vs. S tasks, the WOA, BEO, BDA, and GWO algorithms were better than the others, respectively. For all four classification tasks, the EEG-seizure system achieved an excellent classification ACC of 100%. The proposed EEG-seizure system can be used as automatic software in hospitals and clinics to identify seizure disorders. In the future, the EEG-seizure system will be assessed for the diagnosis of a variety of mental disorders, including Alzheimer's disease, Parkinson's disease, stress, and depression.

References

[1] World Health Organization (WHO) 2022 Epilepsy https://www.who.int/health-topics/epilepsy#tab=tab_1

[2] Akbari H, Sadiq M T, Jafari N, Jingwei T, Mikaeilvand N, Cicone A and Serra-Capizzano S 2023 Recognizing seizure using Poincaré plot of EEG signals and graphical features in DWT domain *Bratisl. Med. J.* **124** 12–24

[3] Sadiq M T, Akbari H, Siuly S, Li Y and Wen P 2022 Fractional fourier transform aided computerized framework for alcoholism identification in EEG *Int. Conf. on Health Information Science* (Berlin: Springer) pp 100–12

[4] Khare S K, Blanes-Vidal V, Nadimi E S and Acharya U R 2023 Emotion recognition and artificial intelligence: a systematic review (2014–2023) and research recommendations *Inf. Fusion* **102** 102019

[5] Sadiq M T, Akbari H, Siuly S, Yousaf A and Rehman A U 2021 A novel computer-aided diagnosis framework for EEG-based identification of neural diseases *Comput. Biol. Med.* **138** 104922

[6] Khare S K, Gadre V M and Acharya R 2023 ECGPsychnet: an optimized hybrid ensemble model for automatic detection of psychiatric disorders using ECG signals *Physiol. Meas.* **44** 115004

[7] Sadiq M T, Akbari H, Rehman A U, Nishtar Z, Masood B, Ghazvini M, Too J, Hamedi N and Kaabar M K 2021 Exploiting feature selection and neural network techniques for

identification of focal and nonfocal EEG signals in TQWT domain *J. Healthc. Eng.* **2021** 6283900

[8] Khare S K and Acharya U R 2023 ADAZD-Net: automated adaptive and explainable Alzheimer's disease detection system using EEG signals *Knowl.-Based Syst.* **278** 110858

[9] Swami P, Gandhi T K, Panigrahi B K, Tripathi M and Anand S 2016 A novel robust diagnostic model to detect seizures in electroencephalography *Expert Syst. Appl.* **56** 116–30

[10] Sharma M and Pachori R B 2017 A novel approach to detect epileptic seizures using a combination of tunable-Q wavelet transform and fractal dimension *J. Mech. Med. Biol.* **17** 1740003

[11] Sharma M, Dhere A, Pachori R B and Acharya U R 2017 An automatic detection of focal EEG signals using new class of time–frequency localized orthogonal wavelet filter banks *Knowl.-Based Syst.* **118** 217–27

[12] Sharma M, Pachori R B and Acharya U R 2017 A new approach to characterize epileptic seizures using analytic time-frequency flexible wavelet transform and fractal dimension *Pattern Recognit. Lett.* **94** 172–9

[13] Yadav V P and Sharma K K 2023 Variational mode decomposition and binary grey wolf optimization-based automated epilepsy seizure classification framework *Biomed. Eng.* **68** 147–63

[14] Khare S K, Gaikwad N B and Bajaj V 2022 VHERS: a novel variational mode decomposition and Hilbert transform-based EEG rhythm separation for automatic ADHD detection *IEEE Trans. Instrum. Meas.* **71** 1–10

[15] Nicolaou N and Georgiou J 2012 Detection of epileptic electroencephalogram based on permutation entropy and support vector machines *Expert Syst. Appl.* **39** 202–9

[16] Zhu G, Li Y and Wen P P 2014 Epileptic seizure detection in EEGs signals using a fast weighted horizontal visibility algorithm *Comput. Methods Programs Biomed.* **115** 64–75

[17] Li Y, Wen P P *et al* 2011 Clustering technique-based least square support vector machine for EEG signal classification *Comput. Methods Programs Biomed.* **104** 358–72

[18] Altunay S, Telatar Z and Erogul O 2010 Epileptic EEG detection using the linear prediction error energy *Expert Syst. Appl.* **37** 5661–5

[19] Joshi V, Pachori R B and Vijesh A 2014 Classification of ictal and seizure-free EEG signals using fractional linear prediction *Biomed. Signal Process. Control* **9** 1–5

[20] Pachori R B and Patidar S 2014 Epileptic seizure classification in EEG signals using second-order difference plot of intrinsic mode functions *Comput. Methods Programs Biomed.* **113** 494–502

[21] Sharma R and Pachori R B 2015 Classification of epileptic seizures in EEG signals based on phase space representation of intrinsic mode functions *Expert Syst. Appl.* **42** 1106–17

[22] Khare S K, Bajaj V and Sinha G 2020 Automatic drowsiness detection based on variational non-linear chirp mode decomposition using electroencephalogram signals *Modelling and Analysis of Active Biopotential Signals in Healthcare, Volume 1* (Bristol: IOP Publishing) p 5–1

[23] Akbari H, Saraf Esmaili S and Farzollah Zadeh S 2020 Detection of seizure EEG signals based on reconstructed phase space of rhythms in EWT domain and genetic algorithm *Signal Process. Renew. Energy* **4** 23–36

[24] Sharma S, Khare S K, Bajaj V and Ansari I A 2021 Improving the separability of drowsiness and alert EEG signals using analytic form of wavelet transform *Appl. Acoust.* **181** 108164

[25] Akbari H and Esmaili S 2020 A novel geometrical method for discrimination of normal, interictal and ictal EEG signals *Trait. Signal* **37** 59–68

[26] Akbari H and Ghofrani S 2019 Fast and accurate classification of F and NF EEG by using SODP and EWT *Int. J. Image Graph. Signal Process.* **11** 29–35
[27] Sadiq M T, Akbari H, Siuly S, Li Y and Wen P 2022 Alcoholic EEG signals recognition based on phase space dynamic and geometrical features *Chaos Solit. Fractals* **158** 112036
[28] Akbari H, Ghofrani S, Zakalvand P and Sadiq M T 2021 Schizophrenia recognition based on the phase space dynamic of EEG signals and graphical features *Biomed. Signal Process. Control* **69** 102917
[29] Khare S K, March S, Barua P D, Gadre V M and Acharya U R 2023 Application of data fusion for automated detection of children with developmental and mental disorders: a systematic review of the last decade *Inf. Fusion* **99** 101898
[30] Andrzejak R G, Lehnertz K, Mormann F, Rieke C, David P and Elger C E 2001 Indications of nonlinear deterministic and finite-dimensional structures in time series of brain electrical activity: dependence on recording region and brain state *Phys. Rev.* E **64** 061907
[31] Gandhi T, Panigrahi B K and Anand S 2011 A comparative study of wavelet families for EEG signal classification *Neurocomputing* **74** 3051–7
[32] Gandhi T K, Chakraborty P, Roy G G and Panigrahi B K 2012 Discrete harmony search based expert model for epileptic seizure detection in electroencephalography *Expert Syst. Appl.* **39** 4055–62
[33] Gandhi T, Panigrahi B K, Bhatia M and Anand S 2010 Expert model for detection of epileptic activity in EEG signature *Expert Syst. Appl.* **37** 3513–20
[34] Gilles J 2013 Empirical wavelet transform *IEEE Trans. Signal Process.* **61** 3999–4010
[35] Akbari H and Sadiq M T 2021 Detection of focal and non-focal EEG signals using non-linear features derived from empirical wavelet transform rhythms *Phys. Eng. Sci. Med.* **44** 157–71
[36] Gilles J 2020 Continuous empirical wavelets systems *Adv. Data Sci. Adapt. Anal.* **12** 2050006
[37] Daubechies I 1992 *Ten Lectures on Wavelets* (CBMS-NSF Regional Conf. Series in Applied Mathematics vol 61) (Philadelphia, PA: Society for Industrial and Applied Mathematics)
[38] Khare S K, Bajaj V and Acharya U R 2023 SchizoNet: a robust and accurate Margenau–Hill time-frequency distribution based deep neural network model for schizophrenia detection using EEG signals *Physiol. Meas.* **44** 035005
[39] Krishnaprasanna R, Baskar V V and Panneerselvam J 2021 Automatic identification of epileptic seizures using volume of phase space representation *Phys. Eng. Sci. Med.* **44** 545–56
[40] Korani W and Mouhoub M 2021 Review on nature-inspired algorithms *SN Oper. Res. Forum* **2** 36
[41] Too J, Abdullah A R and Saad N M 2019 Binary competitive swarm optimizer approaches for feature selection *Computation* **7** 31
[42] Too J, Sadiq A S and Mirjalili S M 2022 A conditional opposition-based particle swarm optimisation for feature selection *Connect. Sci.* **34** 339–61
[43] Korani W and Mouhoub M 2022 Discrete mother tree optimization and swarm intelligence for constraint satisfaction problems *14th International Conference on Agents and Artificial Intelligence, ICAART* (Setúbal: Science and Technology Publications) pp 234–41
[44] Bao F S, Lie D Y-C and Zhang Y 2008 A new approach to automated epileptic diagnosis using EEG and probabilistic neural network *20th IEEE Int. Conf. on Tools with Artificial Intelligence 2* (Piscataway, NJ: IEEE) pp 482–6
[45] Kaya Y, Uyar M, Tekin R and Yıldırım S 2014 1D-local binary pattern based feature extraction for classification of epileptic EEG signals *Appl. Math. Comput.* **243** 209–19

[46] Tzallas A T, Tsipouras M G, Fotiadis D I *et al* 2007 Automatic seizure detection based on time-frequency analysis and artificial neural networks *Comput. Intell. Neurosci.* **2007** 080510
[47] Guo L, Rivero D, Dorado J, Rabuñal J R and Pazos A 2010 Automatic epileptic seizure detection in EEGs based on line length feature and artificial neural networks *J. Neurosci. Methods* **191** 101–9
[48] Orhan U, Hekim M and Ozer M 2011 EEG signals classification using the k-means clustering and a multilayer perceptron neural network model *Expert Syst. Appl.* **38** 13475–81
[49] Samiee K, Kovács P and Gabbouj M 2014 Epileptic seizure classification of EEG time-series using rational discrete short-time Fourier transform *IEEE Trans. Biomed. Eng.* **62** 541–52
[50] Peker M, Sen B and Delen D 2015 A novel method for automated diagnosis of epilepsy using complex-valued classifiers *IEEE J. Biomed. Health Inform.* **20** 108–18

Chapter 9

Prediction of rhythm-based abnormalities in electrocardiograms using time–frequency representations

Sandeep Kumar Singh, Anirvina Sharma, Sunil Athawale, Annapureddy Srija Reddy, Ashwin Kamble and Ankush Jamthikar

Cardiovascular disease (CVD) ranks as a leading cause of death and illness globally, claiming over 17.7 million lives annually. A key strategy in preventing CVD is early screening. However, the high costs associated with healthcare often make imaging technologies a less favored option for initial screening. Instead, physiological signals such as the electrocardiogram (ECG) are preferred for this purpose. ECGs record the heart's electrical activity and reveal patterns pertinent to its conduction system. Traditional methods of screening involve analyzing ECG signals using their graphical representations, but this often results in variability among interpreters. In this chapter, we explore the fundamental principles of ECGs, the heart's conduction system, and traditional interpretation techniques. In addition, we introduce the use of time–frequency representations (TFRs), which provide both temporal and spectral insights into ECG signals. These representations facilitate the use of machine learning techniques to distinguish cardiac abnormalities.

9.1 Introduction

Heart diseases were documented as far back as ancient Egypt, well before the advancements of modern medicine were available to aid civilization [1]. Despite contemporary advancements in cardiac care, heart disease remains one of the primary causes of mortality in the United States. The Journal of the American College of Cardiology reported that in 2022, age-standardized mortality rates for cardiovascular disease (CVD) varied widely, ranging from 73.6 and 432.3 per 100 000 in the high-income Asia Pacific and Eastern Europe, respectively [2]. This underscores the vital importance of the early diagnosis and treatment of heart conditions.

doi:10.1088/978-0-7503-5964-1ch9

The electrocardiogram (ECG) stands as a cornerstone in the arsenal of modern medical diagnostics. Originating with the invention of the electrocardiograph by Dutch physiologist Willem Einthoven in 1902, this breakthrough marked the beginning of an era where technological instruments and methods began to supplement, and often surpass, traditional sensory-based diagnostics and the use of the stethoscope [3]. Today, the 12-lead ECG is the most administered cardiovascular test, with an estimated 200 million ECGs performed globally each year. The ECG plays a crucial role in the clinical assessment and management of numerous CVDs, including acute myocardial infarction, suspected chronic cardiac ischemia, arrhythmias, heart failure, and conditions requiring implantable cardiac devices [4]. The ECG's simplicity, noninvasiveness, speed, and cost-effectiveness contribute to its extensive utility and profound impact on diagnostic medicine. Despite its routine and straightforward acquisition, the interpretation of ECGs requires a depth of expertise that some suggest is becoming rare. Even in an era of computerized ECG analysis, the critical need for skilled clinician review in the diagnostic process remains recognized and valued across healthcare settings [5].

Recently, there has been a notable surge in interest in integrating artificial intelligence (AI) and machine learning (ML) into the realm of ECG interpretation for enhanced accuracy [6–8]. AI involves the use of machine-based data processing to achieve tasks typically requiring human cognitive functions [9]. The overarching aim of AI is to create systems that can emulate human cognitive abilities such as perception, reasoning, learning, planning, and prediction. The development of AI encompasses several layers, including perceptual intelligence, cognitive intelligence, and decision-making intelligence, all underpinned by a robust infrastructure supported by data, storage capacity, computing power, ML algorithms, and AI frameworks [10]. This infrastructure facilitates the training of models that learn from data, thereby advancing AI applications. ML can be categorized into two main types: 'supervised' or 'unsupervised,' depending on the nature of the learning process [11]. This technological progress opens up new avenues for automating and refining ECG analysis, potentially transforming diagnostic practice.

In the context of AI and its application to data interpretation, particularly in ML, the data must be organized into structured feature vectors. A 'feature' is a quantifiable attribute of the input data, which is compiled into a feature vector to mathematically represent the data in a form suitable for computational analysis. In the realm of supervised ML, the training phase involves providing the ML algorithm with a data set that includes both the input features and the corresponding labels (or outputs). During this phase, the algorithm learns to discern patterns by mapping the relationships between the features and the labels, a process known as 'training.' After the model has been adequately trained, it transitions to the 'testing' phase, where it applies what it has learned to make predictions about new, unseen data [9]. This dual-phase process is critical for developing ML models that can effectively interpret and predict based on the data they are fed.

One of the principal challenges in developing these ML models is the scarcity of labeled training data. To address this, various innovative models and techniques have been proposed to enhance the preprocessing, processing, and interpretation of ECG data. Notable among these is the use of contrastive learning through patient contrastive learning of representations (PCLR) [7], which leverages patient-specific data to improve learning accuracy. In addition, self-supervised learning models such as the SimCG-L + vector cardiogram (VCG) + time mask model, referred to as '3KG' [8], help machines learn useful representations without requiring extensive labeled data. Contrastive predictive coding [12] is another method employed to learn high-quality feature representations by predicting the future in latent space. Techniques such as the two-event related moving averages (TERMA) algorithm and the fractional Fourier transform (FrFT) [13] have also been utilized to process and interpret ECG signals more effectively, further showcasing the breadth of approaches being explored to overcome the challenge of limited data labels.

The use of TFRs of ECG signals is a crucial analytical technique in signal processing that provides insights into how the spectral content of an ECG signal evolves over time [14, 15]. This method combines time-domain and frequency-domain information to produce a comprehensive view of the signal's dynamic behavior. Such representations are particularly valuable for analyzing nonstationary signals such as ECGs, for which traditional Fourier transform methods may not capture transient features effectively. Techniques such as the short-time Fourier transform (STFT) and wavelet transforms are commonly used for this purpose. STFT offers a compromise between time and frequency resolution by applying a moving window to the signal, while wavelet transforms provide variable resolution in different frequency bands, making them ideal for detecting transient components and subtle anomalies in ECG signals. These time–frequency methods enhance the detection and characterization of complex cardiovascular conditions, improving diagnostic accuracy and patient outcomes.

The objective of this chapter is to provide a brief overview of several ECG analysis stages. We start by understanding the conduction system, ECG interpretations, and processing, and then we discuss the concept of TFRs for ECG analysis. We also aim to provide a preliminary analysis that utilizes the TFR methods to transform ECG signals into images, which are then used to predict cardiac rhythm-based abnormalities such as atrial fibrillation (AF).

9.2 Physiology and the basics of the ECG

To precisely diagnose abnormalities in an ECG, it is crucial to possess a comprehensive understanding of the characteristics of a normal ECG. Such knowledge provides a fundamental reference point, enabling the detection of anomalies that might indicate cardiac conditions. A concise overview of the heart's structure and functions, its electrical conduction system, and the fundamental principles of ECG interpretation is essential to support this diagnostic process.

9.2.1 Anatomy and physiology

The human heart comprises four hollow chambers encased in muscle and other cardiac tissues. These chambers are segregated by valves that ensure blood flows in the correct direction. The two upper (atria) and two lower chambers (ventricles) receive and pump blood, respectively. The right and left sides of the heart are bifurcated by a tissue wall called the septum, and the functioning of each side is somewhat independent. The heart's electrical system regulates the heartbeat's rate and rhythm [16].

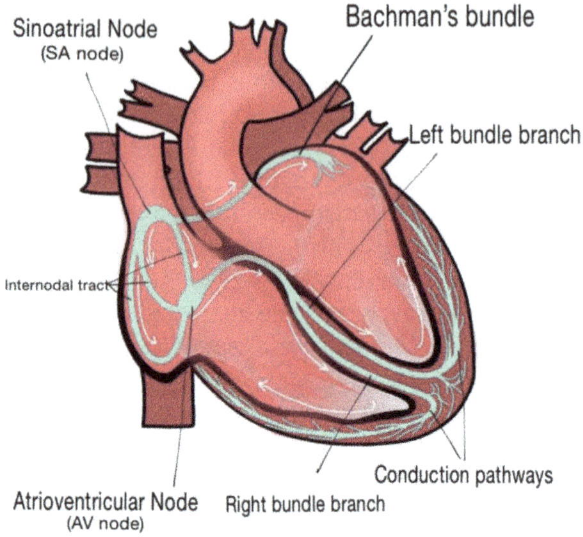

Figure 9.1. Conduction pathway of the heart.

In understanding the cardiac cycle, it is crucial to recognize the sequence of events. The atria contract first, followed by the ventricles. This sequence ensures functional separation of the right and left sides of the heart into two distinct circuits. The cardiac cycle is divided into two phases: diastole and systole. During diastole, the ventricles are filled with blood. In contrast, during systole, the ventricles contract and pump blood out. These phases occur in both sides of the heart [17].

A pulse is electrically triggered by the sinus or sinoatrial (SA) node of the heart muscle located in the right upper chamber, as shown in figure 9.1. The triggered electrical impulses travel through the conduction pathways, causing the atria to contract first and push blood into the ventricles. The signal then reaches the AV node, where it briefly slows down, allowing the atria to finish contracting before the ventricles begin. Thereafter, it passes through the bundle of His, which splits into right and left bundle branches, stimulating the ventricles to contract and pump blood into the body's blood vessels [18].

9.2.2 Basics of the ECG and its interpretation

An ECG captures the electrical activity occurring within the heart. Normally, the electrical pulse is initiated at the SA node. It then moves across the atrium towards the atrioventricular (AV) node, and then passes through the ventricular septum. This impulse prompts the heart's four chambers to contract and relax in a synchronized manner, which is crucial for effective heart function. Analyzing these electrical impulses provides insights into the heart's operational status [19].

The characteristics of a normal ECG are methodically outlined in table 9.1 to facilitate comprehension. This table delineates each component of the ECG, such as the P wave, QRS complex, and T wave, including their typical durations and

Table 9.1. Components of ECG and their characteristics [19, 20].

	Component of ECG	Cardiac cycle representation	Corresponds to	Normal features in ECG	Lead variations
1	P wave	Denotes depolarization of both atria	Atrial contraction	Smooth, rounded, 2.5 mm tall, 0.11 s in duration	Positive in leads I, II, aVF, and V1-V6
2	QRS complex	Ventricular depolarization	Ventricular contraction	Three waves in rapid succession. The Q wave is always negative. The R wave is the first positive deflection in the QRS complex. Duration: 0.06–0.10 s	Typically positive in leads I, II, III, aVL, aVF, V5, V6. Typically negative in leads aVR, V1, V2
3	ST segment	Period of zero potential between ventricular depolarisation and repolarization	Nil	Flat—negligible negative or positive amplitude	Similar in all leads
4	T wave	Ventricular repolarization	Ventricular relaxation	Slightly asymmetric; the peak of the wave is closer to its end	Usually positive in leads I, II, V2-V6. Usually negative in aVR. The T wave generally follows the same direction as the QRS complex that precedes it
5	U wave	Unknown	Unknown	Very small deflection between the T wave and the next P wave	Same as the T wave

features. This structured information aids in the interpretation and recognition of standard ECG patterns.

Traditional ECG analysis involves a detailed, manual review of the ECG trace by a trained medical professional. This method depends heavily on the practitioner's expertise, which is developed through extensive medical training and characterized by a precise ability for visual interpretation. However, the reliability of this approach can be influenced by several factors, such as ECG machine malfunctions, incorrect placement of electrodes, the presence of artifacts, and external noise from other equipment. Despite these potential complications, manual ECG analysis remains a fundamental practice in cardiac diagnostics.

Let us delve into the traditional systematic method of ECG interpretation, which offers a structured approach to analyzing ECGs. This method ensures comprehensive evaluation of all critical elements of heart function for accurate interpretation. In this process, the electrocardiograph operates at a standard speed of 25 mm per second.

Each second in the time (x-) axis is divided into five large squares of 0.2 s each. Each of these large squares is subdivided into five smaller squares of 0.04 s each. This detailed scaling allows clinicians to measure the timing of various cardiac events precisely, facilitating a thorough and systematic analysis of the electrical activity of the heart [21, 22], as we can see in figure 9.2.

(1) Standardization: the initial step in ECG interpretation involves confirming the calibration of the ECG. Check for a rectangle, often found at the beginning or the end of the ECG trace, which forms a 90° angle. This rectangle serves as a reference to verify that the ECG is standardized

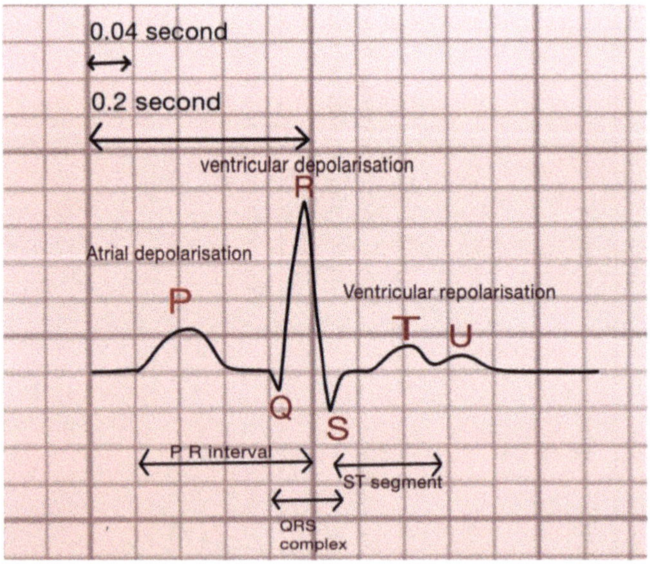

Figure 9.2. Components of an ECG trace.

correctly. The standard calibration should measure 10 mm per mV in height, and the paper speed should be set to 25 mm per second. Ensuring these parameters are accurately set is crucial for the correct interpretation of the ECG.

(2) Rhythm: once the ECG is confirmed to be calibrated, the next step is to assess the rhythm. Determine whether the heart rhythm is regular or irregular by examining the RR intervals. Regular rhythms show RR intervals that are consistently equidistant, whereas irregular rhythms display RR intervals that vary. Accurately identifying the rhythm type is fundamental in diagnosing potential cardiac abnormalities.

(3) Rate: following the assessment of rhythm, the next crucial step is to calculate the heart rate. Since an ECG graphically represents cardiac signals over time, the heart rate can be determined using the RR intervals. Typically, for adults, a normal heart rate lies within the range of 50 to 100 beats per minute [23]. Correspondingly, a normal RR interval should fall between 0.6 and 1.2 s. An RR interval shorter than 0.6 s indicates tachycardia, suggesting a faster-than-normal heart rate. Conversely, an RR interval exceeding 1.2 s is indicative of bradycardia, reflecting a slower-than-normal heart rate. Accurately calculating the heart rate is essential for diagnosing and managing various cardiac conditions.

(4) PR interval: after determining the heart rate, the next focus should be on the PR interval. This interval reflects the time taken for the electrical impulse to travel from the atria to the ventricles. It is crucial to assess whether the PR interval is normal or prolonged; and whether it remains consistent throughout the ECG. A normal PR interval typically measures less than 200 milliseconds [24]. Consistency in the PR interval across the ECG is important, as variations can indicate underlying cardiac abnormalities such as first-degree heart block.

(5) QRS interval analysis is an essential step in ECG interpretation, focusing on ventricular contractility and the cardiac axis. A normal QRS complex typically measures between 0.10 and 0.11 s, indicating efficient ventricular depolarization [21]. A wider complex may suggest a conduction delay or other ventricular abnormalities. The cardiac axis is determined by examining the QRS complexes in leads I and aVF. A normal cardiac axis shows positive QRS complexes in both leads. Deviations are categorized as follows: left axis deviation is indicated by a positive QRS in lead I and a negative QRS in lead aVF, representing an axis between 0° and −90°. The right axis ranges from + 90° to + 180° featuring a negative QRS in lead I and positive in lead aVF. An extreme axis deviation, or indeterminate axis, occurs when both QRS complexes are negative in leads I and aVF, ranging from −90° to 180° [22]. Analyzing the QRS interval provides critical insights into ventricular function and overall heart orientation.

(6) ST segment: after evaluating the QRS interval, attention shifts to the ST segment, which is an isoelectric line that ideally aligns with the PR interval on the ECG. It is crucial to assess the ST segment because any elevation or

depression of this segment by 1 mm or more, particularly measured at the *J* point, is considered abnormal [22]. Changes in the ST segment are significant as they can indicate acute myocardial ischemia or other forms of cardiac stress. Careful examination of this segment helps in detecting and diagnosing potentially serious conditions early, facilitating timely intervention.

(7) T wave—typically, the T wave has a height less than 10 mm. Besides, its size is approximately one-eighth or less than two-thirds of that of the R wave [22].

(8) Additional information—finally, we should look at the ECG as a whole and look for any additional waves or any abnormal deviation from a normal ECG [21].

The significance of ECGs in medical diagnostics is well-established, yet interpreting them remains challenging. One key issue is the dependence on visual analysis, which can vary significantly in accuracy. Cook *et al* [25] examined the accuracy of ECG interpretations by physicians in controlled environments, analyzing 78 studies. Their findings revealed a broad range of accuracy, from as low as 4% to as high as 95%. The median accuracy was notably modest at 54%, though it generally improved with advanced training and specialization. Traditional ECG interpretation methods enable various cardiac diseases to be classified by identifying specific abnormalities in ECG components. Some common cardiac conditions that can be diagnosed through careful ECG analysis are tabulated in table 9.2.

Table 9.2. Abnormal ECG findings and their characteristics.

	Type	Abnormality	Abnormal ECG findings [26]
1	Conduction abnormalities	First-degree AV block	PR interval > 200 milliseconds, rhythm is always regular.
		Second-degree AV block	Mobitz type I: progressive lengthening of PR interval along with decreasing RR interval. A pause typically less than twice the duration of the immediately preceding RR interval. Mobitz type II: some intermittent P waves are not followed by a QRS complex, with no changes in the preceding PR or RR interval.
		Third-degree AV block	There is no consistent relationship between the P wave and the QRS complex; not every P wave is followed by a QRS complex.

		Right bundle branch block (RBBB)	QRS duration > 120 ms, RSR pattern seen in V1-V3 (M-shaped QRS complex). A broad, slurred S wave in leads I/aVL/V5/V6.
		Left bundle branch block (LBBB)	QRS duration > 120 ms, dominant S wave seen in V1, a broad notched M-shaped R wave seen in I/aVL/V5/V6 leads.
2	Rhythm abnormalities	Sinus rhythms	
		Sinus arrhythmia	Variation seen in PP interval > 120 ms, PP interval gradually increases and decreases in cyclical manner, P wave is normal and sinus in nature, constant PR interval.
		Sinus bradycardia	RR interval of more than 1.2 s in adults, U wave appears prominent in V1-V6.
		Sinus tachycardia	RR interval of less than 0.6 s in adults, P waves are concealed in T waves (camel hump appearance).
		Ventricular rhythm	
		Junctional escape	Narrow QRS < 120 ms, no relation between QRS and atrial activity (which could be either P wave, or atrial flutter, or atrial fibrillatory waves).
		Ventricular escape	Broad QRS > 120 ms, either LBBB or RBBB may be present, heart rate is generally between 20–40 beats per minute, with absence or scarcity of P waves.
		Accelerated idioventricular rhythms	Rate is seen between 60–120 beats, three or more ventricular complexes are seen after the P wave, QRS > 120 ms, presence of fusion and capture beats.
3	Tachycardia	Supraventricular tachycardia	
		Atrial tachycardia	Atrial rate > 100 beats per minute, P morphology and cardiac axis deviates from the normal, baseline is isoelectric, QRS complexes are normal in nature.
		Atrial flutter	Narrow QRS complex, rate of P waves is usually > 300 min^{-1}, isoelectric baseline is lost, saw-tooth pattern present in leads II, III, aVF, rate of QRS complex is < 150 min^{-1}.

(Continued)

Table 9.2. (*Continued*)

	Type	Abnormality	Abnormal ECG findings [26]
		Ventricular tachycardia	Very broad QRS complex which is > 160 ms, rate is regular, notching is present near the nadir of the S wave, RS interval > 100 ms.
4	Fibrillation	AF	Irregularly irregular rhythm is a classic finding, P waves are absent, isoelectric baseline is lost, QRS rate is variable, fibrillation waves present which are either fine (< 0.5 mm in amplitude) or coarse (> 0.5 mm in amplitude) in nature, fibrillation waves may mimic P waves.
		Ventricular fibrillation	Disorganized irregular deflections, no identifiable P wave, QRS complex, or R wave is seen, the rate varies between 150–500 min^{-1}, amplitude decreases with duration.
5	Device	Pacemaker	Vertical spikes of short duration, usually 2 mm, called pacing spikes are seen. The location depends on the type of pacemaker.
6	Myocardial	Myocardial ischemia	ST segment is usually downsloping or seen as a flat depression > 0.2 mm.
		Myocardial infarction	ST segment is elevated from the baseline, lead variation is seen depending on the location of infarct (anterior wall MI: V2-V5, septal MI: V1-V2, anteroseptal MI: V1-V4, anterolateral MI: V3-V6 + I + aVL).
7	Pericardial disease	Pericarditis	As time progresses, diffuse ST elevation with PR depression is observed, followed by T wave flattening, then deep symmetrical T wave inversion, and finally resolution.
		Pericardial effusion	Low QRS voltage/amplitude is seen, a raised heart rate of >100 min^{-1}, QRS complexes are conducted normally but alternate in height.

8	Electrolyte derangements	Hyperkalaemia	T wave is usually peaked, P wave flattening/widening is seen along with PR prolongation, bradyarrhythmia or conduction blocks may or may not be present, QRS widening is also observed.
		Hypokalaemia	P wave amplitude is increased, along with prolongation of PR interval, widespread ST depression, and T wave flattening/inversion. T & U waves are fused together (apparent long QT interval).
		Hypercalcemia	Shortening of QT interval is seen, Osborne wave which is a positive deflection seen at J point in the precordial and the true limb leads.
		Hypocalcemia	QT interval prolongation is present, AF may or may not be present.
9	Inherited channelopathy	Wolff–Parkinson-White syndrome	Delta waves are seen which are described as having a slurred upstroke in the QRS complex; associated shortening of the PR interval is also present.
11	Other inherited disorders	Arrhythmogenic right ventricular dysplasia	T wave inversion is seen in V1-V3 leads in absence of an RBBB, Epsilon wave described as a small deflection buried in the end of the QRS complex is also present, QRS widening seen in V1-V3, and prolonged S wave upstroke of 55 ms seen in V1-V3.
12	Drug toxicity	Sodium channel blockade	QRS > 100 ms seen in lead II, terminal R wave > 3 mm present or the R/S ratio of > 0.7 is seen in the aVR lead, sinus tachycardia may or may not be present.

9.3 Search strategy

In this chapter, we retrospectively explore the evolution and advancements in the use of AI for automated ECG interpretation. To develop a thorough understanding, we conducted a systematic search across key academic databases, specifically PubMed and Google Scholar. Our search strategy involved key terms such as 'AI and ECG,' 'ML and ECG,' and 'DL and ECG' to capture all pertinent literature. We initiated the search without any filters to include articles where these specified keywords

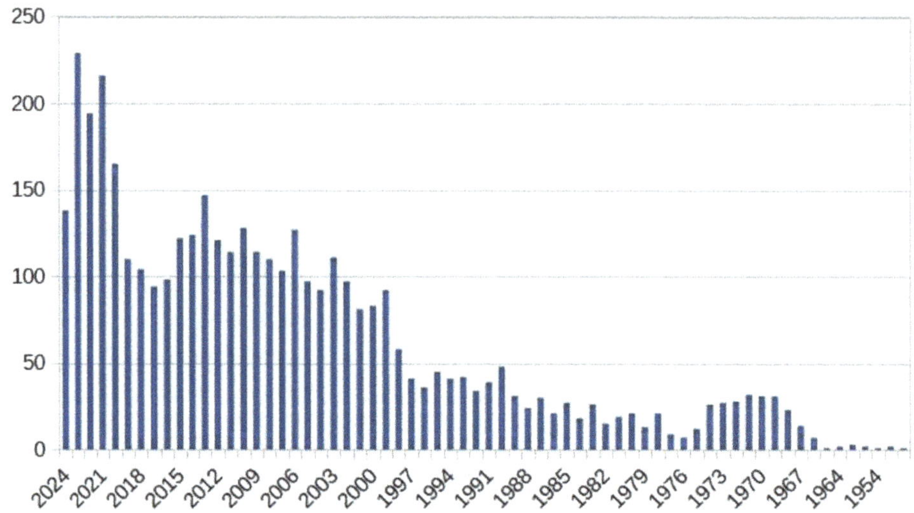

Figure 9.3. Distribution of research articles on the topic of AI and ECG.

appeared anywhere in the text, whether in the abstract or the main body. This approach ensured the comprehensive inclusion of relevant studies, providing a broad perspective on the topic.

When analyzing the output from the PubMed database using the keywords 'AI and ECG,' we observe a total of 3559 results; see figure 9.3. The earliest article in this collection dates to 1951. Over the decades, there has been a notable increase in publication volume within this field. Specifically, between the late 1990s and early 2000s, the number of articles published annually ranged from 50 to 100. However, this figure has seen a significant rise since 2020, with more than 150 articles published per year, and nearly 250 articles were released just last year. This surge underscores the rapid growth of AI as a field, a trend that is expected to continue as both the methodologies and their applications are further refined. Similar trends were observed when employing the search terms 'ML and ECG' and 'DL and ECG.' Notably, the search for 'ML and ECG' yielded the highest volume of publications, with annual submissions peaking at 7000 articles, highlighting the expanding scope of research in this area.

In addition to exploring the historical development and current landscape of AI applications in automated ECG interpretation, this study also delves into the methodologies associated with TFR in ECG analysis. To ensure a thorough examination, our research strategy was broadened to include the keywords 'TFR and ECG' across the selected academic databases. This targeted approach facilitated a review of both historical and contemporary uses of TFR techniques in ECG data analysis. The search yielded 143 results, with the earliest article dating back to 1989. Despite its innovative potential, the application of TFR in electrocardiography is still an emerging field, garnering limited attention and research compared to more conventional methods. This finding underscores the novelty and untapped potential of TFR in enhancing ECG interpretation through detailed temporal and spectral analysis.

9.4 Acquisition and preprocessing

9.4.1 ECG acquisition and anatomical placement of electrodes

In the configuration of an ECG machine, electrode placement is critical and involves ten leads, which are divided into two main groups: six chest leads and four limb leads. The chest leads, also referred to as 'V' leads, are numbered from V1 to V6 and are placed in specific positions across the chest to capture the heart's electrical activity from different angles. The limb leads, on the other hand, are attached to the extremities—specifically, the wrists and ankles. These leads help record the heart's electrical signals from the frontal plane. For a visual guide on how these leads are accurately placed, refer to figure 9.4. This setup is instrumental in providing a comprehensive view of the heart's electrical function, which is crucial for diagnosing various cardiac conditions.

In the arrangement of limb leads on an ECG machine, one of the wires functions as a neutral lead, like a grounding wire in electrical setups. Its primary role is to complete the electrical circuit, although it does not directly contribute to the ECG readings themselves. This setup is essential for the proper functioning of the ECG machine, as it helps to stabilize and ensure the accuracy and consistency of the cardiac signals that are recorded. This neutral lead effectively helps mitigate potential interference and noise, providing clearer and more reliable ECG results [27].

In terms of electrical characteristics, limb leads on an ECG exhibit both unipolar and bipolar properties. The unipolar leads include aVR, aVL, and aVF, as well as the chest leads. This configuration captures electrical activity relative to a central reference point, which is instrumental in providing detailed insights into the patterns of cardiac depolarization.

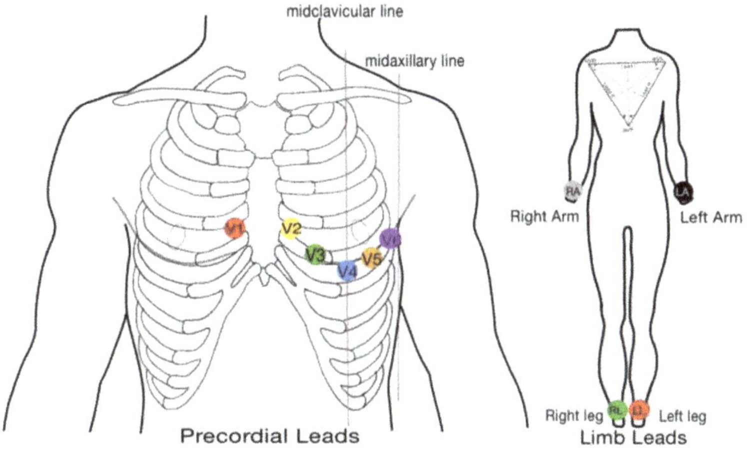

Figure 9.4. ECG lead placement.

Conversely, the bipolar leads are derived from the limb leads and form what is known as 'Einthoven's Triangle.' This geometric arrangement consists of leads aVR and aVL, which originate from the right and left wrists or shoulders, respectively, and aVF, which is derived from the left ankle or lower abdomen. The interplay between these leads results in bipolar recordings, specifically identified as leads I, II, and III.

By integrating both unipolar and bipolar perspectives, the ECG system offers a comprehensive view of cardiac electrical activity. This dual approach enhances the precision in diagnosing and monitoring various cardiac conditions, making it an essential tool in cardiovascular healthcare.

9.4.2 Capturing cardiac activity: understanding the recording process of ECG signals

Our body's complex communication network depends heavily on the electrical and chemical signals exchanged between nerve and muscle cells. A critical aspect of this system is the regulation of our heartbeat, controlled by regular electrical impulses. These impulses originate from a cluster of cells in the right atrium known as the SA node. From there, they spread through the heart muscle, initiating the coordinated contraction of the heart's chambers. For a visual representation of this electrical pathway, see figure 9.1. Interestingly, the transmission of these electrical signals through the heart can also be detected on the skin's surface. An ECG is a diagnostic tool designed to capture these variations in electrical signals, or voltage, across different areas of the skin. By graphically displaying these changes, an ECG provides a visual map of the heart's electrical activity. This visualization offers critical insights into the heart's operational status and overall health.

9.4.3 Preprocessing methods

In ECG, preprocessing plays a pivotal role in refining raw data by eliminating noise and artifacts, thereby enhancing the signal-to-noise ratio. This crucial step ensures the accurate analysis of the heart's electrical activity. This chapter delves into a variety of preprocessing techniques commonly employed in ECG signal processing. Among these are the wavelet transform and its inverse, which are used to decompose and reconstruct the ECG signal, allowing for detailed analysis and noise reduction. Thresholding is another technique used to differentiate between relevant signal components and noise. In addition, baseline wander removal is essential for correcting low-frequency variations in the signal. Together, these preprocessing methods significantly improve the quality and accuracy of ECG signals, which is vital for both clinical diagnostics and research applications.

(1) *Wavelet transform for denoising*

Denoising is a crucial preprocessing step in ECG signal processing that enhances the signal-to-noise ratio. The wavelet transform method, a popular choice for this task, decomposes the ECG into various frequency components using wavelet functions. This allows for effective differentiation and removal of noise while preserving vital signal features. Capturing both high- and low-frequency components, the wavelet transform provides a comprehensive representation of the ECG, significantly improving its clarity, accuracy, and clinical interpretability.

(2) *Inverse wavelet transform for signal reconstruction*

After denoising the ECG signal with wavelet transform, the next step involves reconstructing the signal in its original time domain. This is achieved using the inverse wavelet transform, which reverses the frequency components obtained during the wavelet transform to recreate the denoised ECG signal. This approach ensures that essential information is preserved throughout the denoising process, making the signal suitable for further analysis and interpretation. By maintaining the integrity of the reconstructed signal, it ensures that the signal can be effectively used for detecting abnormalities and facilitating accurate diagnoses.

(3) *Thresholding for noise removal*

Thresholding is a prevalent denoising technique in ECG signal preprocessing. This method sets a specific threshold value and eliminates any signal components falling below this threshold, effectively filtering out noise while retaining critical ECG features. This enhances signal quality and interpretability. There are various thresholding algorithms, such as hard and soft thresholding, which can be chosen based on the ECG signal's characteristics. The use of thresholding reduces noise interference, thereby rendering the ECG signal clearer and more suitable for precise analysis and diagnosis.

(4) *Baseline wander removal*

Baseline wander, caused by low-frequency drifts in ECG signals due to patient movement, electrode placement, or external factors, can distort the signal and impact analytical accuracy. Techniques such as high-pass filtering and polynomial fitting are employed to remove these drifts and stabilize the signal. High-pass filtering eliminates the low-frequency components causing baseline wander, whereas polynomial fitting models the signal and subtracts the drift from it. Implementing these techniques prepares the ECG for further processing and ensures precise interpretation of cardiac activity.

9.5 Time–frequency representations

ECG signals are nonstationary in nature because their frequency content changes over time due to the dynamic nature of cardiac activities. Time–frequency analysis (TFA) plays a pivotal role in signal processing applications, particularly in the analysis of ECG signals due to their nonstationary nature [28, 29]. TFA provides a detailed representation of how the spectral content of an ECG signal evolves over time, making it an invaluable tool for analyzing and interpreting ECG signals.

Several methods are available for generating TFR images of signals, each with its own advantages and disadvantages. In addition, the ability to capture the spectral variation in ECGs makes the use of TFR extremely favorable when analyzing nonstationary signals. Two of the most widely used techniques are the wavelet and STFT. These techniques help researchers see and measure how the signal's frequency components vary over time. This is useful for identifying and understanding various heart conditions in ECG signals.

9.5.1 Short-time Fourier transform

The STFT is a widely used method for TFA. In STFT, the signal is segmented into overlapping and fixed-length windows, a process known as windowing. Once the signal is segmented, a Fourier transform is applied to each windowed segment to obtain the frequency spectrum for that specific time interval. The magnitudes of the resulting complex numbers are then plotted as a function of time and frequency, creating a spectrogram that shows how the frequency content of the signal changes over time. Consider a time-varying signal $x(t)$. The following equation illustrates the analytical representation of its STFT:

$$S_x(t, f) = -\int_{-\infty}^{+\infty} x(v)h \times (t - v)e - (j2\pi f\nu \; d\nu) \tag{9.1}$$

where ν and f represent the factor relative to the sliding window and the respective frequency, respectively, and $h(\cdot)$ depicts the window function. STFT is simple to implement and provides a clear and intuitive visual representation of the time–frequency characteristics of a signal, making it easier for researchers and clinicians to interpret and analyze the data. This clarity is particularly useful in applications where a quick and easy-to-understand visualization of frequency changes over time is needed.

However, STFT also has limitations. One of its significant drawbacks is its fixed resolution. In particular, due to the fact that time and frequency are inversely proportional, improper selection of the window size significantly impacts or degrades either the time or frequency resolution. A shorter window leads to enhanced (degraded) time (frequency) resolution and vice versa. This trade-off makes STFT less suitable for signals with rapidly changing frequencies, as it cannot accurately capture both the temporal and spectral details simultaneously.

9.5.2 Wavelet transform

Wavelet transform overcomes some of the limitations of STFT by providing multiresolution analysis. It uses a set of basis functions, called wavelets, which are localized in both time and frequency. Wavelets are functions that can be dilated and translated to capture different aspects of the signal. By dilating the wavelet, low-frequency components are captured, and by translating it, high-frequency components are captured. This ability to adjust the wavelet makes it a versatile tool for analyzing various signal features across different time and frequency scales. Unlike STFT, which uses frequency shift, complex wavelet transform (CWT) adopts frequency or time to transform the signal of interest. The CWT of $x(t)$ is given by

$$C_x(\delta, \alpha) = \frac{1}{\sqrt{\alpha}} \int_{-\infty}^{\infty} x(t)\psi \times \left(\frac{t - \delta}{\alpha}\right) dt \tag{9.2}$$

where δ, a, and $\psi(\cdot)$ represent the translation and scaling parameters and the mother wavelet, respectively.

Wavelet transform has several advantages, including adaptive resolution. High-frequency components are analyzed with high time resolution, while low-frequency components are analyzed with high frequency resolution. This adaptability makes wavelet transform suitable for analyzing signals with abrupt changes and nonstationary characteristics. However, the performance of wavelet transform depends on the choice of the mother wavelet, which may require domain-specific knowledge. In addition, wavelet transform can be computationally more intensive than the STFT.

This paper explores the application of STFT and wavelet transform for the time–frequency analysis of ECG signals. By comparing these methods, we aim to highlight their respective advantages and limitations and demonstrate their utility in the context of ECG signal analysis.

TFR images were generated using the STFT to analyze the frequency content of the signals over time. In the TFR images, the x-axis represents time, and the y-axis represents frequency, while the color intensity indicates the amplitude of the signal at each time and frequency point. Figures 9.5 and 9.6 show the TFR images generated for AF and normal conditions, respectively. For the ECG signals of normal individuals (figure 9.6), the energy distribution is concentrated and stable, reflecting the regular and rhythmic heartbeats typical of healthy cardiac function. In contrast, the TFR images for individuals with AF (figure 9.5) display irregular and chaotic frequency patterns.

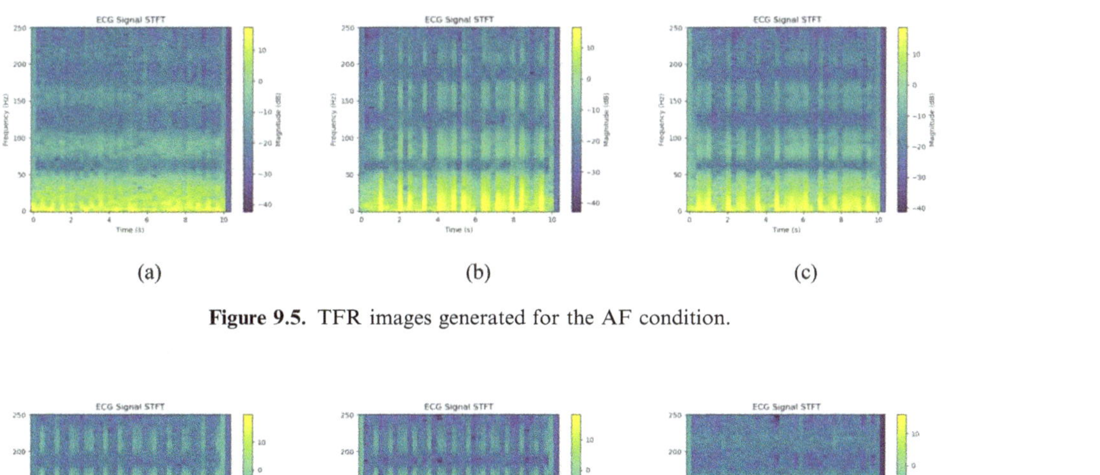

(a) (b) (c)

Figure 9.5. TFR images generated for the AF condition.

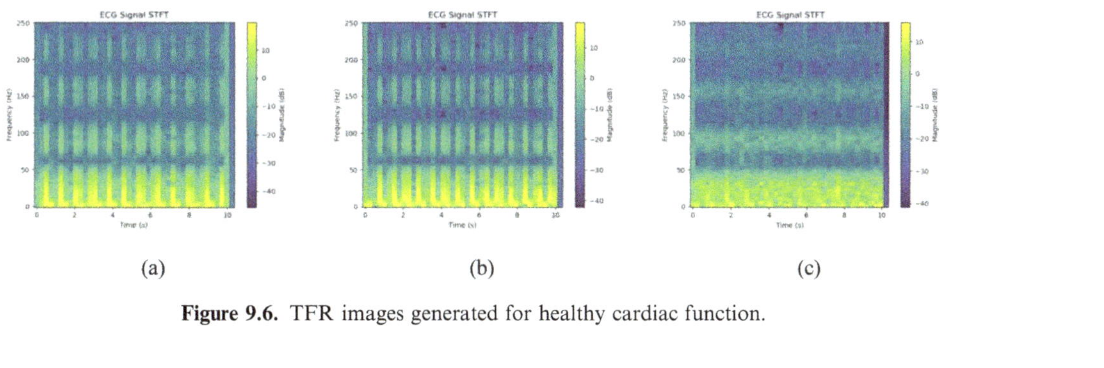

(a) (b) (c)

Figure 9.6. TFR images generated for healthy cardiac function.

9.6 Role of AI in ECG analysis

In recent years, the integration of AI into healthcare has witnessed remarkable strides, particularly in the realm of cardiac abnormality assessment using ECG signals. AI, a burgeoning field in computer science, works similarly to human intelligence and has the prime objective of developing systems capable of performing tasks with similar or higher precision to that of humans. In healthcare, AI applications span diverse areas, including image analysis, natural language processing, and medical diagnostics. The evolution from rule-based systems to ML and deep learning (DL) techniques has significantly enhanced our ability to extract meaningful information from complex data sets, such as ECG signals. The widespread availability of comprehensive, open-access healthcare databases has been a pivotal factor in the development and application of AI across a diverse range of healthcare domains [30].

AI uses computational algorithms, which constitute the set of processes embedded in digital tools and used to execute a series of operations with a specific objective. While the logical rules of explicit algorithms are precisely defined by the designers, the logic of implicit algorithms comes from an architecture (which describes the logical connections between the parameters established for the model) defined by learning based on real scenarios. The training therefore works to find the relationships that exist between the (measured) input variables and the desired final result [31].

Advancements in artificial intelligence offer significant opportunities to mitigate medical errors within the healthcare sector. Specifically, the application of ML and DL methods for the automatic prediction of heart diseases shows considerable promise. These ML techniques necessitate expert involvement for feature extraction and selection, identifying the most pertinent features before the classification phase. Feature extraction reduces the number of features in a data set by transforming or projecting the data into a new, lower-dimensional space. This process preserves the essential information in the original data.

9.6.1 Supervised AI algorithms for CVD detection

Supervised AI algorithms have emerged as powerful tools for CVD detection, offering promising solutions to address this global health challenge. Supervised AI algorithms are trained on labeled data, where the labels indicate the presence or absence of a CVD. By learning from these labeled examples, supervised AI algorithms can make predictions on new data, aiding in the early detection of CVDs. The most used supervised AI algorithms for CVD detection are briefly discussed below:

- ***Logistic regression***: a statistical model that predicts the probability of a binary outcome, such as the presence or absence of a CVD.
- ***Support vector machines (SVMs)***: these classify data points by creating hyperplanes that optimally separate data points belonging to different classes.
- ***Random forests (RF)***: these provide more accurate prediction by combining multiple decision trees using learning algorithms.

- ***Neural networks***: inspired by the structure of the human brain, neural networks are complex algorithms that can learn from large data sets and identify intricate patterns.

For example, [32] predicted coronary artery disease (CAD) by adopting an SVM, an artificial neural network (ANN), and an RF. The Isfahan cohort study data set was used for training and prediction. The study extracted 19 features from 11 495 records. The results indicated that all three algorithms produced similar outcomes, with SVM achieving the highest accuracy of 89.73%. The ANN algorithm achieved high values for the area under the curve (AUC), sensitivity, and accuracy, which demonstrates its dominance in such applications. Key features correlated with the target class included age, sex, history of stroke, palpitations, and heart diseases. The study concluded that ML algorithms can effectively and accurately detect CAD.

9.6.2 Unsupervised AI algorithms for CVD detection

Alongside supervised AI algorithms, unsupervised AI techniques are gaining prominence in the field of CVD detection. Unlike supervised algorithms that rely on labeled data, unsupervised AI algorithms explore unlabeled data sets to identify hidden patterns and structures that may be indicative of CVDs. This ability to uncover hidden patterns makes unsupervised AI a valuable tool for early CVD detection and risk stratification. The most used unsupervised AI algorithms for CVD detection are briefly discussed below:

- ***K-means clustering*** groups data points into clusters based on their similarity, allowing for the identification of distinct patient subgroups with unique CVD risk profiles.
- ***Hierarchical clustering*** creates a hierarchical representation of data points, revealing relationships and subgroups at different levels of granularity.
- ***Principal component analysis (PCA)*** reduces the dimensionality of complex data sets by identifying the most significant patterns and transforming data into a lower-dimensional space.
- ***Anomaly detection*** identifies data points that deviate significantly from the expected patterns, potentially indicating CVD-related abnormalities.

9.6.3 Combining supervised and unsupervised AI algorithms for enhanced CVD detection

The use of both supervised and unsupervised algorithms provides a powerful approach to detecting CVD. Supervised algorithms make predictions using labeled data, while unsupervised algorithms find hidden patterns in unlabeled data. Together, they offer a more complete understanding, leading to earlier diagnoses and better patient outcomes. Combining these methods has the potential to transform CVD detection and treatment. By using the strengths of both types of learning, new insights can be discovered, allowing for earlier diagnoses and personalized treatment plans. As AI technology advances, the integration of these hybrid models will play a crucial role in combating CVD, contributing to a healthier future for everyone.

9.7 Preliminary analysis for predicting ECG rhythm-based abnormality

For this pilot study, we utilized a publicly available 12-lead ECG database from Physionet to predict AF using TFR images [33]. The database comprises ECG recordings from 45 152 patients, sampled at a rate of 500 Hz. We specifically selected the lead 1 ECG signals from 1000 patients, evenly split between 500 individuals diagnosed with AF and 500 exhibiting normal sinus rhythm. These ECG signals were segmented into three subsets: training, validation, and testing, to facilitate model development and evaluation. TFR images were generated from these signals using the STFT technique. Subsequently, these images were employed to train a convolutional neural network (CNN) based on the AlexNet architecture.

The TFR images display prominent high-frequency components and a broad dispersion of energy across various frequency ranges, indicative of the erratic electrical activity and uncoordinated atrial contractions typical of AF. Upon examining the TFR images (figure 9.5 for AF and figure 9.6 for normal sinus rhythm), distinct differences in frequency characteristics and temporal patterns between normal individuals and those with AF are apparent. These distinctions are crucial for enabling precise diagnosis and assessment of the condition.

We trained our AlexNet model over 100 epochs. Following the training phase, we evaluated the model's performance using several metrics. The ROC curve was particularly scrutinized to assess the model's capability to differentiate between classes effectively. In addition, we analyzed the training and validation loss to gauge how well the model learned from the data. These measures are critical to understanding the model's accuracy and overall effectiveness in diagnosing conditions based on the input data. In addition to basic metrics, we calculated the accuracy, sensitivity (recall), specificity, and F1-score to comprehensively assess the overall performance of our models. By comparing these metrics, we were able to identify the model that performed best on our data set. Training and validation accuracy, as well as loss, are crucial metrics for evaluating the performance of a CNN model. Training loss quantifies the model's error on the training data, reflecting how effectively it learns from the data. Conversely, validation loss measures the model's error on a separate validation data set, indicating its ability to generalize to new, unseen data. Ideally, as the model learns, the training loss should decrease, and the validation loss should initially decrease and then stabilize.

Figure 9.7(a) illustrates the training and validation accuracy over the course of the training epochs for AlexNet. The x-axis represents the number of epochs, while the y-axis indicates the accuracy percentage. Initially, both training and validation accuracies start at lower levels—50% and 48%, respectively—and exhibit a steady

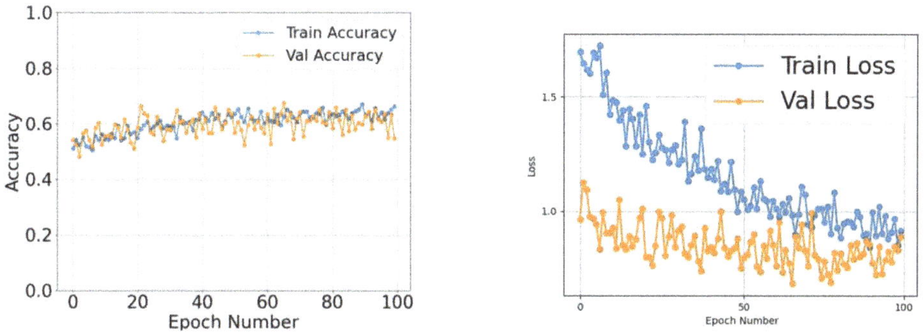

(a) Train and Validation Accuracy for AlexNet (b) Train and Validation Loss for AlexNet

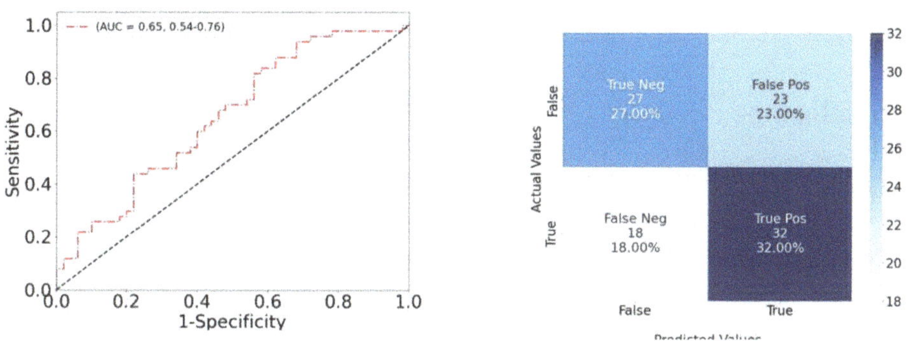

(c) Train and Validation Loss for AlexNet (d) Train and Validation Accuracy for AlexNet

Figure 9.7. Training and validation loss and accuracy for AlexNet.

upward trend. As training progresses, the training accuracy nears saturation at 65%, and the validation accuracy stabilizes at around 60%. This graphical representation provides a clear visual of the model's learning trajectory and its stabilization in performance over time.

Figure 9.7(b) depicts loss values versus number of epochs, providing a detailed view of the training and validation losses throughout the training process. Initially, both training and validation losses start relatively high. As training progresses, these losses consistently decrease, reflecting a minimization of errors on the training set and an improvement in the ability to generalize to new data.

The receiver operating characteristic (ROC) curve is a graphical representation of the diagnostic power of a binary classification system. The ROC curve presents the true positive rate (sensitivity) against the false positive rate (1—specificity) at different threshold settings. The AUC of each model provides a scalar value that summarizes overall performance. Higher AUC values indicate better model performance. Figure 9.7(c) depicts the ROC curve for our analysis. Although the AUC values are low, our analysis shows the capability of our model to discriminate between ECG-based abnormalities using the TFR images. Figure 9.7(d) shows the

Table 9.3. Model metrics.

Metric	Validation	Testing
Loss	0.76	0.73
Recall	0.63	0.33
Precision	0.64	0.41
F1-score	0.63	0.37
ACC	0.61	0.66
AUC	0.63	0.6548

confusion matrix for the test data processed by the trained model, i.e. the discrimination performed by the model on the test data. The performance of the model on the internal validation and test data is also shown in table 9.3.

9.8 Conclusions

This study explored the application of ML algorithms for the classification of AF and normal conditions. TFRs of ECG signals were generated using the STFT, providing valuable insights into the distinct characteristics of normal and AF conditions. The analysis of the TFR images demonstrated clear differences in frequency patterns between the two conditions, highlighting the potential of this approach in aiding accurate diagnosis and assessment. The integration of TFR images with ML algorithms provided a robust framework for distinguishing between normal and AF conditions. The results underscore the importance of leveraging advanced ML models and TFR images to enhance diagnostic accuracy. Future work could focus on further optimizing the model, incorporating additional features, and exploring more sophisticated techniques to improve generalization and robustness.

References

[1] History of heart disease: Ancient egypt to cutting edge surgery *Baystate Health* [Online]. https://baystatehealth.org/articles/history-of-heart-disease (accessed 19 May 2024)

[2] Mensah G A *et al* 2023 Global burden of cardiovascular diseases and risks, 1990–2022 *J. Am. Coll. Cardiol.* **82** 2350–473

[3] Fye W B 1994 A history of the origin, evolution, and impact of electrocardiography *Am. J. Card.* **73** 937–49

[4] Reichlin T, Abächerli R, Twerenbold R, Kühne M, Schaer B, Mueller C, Sticherling C and Osswald S 2016 Advanced ECG in 2016: is there more than just a tracing? *Swiss Med. Wkly.* **146** w14 303–w3

[5] Rafie N, Kashou A H and Noseworthy P A 2021 ECG interpretation: clinical relevance, challenges, and advances *Hearts* **2** 505–13

[6] Nezamabadi K, Sardaripour N, Haghi B and Forouzanfar M 2023 Unsupervised ECG analysis: a review *IEEE Rev. Biomed. Eng.* **16** 208–24

[7] Diamant N, Reinertsen E, Song S, Aguirre A D, Stultz C M and Batra P 2022 Patient contrastive learning: a performant, expressive, and practical approach to electrocardiogram modeling *PLoS Comput. Biol.* **18** e1009862
[8] Gopal B, Han R, Raghupathi G, Ng A, Tison G and Rajpurkar P 2021 3KG: Contrastive learning of 12-lead electrocardiograms using physiologically-inspired augmentations *Proceedings of Machine Learning for Health* (PMLR) 156–67 https://proceedings.mlr.press/v158/gopal21a.html
[9] Feeny A K *et al* 2020 Artificial intelligence and machine learning in arrhythmias and cardiac electrophysiology *Circ. Arrhythmia Electrophysiol.* **13** e007952
[10] Xu Y *et al* 2021 Artificial intelligence: a powerful paradigm for scientific research *Innovation* **2** 100179
[11] Bi Q, Goodman K E, Kaminsky J and Lessler J 2019 What is machine learning? A primer for the epidemiologist *Am. J. Epidemiol.* **188** 2222–39
[12] van den Oord A, Li Y and Vinyals O 2018 Representation learning with contrastive predictive coding arXiv:1807.03748
[13] Aziz S, Ahmed S and Alouini M-S 2021 ECG-based machine-learning algorithms for heartbeat classification *Sci. Rep.* **11** 18738
[14] Daydulo Y D, Thamineni B L and Dawud A A 2023 Cardiac arrhythmia detection using deep learning approach and time frequency representation of ECG signals *BMC Med. Inform. Decis. Mak.* **23** 232
[15] Zhang J, Tian J, Cao Y, Yang Y and Xu X 2020 Deep time–frequency representation and progressive decision fusion for ecg classification *Knowl.-Based Syst.* **190** 105402
[16] *How the Heart Works—How the Heart Beats* (NHLBI, NIH) [Online] https://nhlbi.nih.gov/health/heart/heart-beats (accessed 19 May 2024)
[17] Physiology, cardiac cycle *StatPearls—NCBI Bookshelf* [Online] https://ncbi.nlm.nih.gov/books/NBK459327/ (accessed 19 May 2024)
[18] Anatomy and function of the electrical system *Stanford Medicine Children's Health* accessed 19 May 2024 https://www.stanfordchildrens.org/en/topic/default?id=anatomy-and-function-of-the-electrical-system-90-P01762
[19] The basics of ECG ACLS Medical Training 2024 [Online] https://www.aclsmedicaltraining.com/basics-of-ecg (accessed 19 May 24).
[20] Physiology, cardiac cycle—ncbi.nlm.nih.gov https://ncbi.nlm.nih.gov/books/NBK459327/ (accessed 01 June 2024).
[21] Fauci A, Braunwald E, Kasper D, Hauser S, Longo D, Jameson J and Loscalzo J 2008 *Harrison's Principles of Internal Medicine* 17th edn (McGraw-Hill)
[22] Sattar Y and Chhabra L 2023 Electrocardiogram https://www.ncbi.nlm.nih.gov/books/NBK549803/
[23] Cadogan M and Buttner R ECG rate interpretation—litfl.com https://litfl.com/ecg-rate-interpretation/ (accessed 24 May 2024)
[24] Aro A L, Anttonen O, Kerola T, Junttila M J, Tikkanen J T, Rissanen H A, Reunanen A and Huikuri H V 2013 Prognostic significance of prolonged PR interval in the general population *Eur. Heart J.* **35** 123–9
[25] Cook D A, Oh S-Y and Pusic M V 2020 Accuracy of physicians' electrocardiogram interpretations: a systematic review and meta-analysis *JAMA Int. Med.* **180** 1461–71
[26] EKG library • LITFL • ECG library basics https://litfl.com/ecg-library/ (accessed 06.02.2024).

[27] Limb leads—ECG lead placement—normal function of the heart—cardiology teaching package—practice learning—division of nursing—The University of Nottingham (accessed 01.06.2024) https://www.nottingham.ac.uk/nursing/practice/resources/cardiology/function/limb_leads.php

[28] Pachori R B and Nishad A 2016 Cross-terms reduction in the Wigner–Ville distribution using tunable-Q wavelet transform *Signal Process.* **120** 288–304

[29] Gupta V and Pachori R B 2021 FBDM-based time-frequency representation for sleep stages classification using EEG signals *Biomed. Signal Process. Control* **64** 102265

[30] Jiang F, Jiang Y, Zhi H, Dong Y, Li H, Ma S, Wang Y, Dong Q, Shen H and Wang Y 2017 Artificial intelligence in healthcare: past, present and future *Stroke Vasc. Neurol.* **2** 230–43

[31] Jean A 2020 A brief history of artificial intelligence *Med. Sci.* **36** 1059–67 (in French)

[32] Saeedbakhsh S, Sattari M, Mohammadi M, Najafian J and Mohammadi F 2023 Diagnosis of coronary artery disease based on machine learning algorithms support vector machine, artificial neural network, and random forest *Adv. Biomed. Res.* **2023** 1–8

[33] Zheng J, Guo H and Chu H 2022 A large scale 12-lead electrocardiogram database for arrhythmia study (version 1.0.0) *PhysioNet*

Chapter 10

Real-time implementation of ECG beat identification using Hilbert transform and artificial neural network

Vikas Kumar Sinha and Govind Prasad

In the last few decades, biomedical science has encountered a significant hurdle related to R peak detection in electrocardiogram (ECG) data. To overcome this difficulty, an algorithm was developed to improve QRS detection accuracy. This algorithm precisely locates the R peaks of the ECG signal by employing the fractional-order differential (FOD) and Hilbert transform (HT), which helped to achieve 99.85% positive predictivity. Standard ECG records from the Massachusetts Institute of Technology Beth Israel Hospital (MIT-BIH) arrhythmia database were used. The algorithm's performance was evaluated using an artificial neural network (ANN) classifier, which obtained impressive accuracy, sensitivity, and F1-scores of 97.24%, 70.47%, and 0.56, respectively. Employing the algorithm's output as training data, this classifier could discriminate between normal and pathological ECG signals. According to these results, the proposed approach is expected to be an effective tool for processing and analyzing ECG signals, which will increase the ability of the biomedical science to identify cardiovascular disease. The examination and interpretation of ECG signals are critical components of clinical processes, and the significance of technology in diagnosing cardiac issues cannot be overemphasized. Assessing cardiac health requires automatic machine estimation, which primarily utilizes ECG data. An essential part of ECG analysis is the R peak, a focal point for analyzing healthy and abnormal cardiac rhythms in individuals, including patients.

10.1 Introduction

An electrocardiogram (ECG) is a tool which can be used for cardiology tests. It records the electrical activity of the human heart over time, which helps to detect various abnormalities and cardiac diseases by deciphering the heart's status.

doi:10.1088/978-0-7503-5964-1ch10

To detect the QRS complex, the time between successive R peaks is required. However, the detection of ECG signals is not simple, as noise interference from several sources affects the QRS complex. Some significant causes of these low- and high-frequency noise signals are artifacts, interference, wandering baselines, and apparatus problems. Noise occurs due to poor contact made by electrodes, interference from other signals, broken wires or cables, faulty equipment, etc. In cardiology, an electrocardiogram is a vital diagnostic tool that records the complex electrical dynamics of the human heart over time. Measuring an individual's heart rate and identifying abnormalities or heart problems is essential. The ability to precisely detect the QRS complex depends on measuring the interval between consecutive R peaks, a vital statistic for evaluating heart function. Nevertheless, detecting ECG signals is not straightforward and is full of obstacles arising from multiple interference sources.

The high-frequency and low-frequency noise signals can be produced by numerous sources of interference, wandering baselines, artifacts, and problems with the equipment, all of which can minimize the fidelity of the QRS complex. Inadequate electrode contact that introduces undesirable impulses, damaged wires or connections, and equipment malfunctions can all cause these interruptions. Therefore, robust signal processing techniques and careful attention to detail are required to identify the underlying signal within this noise. Clinical professionals can gain significant insights into cardiac health by overcoming these difficulties, which could eventually lead to more precise diagnoses and targeted therapies.

The comprehension and diagnosis of cardiac disorders rely extensively on the temporal dynamics of cardiac electrical activity. Ventricular depolarization gives rise to the subsequent QRS complex, which starts the contraction phase that pumps blood out of the heart. This intricate procedure starts 0.16 s after the P wave [1]. The characteristic T wave appears as the ventricular muscle fibers repolarize, indicating the relaxation phase. It is noteworthy that, according to [2], this essential electrical event occurs right before the completion of ventricular contraction and has a width of approximately 0.16 s. Table 10.1 shows the typical ECG signal parameters of the typical ECG waveform shown in figure 10.1(b). The P wave, QRS complex,

Table 10.1. Typical ECG signal parameters.

Parameters	Values of a normal ECG
Heart rate	60–100 bpm
P wave	Amplitude: 0.25 ± 0.05 mv Interval: 110 ± 20 ms
Q wave	25% of R
R wave	1.60 mV
S wave	0.1–0.5 mv
RR Interval	0.6–1.2 mV
T wave	0.1–0.5 mV
ST segment	Period: 80–120 ms

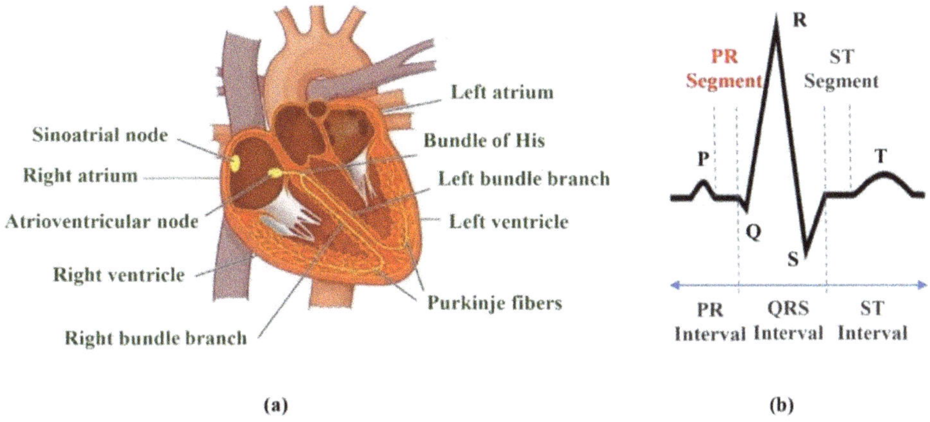

Figure 10.1. (a) Internal structure of the heart and (b) typical ECG signal.

Table 10.2. Parameters of the various artifacts observed in ECG signals [5].

Artifact	Frequency band (in Hz)	Amplitude	Reason
Baseline wander	0.15–0.3 Hz (< 1 Hz)	15% of peak-to-peak ECG amplitude	Respiration
Power-line interference	50/60 Hz	50% of peak-to-peak ECG amplitude	Capacitive and inductive coupling
Motion artifacts	1–10 Hz	500% of peak-to-peak ECG amplitude	Variations in charge distribution at the interface between the skin and the electrode
EMG Interference	5–500 Hz	10% of peak-to-peak ECG amplitude	Contraction of any muscle other than cardiac muscle

and T wave are three complex wave patterns that work collectively and form the basis for identifying and understanding different heart rhythms. The practitioner must recognize specific ECG patterns in clinical practice quickly. In cardiac care, this skillful detection helps medical practitioners rapidly assess and comprehend their patients' cardiovascular health, allowing immediate action and well-informed decision-making. The comprehensive monitoring and analysis of these time-related characteristics in cardiac activity significantly accelerates the diagnosis process and improves patient outcomes.

Table 10.2 shows the parameters of various artifacts in terms of frequency band and amplitude. A modified moving average filter has been presented [3] as a solution to baseline wander, muscle interference, power-line noise, and electrode motion artifact issues, improving noise reduction. Digital filters that ignore baseline wander noise, such as high-pass filters with low cutoff frequencies, are valuable additions to the moving average filter. In particular, notch filters are successful in reducing interference from power lines. In [4], researchers developed a nonlinear adaptive notch filter that could effectively reduce noise in fluctuating power-line interface frequencies, offering a reliable remedy for this ubiquitous problem. Adaptive filters have proven to be advantageous tools for minimizing motion artifacts; furthermore, filter parameters can be precisely adjusted for optimum outcomes. One common tactic is to set all noise-representing components to zero, which maintains the denoised signal. Wavelet transforms (WTs) and Hilbert transforms (HT) are two other approaches that can handle different kinds of noise in addition to baseline wander; they expand the range of tools that can be employed to improve the precision of diagnostic procedures.

This chapter examines the complex systems that govern heart function and considers their significance in preserving human life. Researchers have analyzed several lead types employed for cardiac activity monitoring, emphasizing their importance in identifying and monitoring cardiac electrical signals. In addition, this chapter describes the application of precise R peak identification in ECG signals, which is an essential step in assessing heart rhythms and detecting anomalies as shown in figure 10.2. Furthermore, we explore the application of ANNs for classifying arrhythmia beats, utilizing advanced computational methods to accurately distinguish between normal and pathological cardiac rhythms. Our research aims to improve our knowledge and treatment of cardiovascular disorders by contributing to the development of diagnostic techniques in cardiology through our intensive research (figure 10.2).

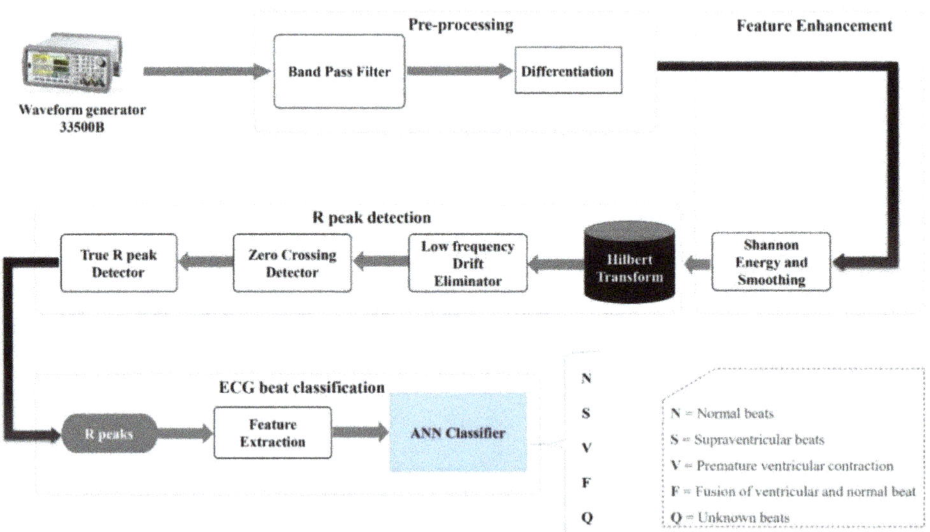

Figure 10.2. Framework of ECG signal R peak detection, feature extraction, and classification.

10.2 Artifacts/noises affecting ECGs

Electronic health systems are built on a framework of technology, infrastructure, and procedures that facilitate the collection, storage, and exchange of electronic healthcare records (EHRs) and other important patient data. These systems are designed primarily to improve the quality and efficiency of healthcare, simplify administrative tasks, and strengthen decision-making based on evidence [6]. At the core of electronic health systems is the adoption of EHRs, which serve as a digital platform for storing and retrieving patient information.

These EHR systems have replaced traditional paper-based systems, improving the efficiency, accuracy, and accessibility of patient information. Electronic health systems are based on the principles of technology and information management [7]. They seamlessly integrate patient data, clinical documentation, and management functions to streamline healthcare workflows and improve patient outcomes.

While removing noise from several sources is difficult, ECG signals are crucial in assessments of heart health. Key interferences include ambient and electrode contact issues, baseline wander, power-line interference, motion artifacts, and muscle noise. When power-line interference occurs, unwanted frequencies from the electrical grid are introduced, while baseline wander causes progressive baseline alterations that may obscure cardiac data. The patient's movements cause motion artifacts, and muscle noise muddies signals during exercise. Effective ECG signal processing necessitates strong and creative ways to reduce ambient noise and thus evaluate and diagnose the heart accurately. As biological signal processing technology develops, ongoing efforts are necessary to minimize these interferences and preserve the reliability of ECG-based diagnostic tools.

10.3 Related works

This section provides an extensive summary of several filtering techniques employed to denoise ECG signals. In the last decade, a wide variety of filtering techniques have been presented, exhibiting significant variations in outcomes and parameter values. The following discussion explains recent developments in ECG signal filtering. A critical study [8] concentrates on identifying the QRS complex in the ECG waveform —a step in the analysis of the ECG that is more significant than detecting other signal components, beat segments, or morphological features. A unique minimal preprocessing method for QRS complex recognition is provided, emphasizing efficiency. This technique employs a two-stage filtering strategy for preprocessing that combines a median filter and a Savitzky–Golay (SG) smoothing filter. The root mean square value of the ECG wave can be utilized to analyze the technique's effectiveness and provides a quantitative way to measure the filtering process. This two-step filtering technique improves signal quality and enables more precise and dependable QRS complex identification by reducing noise. By highlighting the significance of efficient preprocessing approaches for precise QRS complex identification, the study adds to the ongoing efforts to improve ECG signal processing techniques.

The study described in [9] addresses the automatic detection and localization of myocardial infarction (MI) in ECG signal processing. A vital study component is the meticulous preprocessing of ECG signals utilizing a sequential approach. The first critical preparatory phases are signal identification and definition of the QRS complex. WT is subsequently employed to successfully denoise the signal, removing undesirable artifacts and improving the signal's quality. After discussing the preprocessing, this chapter analyzes the predictive power of different ECG signal characteristics, including data for the Q wave, T wave, and ST-level elevation extracted from 12-lead ECG signals. By determining whether myocardial infarction is present or absent, this perceptive analysis aims to provide critical diagnostic data. The final phase of the research involves employing the unique features discovered and retrieved during the signal processing phases to operate a *k*-NN (*k*-nearest neighbors) classifier for classification difficulty. The experimentation is carried out using the Physikalisch-Technische Bundesanstalt (PTB) database, an established resource available via PhysioBank, to validate the proposed approach. Using this database, the research gains a robust empirical component that grounds the results in real-world conditions and improves the discipline of automated MI detection and localization.

A critical mathematical tool in signal processing, the fast Fourier transform (FFT) reliably converts information into the frequency domain, rendering it particularly helpful for examining stationary signals. Even with its capability in this domain, the FFT cannot meet the challenge of handling nonstationary signal analysis. This constraint is addressed by introducing the short-time Fourier transform (STFT), which provides a fundamental time–frequency analysis with a constant resolution influenced by the window size. This trade-off affects both time and frequency resolution. WT was developed as an improved way to overcome the limitations of STFT. WT is used because of its capacity to reduce noise and compress signals. It also improves the versatility of signal analysis [10], marking a significant development in the discipline.

Discrete WT (DWT) is a signal processing technique widely recognized for its efficiency in multiresolution analysis and minimal computational cost [10]. DWT employs two essential filters: the low-pass filter and the high-pass filter (HPF); both use a cutoff frequency set at half the input signal's bandwidth. This method produces the WT's first level by integrating filtering and downsampling by a factor of two. The decomposition level is restricted to $\log_2 N$ for optimal analysis, where N is the signal length. Two filters upsample the original signal by a factor of two with zero insertion throughout the reconstruction phase [11]. Table 10.3 briefly describes studies of R peak detection, while table 10.4 lists studies of arrhythmia classification. ECG signals are decomposed into different sub-bands (SBs) via three well-known decomposition techniques: variational mode decomposition, empirical mode decomposition, and tunable Q WT. Using two validation procedures, various characteristics can be obtained from the multiple SBs and identified via optimizable ensemble techniques [12].

Table 10.3. Published studies of QRS complex detection.

Author	System used for implementation	Technique	Database	Performance (%)
Rakshit *et al* [13]	MATLAB	Hilbert transform	MITDB	99.83
Deepu *et al* [14]	0.35-m CMOS process	Adaptive thresholding	MITDB	99.81
Pandit *et al* [15]	MATLAB	Max-min difference algorithm	MITDB	99.66
Sahoo *et al* [16]	MATLAB	Hilbert Transform	MITDB	99.72
Manikandan *et al* [17]	MATLAB	Hilbert Transform	MITDB	99.80
Kaur *et al* [18]	MATLAB	Hamming self-convolution window	MITDB	99.65
Nayak *et al* [19]	MATLAB	Hilbert Transform	• The MIT-BIH arrhythmia database (MITDB) • QT database • MIT-NSD • MIT-BIH ST change database	• 99.84 • 99.93 • 90.15 • 99.83
Madeiro *et al* [20]	MATLAB	Hilbert transform + WT	• MITDB • QTDB	• 99.18 • 99.65
Nayak *et al* [21]	MATLAB	Hilbert transform	MITDB	99.88
Thurner *et al* [22]	MATLAB	CPTW	INCARTDB	99.57
Rahul *et al* [23]	MATLAB	Dynamic thresholding	• MITDB • Fantasia database • MIT-NSD • Fetal ECG database • ESTDB	• 99.68 • 99.87 • 93.81 • 98.66 • 99.52
Tueche *et al* [24]	ESP-WROOM-32microcontroller	CPTW	• MITDB • MITPRDB • MIT-NSD	• 99.69 • 99.71 • 99.93
Zidelmal *et al* [25]	MATLAB	S-transform + Shannon energy	MITDB	99.91
Mukhopadhyay *et al* [26]	MATLAB	InTrigTh algorithm	MITDB	99.88
Yakut *et al* [27]		Adaptive thresholding	• MITDB • Fantasia database • MIT-NSD • QTDB • ESTDB	• 99.83 • 99.98 • 94.52 • 99.46 • 98.63
Xiong *et al* [28]	MATLAB	Hilbert transform	MITDB	99.72

(*Continued*)

Table 10.3. (*Continued*)

Author	System used for implementation	Technique	Database	Performance (%)
Nayak *et al* [6]	MATLAB	Hilbert transform	• MITDB • EDB • MIT-NSD • SVDB • AFTDB • TWADB	• 99.90 • 99.80 • 95.20 • 99.90 • 99.80 • 99.50
Tekeste *et al* [7]	65 nm low-power process	A-CLT	MITDB	99.37

Note: A-CLT: absolute curve length transform; MIT-NSD: MIT-BIH Noise Stress Test Database; INCARTDB: St.-Petersburg Institute of Cardiological Technics 12-lead Arrhythmia Database; ESTDB: European ST-T Database; MITPRDB: miRNA target prediction and functional annotations; SVDB: supraventricular arrhythmia database; AFTDB: MIT-BIH Atrial Fibrilation Database; TWADB: T-Wave Alternans Challenge Database; ESP-WROOM: Espressif Wireless Room.

Table 10.4. Published studies of arrhythmia classification.

Author	Implemented on system	Technique	Database	Performance (in %)
Sadhukhan *et al* [29]	• Arduino Mega 2560 board • MATLAB	Threshold-based classification	PTB diagnostic ECG database	95.60
Chen *et al* [30]	SMIC 40 nm LL HVT	WT + weak linear classifier + support vector machine (SVM)	MITDB	98.20
Pławiak [31]	MATLAB	Probabilistic neural network (PNN), radial basis function neural network, SVM and *k*-NN	MITDB	98.85
Raj *et al* [32]	32-bit Microcontroller	Pan–Tompkins algorithm (PTA), SVM	MITDB	96.14
Raj [33]	32-bit microcontroller	PTA, SVM	MITDB	95.68
Raj *et al* [34]	ARM9 board	PTA, ANN	MITDB	97.40
Raj *et al* [35]	MATLAB	PTA, least squares twin SVM	MITDB	99.11
Thomas *et al* [36]	MATLAB	Dual tree complex WT	MITDB	94.64
Das *et al* [37]	MATLAB	Multilayer perceptron neural network	MITDB	97.54
Marsili *et al* [38]	MATLAB	Shannon entropy	MITDB	98.00

Martis *et al* [39]	MATLAB	Discrete WT (DWT) + PNN	MITDB	99.28
Allam *et al* [40]	MATLAB	Stockwell transform + 2D-ResNet	MITDB	99.73
Mar *et al* [41]	MATLAB	Multi-layer perceptron	MITDB	89.00

Note: ANN: artificial neural network; SMIC: semiconductor manufacturing international corporation; LL: low leakage; HVT: high voltage threshold.

10.4 Methodology

In this chapter, we propose the use of the Arduino Mega 2560 microcontroller for ECG signal-processing development. Our approach provides real-time R peak identification and uses the ANN classifier to identify ECG beats based on the Association for the Advancement of Medical Instrumentation (AAMI) standard. First, the Arduino Mega 2560 is an excellent fit for real-time signal processing applications due to its many GPIO pins and capabilities. To provide high temporal resolution for precise detection and classification, the aim is to process ECG signals recorded at 360 Hz. Preprocessing the ECG signal to eliminate noise and baseline drift is the first step in our process. Next, we use the Arduino to find R peaks and significant points of interest for ECG analysis. Fortunately, the timing of cardiac events can be precisely determined by detecting these peaks in real time. Next, using the AAMI standard, an ANN classifier is trained to categorize ECG beats into various groups, including atrial fibrillation, normal, and premature ventricular contractions. The ANN uses features taken from the ECG signal to classify beats accurately. The system under consideration integrates hardware and software elements to facilitate dependable and effective ECG signal processing on a platform with limited resources, such as the Arduino Mega 2560.

The MITDB, which includes a variety of pathological and normal ECG signal types collected at 360 Hz, is the essential data set employed in this work [42]. The unprocessed ECG data is carefully analyzed using a band-pass filter to separate the QRS complex, which lies between 5 and 22 Hz. The first derivative of the ECG waveform, i.e. the differentiation of the ECG, is obtained and used as a step toward further processing. For precision QRS segmentation, a predetermined window of $\pm$ 356 ms is defined around each R peak, and the R peaks are recognized precisely [17]. This extensive processing pipeline ensures the extraction of significant data, thus supporting an in-depth analysis of the ECG signals.

10.4.1 Preprocessing

In this section, the preprocessing of the signal is performed. The raw ECG signal is first passed through a band-pass filter set to a frequency range of 5–22 Hz to filter the QRS complex of the ECG signal. After filtration, the signal is fed to the following block to differentiate the signal, as shown in figure 10.3. Here, a fractional-order differentiator is used instead of a conventional differentiator (the order of differentiation is 0.5).

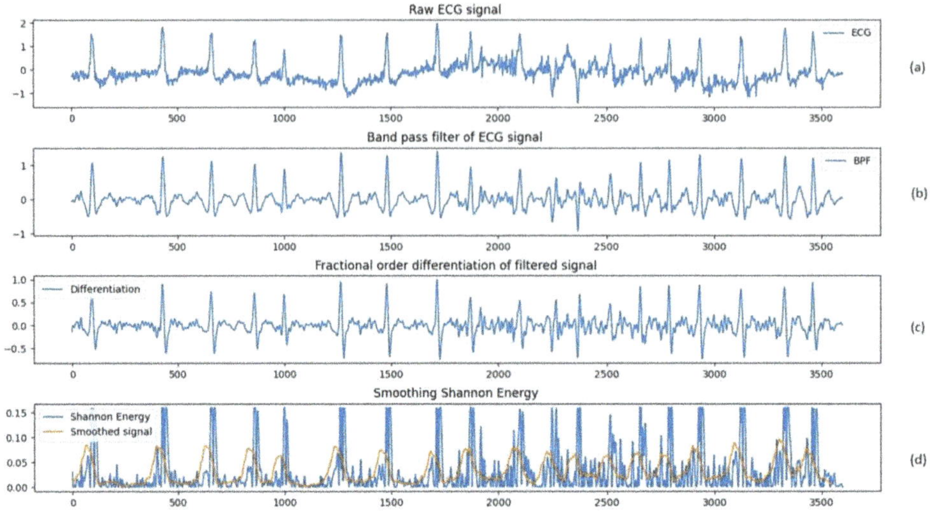

Figure 10.3. (a) Raw ECG signal. (b) Signal filtered by a Chebyshev type I band-pass filter. (c) Fractional-order differentiation of the filtered signal. (d) Shannon energy calculated for applied ordinarily differentiated ECG signal.

10.4.2 Feature enhancement

Following preprocessing, this stage applies feature enhancement. The amplitude normalizer converts the signal to lie within the range of -1 to $+1$ as follows:

$$a[n] = \frac{d[n]}{\mathrm{Max}(|d[n]|)} \tag{10.1}$$

where $a[n]$ and $d[n]$ represent the normalized and differentiated signals, respectively. The Shannon energy is given by

$$g[n] = -((a[n])^2 \log(a[n])^2). \tag{10.2}$$

The normalized signal is subjected to the Shannon energy calculation, resulting in the enhanced feature signal $S[n]$:

$$S[n] = \frac{1}{N}\sum_{m=1}^{N} g[n - (X - m)] \tag{10.3}$$

where the length of the smoothing window, X, is set to 55 in this study.

10.4.3 QRS complex detection

In this study, we use the HT to identify the local maxima within the enhanced QRS features. We examine whether the transformation efficiently represents the ECG signal, denoted by $S(t)$.

This study identifies and analyzes local maxima in the QRS complex, an integral part of ECG signal processing. The technique systematically extracts relevant information from ECG signals, enabling a deeper analysis of heart activity and possible abnormalities:

$$\overline{S}(t) = \frac{1}{\pi}\int_a^b S(\tau)\frac{1}{t-\tau}d\tau. \tag{10.4}$$

Since the independent variable is unchanged during this transformation, $\overline{S}(t)$, the resultant output, remains dependent on time, as shown by equation 10.4. Moreover, by convolution with $\frac{1}{\pi t}$, $\overline{S}(t)$ is a linear function of $S(t)$. The concept of the analytic signal or pre-envelope of a real signal $S(t)$ can be described by the expression:

$$y(t) = S(t) + j\overline{S}(t). \tag{10.5}$$

The envelope $B(t)$ of $y(t)$ is defined by

$$B(t) = \sqrt{S^2(t) + \overline{S}^2(t)}. \tag{10.6}$$

It can be seen that $B(t)$ is always a positive function. Hence, the maximum contribution to $B(t)$ occurs at points where the Hilbert transform gives $S(t) = 0$. The application of the HT to identify R peaks in ECG signals is addressed in this section. As a result of the HT's odd symmetry feature, the appropriate HT crosses the zero axis at each inflection point of the input ECG signal [19]. Figure 10.4 illustrates this characteristic. A zero crossing detector is implemented to detect zero crossings (ZCs) in the HT signal, as shown in figure 10.4(d), thus identifying local maxima corresponding to enhanced QRS characteristics.

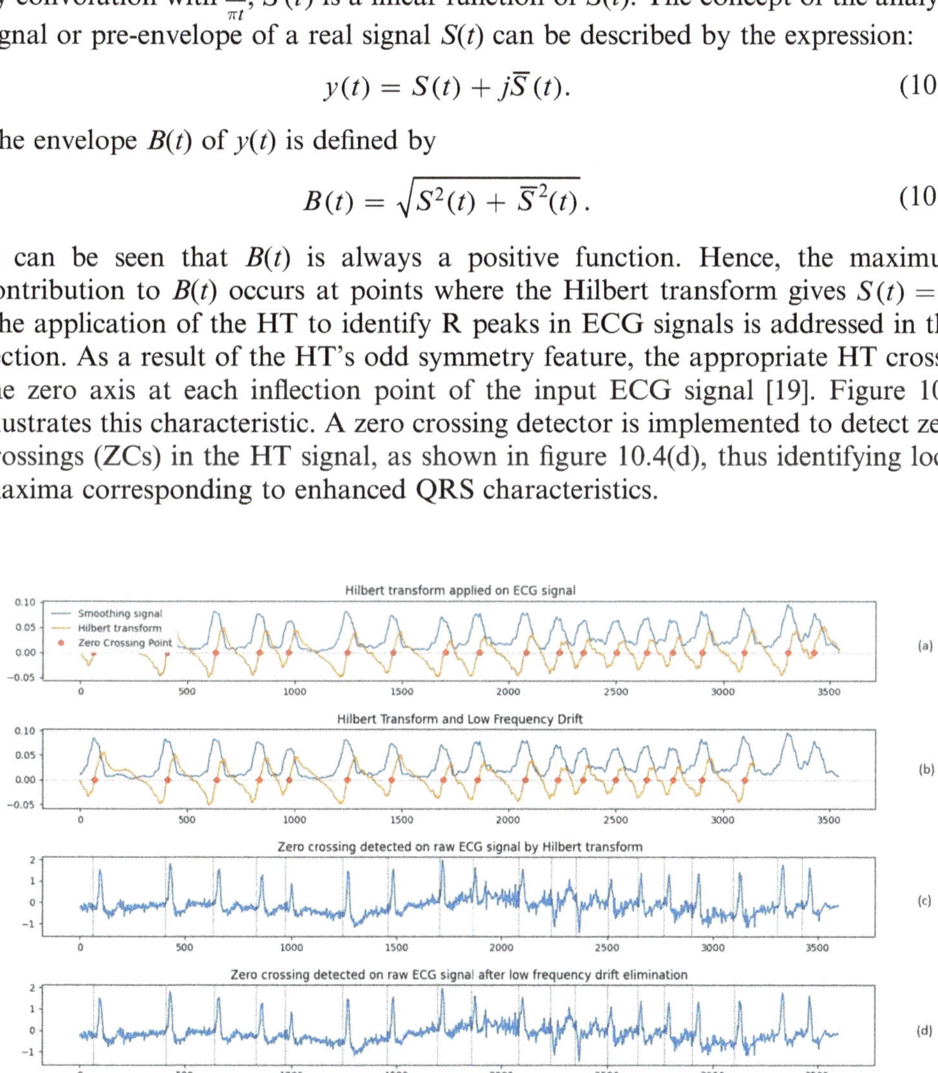

Figure 10.4. (a) Hilbert transform for an applied ordinary differentiator. (b) Hilbert transform with low-frequency drift eliminator for the applied fractional-order differentiation. (c) Zero crossings detected using only the Hilbert transform for the applied fractional-order differentiation. (d) Zero crossings detected by Hilbert transform with a low-frequency drift eliminator for the applied fractional order differentiation.

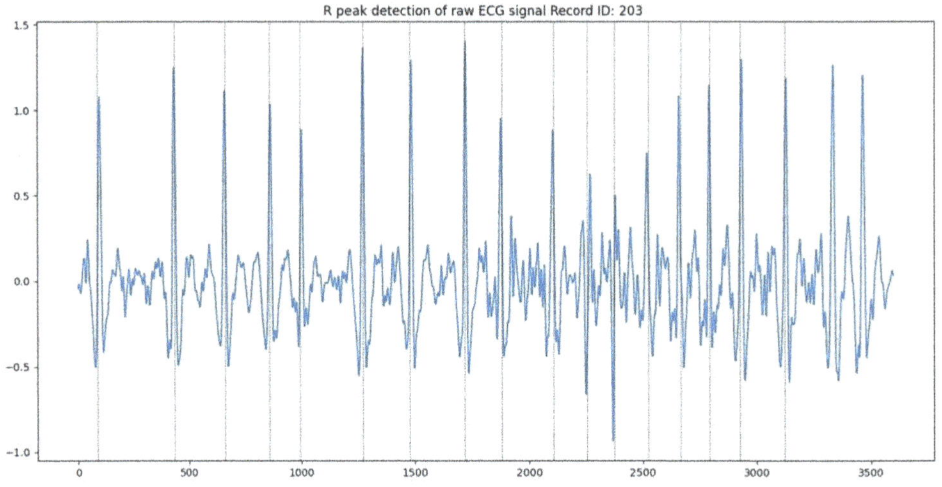

Figure 10.5. True R peak detection for ECG record ID: 203 achieved using fractional-order differentiaton and a Hilbert transform.

The actual R peak locations, shown by the black vertical lines in figure 10.5, can be identified by examining the input ECG record's absolute maximum amplitude within a narrow region of ± 25 samples surrounding each ZC. As shown in figure 10.4(d), it is empirically demonstrated that, in certain instances, the ZC positions of the HT sequence can vary slightly from the exact positions of the heartbeats. A rectification technique is used to address this. Following ZC point identification, the maximum points of the raw ECG signal are searched within the same ± 25 sample interval surrounding each ZC. As seen in figure 10.5, this modification step results in a more precise detection of the R peak time instants. The amplitude variation, timing, and sign of the peak difference between consecutive beats are a few of the parameters affecting ZC point variation. A filter length of $K = 400$ is applied to the HT output using a moving average filter to alleviate this problem. Specifically, this preprocessing step successfully detects R peaks within the MITDB context.

10.4.4 Feature extraction

These preprocessed data can be redefined by considering feature vectors representing the raw data's main characteristics and behavior. This study considers two types of features: temporal features and statistical features. The RR interval is regarded as a temporal feature that is based on the preceding and following RR intervals. The statistical features are extracted for a range of 356 ms across the R peak of the ECG signal. The following statistical parameters are used in constructing the feature matrix: the mean, variance, standard deviation, mean absolute value (MAV), sum of mode, harmonic mean, kurtosis, simple squared integral (SSI), RMS value, and Lyapunov exponent [36, 43, 44], as described in the following sections (S_i = signal, N = number of samples).

10.4.4.1 Mean

The mean of the segment of the ECG signal or given data set is calculated as follows [45]:

$$\text{mean} = \frac{1}{N}\sum_{j=1}^{N} S_j. \tag{10.7}$$

10.4.4.2 Variance

The variance measures the degree by which the amplitude values of the signal fluctuate or disperse over time. Greater variability in heartbeats, indicating disturbances in cardiac rhythm, is characterized by a higher variance. It is essential to monitor variations in ECG readings to identify arrhythmias and evaluate the stability of the heart's electrical activity [46]:

$$\text{var} = \frac{1}{N}\sum_{i=1}^{N} (S_i - \text{mean})^2. \tag{10.8}$$

10.4.4.3 Standard deviation

A statistical measure called standard deviation is used to quantify the dispersion of RR intervals, which shows the variability in heart rate. More significant abnormalities in heart rate patterns can be detected by a higher standard deviation, which may be indicative of cardiac disorders or failure of the autonomic nervous system:

$$\text{std} = \sqrt{\frac{1}{N}\sum_{i=1}^{N} (S_i - \text{mean})^2}\,. \tag{10.9}$$

10.4.4.4 Mean absolute value

The following formula gives the mean of a segment of the ECG signal [43]:

$$\text{MAV} = \frac{1}{N}\sum_{i=1}^{N} |S_i| \tag{10.10}$$

10.4.4.5 Sum of mode

The following formula estimates the sum of the nonnegative values of the data set [43]:

$$\text{SOM} = \sum_{i=1}^{N} |S_i|. \tag{10.11}$$

10.4.4.6 Harmonic mean

The harmonic mean, which uniformly distributes the weight of each data point, is a reliable technique for determining the averages of ratios and rates [43]. While it can reduce the effects of extreme numbers, it is appropriate for presenting an accurate representation of the general pattern. In light of this, the harmonic mean is an advantageous metric when analyzing data sets with different scales or when accurately determining rates and ratios is critical:

$$\text{harmonic mean} = \frac{N}{\sum_{i=1}^{N}\frac{1}{S_i}}. \tag{10.12}$$

10.4.4.7 Kurtosis

Kurtosis measures whether the distribution of an ECG signal is peaked or flat. Sharper peaks are indicated by higher kurtosis, which may suggest abnormalities in heart activity [46, 47]:

$$\text{kurtosis} = \frac{\frac{1}{N}\sum_{i-1}^{N}(S_i - \text{mean})^4}{\left(\sqrt{\frac{1}{N}\sum_{i-1}^{N}(S_i - \text{mean})^4}\right)^4}. \tag{10.13}$$

10.4.4.8 Simple squared integral

The SSI is calculated by integrating a squared data set [43]:

$$\text{SSI} = \frac{1}{N}\sum_{i=1}^{N}(S_i)^2. \tag{10.14}$$

10.4.4.9 RR interval ratio

The RR interval ratio measures the variability between consecutive R waves in an ECG [48]. Higher or lower heart rate variability is indicative of abnormal cardiovascular health. Monitoring the RR interval ratio can reveal details about the general physiological flexibility of the heart:

$$\text{RRI} = \frac{R_{i+1} + R_i}{R_i + R_{i-1}}. \tag{10.15}$$

10.4.4.10 Root mean square

In the context of an ECG, the root mean square (RMS) is the square root of the average of the squared data points. It gives an overview of signal strength or cardiac activity intensity and assists in signal assessment [45]. This tool helps us to understand the properties of the ECG waveform and recognize abnormalities:

$$\text{RMS} = \sqrt{\frac{1}{N}\sum_{i=1}^{N}(S_i)^2}. \tag{10.16}$$

10.4.4.11 Lyapunov exponent

The ECG, like other physiological signals such as the photoplethysmogram (PPG) and the electroencephalogram (EEG), displays signs of chaos in the shape of its higher derivative. Lyapunov exponents represent the separation rate of infinitesimally close trajectories [44] and are thus better metrics for representing the chaotic behavior of a time-series signal. If λ denotes the Lyapunov exponent, the sampling frequency, 360 Hz, can be employed to calculate the absolute value of the greatest Lyapunov exponent for each segment of an ECG:

$$\delta x(t) = e^{\lambda t}\,|\delta x_0|. \tag{10.17}$$

10.4.4.12 Teager energy operator

A prominent tool for nonlinear energy tracking in speech applications is the Teager energy operator (TEO). Rather than depending exclusively on measuring the signal's energy, the TEO can also measure the energy of the system that generated it, including mechanical and physical aspects. In real-time applications, TEO's high temporal resolution allows it to capture quick changes in a signal's energy. Utilizing just three samples, its operation is almost instantaneous. The efficacy of TEO is derived from its ability to identify variations in the energy required to generate signals with the same amplitude but different frequencies. Higher-frequency tones require more energy, which TEO's output aptly reflects. Furthermore, TEO can track a signal's instantaneous frequency, amplitude envelope, and energy [49–51].

TEO's typically positive outcome when simulating energy from a single source is one of its significant characteristics. On the other hand, intervals of negative energy can appear when TEO models energy from several sources. This property can detect deviations from the typical sinus rhythm or disruptions in the pathways that generate and conduct impulses:

$$\mathrm{TEO}_i = S_i^2 - S_{i-1}S_{i+1}. \tag{10.18}$$

10.4.4.13 QRS area ratio

The QRS area ratio (QAR) across the R peak location can be defined as follows [30]:

$$\mathrm{area}_L = \sum_{k=1}^{N} |\mathrm{coef}(i-k)| \tag{10.19}$$

$$\mathrm{area}_R = \sum_{k=1}^{N} |\mathrm{coef}(i+k)| \tag{10.20}$$

$$\mathrm{QAR} = \frac{\max(\mathrm{area}_L, \mathrm{area}_R)}{\min(\mathrm{area}_L, \mathrm{area}_R)}. \tag{10.21}$$

In the context provided, area_L and area_R denote the left and right areas around the R peak. The terms coef($i-k$) and coef($i+k$) represent the kth detailed coefficients before and after the R peak. The parameter N signifies the number of points utilized for summation, which is set explicitly to eight in this scenario due to its demonstrated high classification efficiency while minimizing hardware overhead. This value of N ensures optimized performance in ECG signal analysis and classification tasks, balancing computational efficiency and accuracy.

In this way, the feature is extracted from the raw ECG signal, expressed above, using equations 10.7 to 10.21.

10.5 Theory of ANN

Machine learning models that emulate the composition and operations of the human brain are known as ANN classifiers. ANNs are composed of artificial neurons that are layered and connected. They process input data, extract features, and develop predictions. Their ability to identify complex patterns in data and generate accurate estimates in various disciplines, such as image recognition, natural language processing, and time-series prediction, has resulted in the enormous popularity of these classifiers.

The ANN classifier, a computing unit that applies elementary computations to input data, is the fundamental building block of ANNs, as shown in figure 10.6. After receiving inputs from the previous layer, each neuron transforms the data using an activation function and delivers its outcome to the following layer. An input layer, one or more hidden layers, and an output layer comprise an ANN classifier's architecture. Raw data characteristics are given to the input layer, and the hidden layers gradually extract higher-level representations of the input. The output layer finally produces the anticipated class labels or probabilities. Optimizing an ANN classifier's weights and biases to minimize a specific loss function is referred to as training. Typically, gradient-based optimization techniques, such as the Adam optimizer and stochastic gradient descent (SGD), can be utilized. To minimize prediction errors, the model iteratively modifies its parameters during training based on the gradients of the loss function related to the parameters. The choice of activation function, which adds nonlinearity to the network and allows it to learn complicated mappings between inputs and outputs, is one of the essential elements of the ANN classifier. Regular activation functions include rectified linear units (ReLUs), tanh, sigmoid function, and variations. These functions control each neuron's output and are critical in determining the rate at which the model learns, whether or not it captures complex patterns in the data, and how it develops overall.

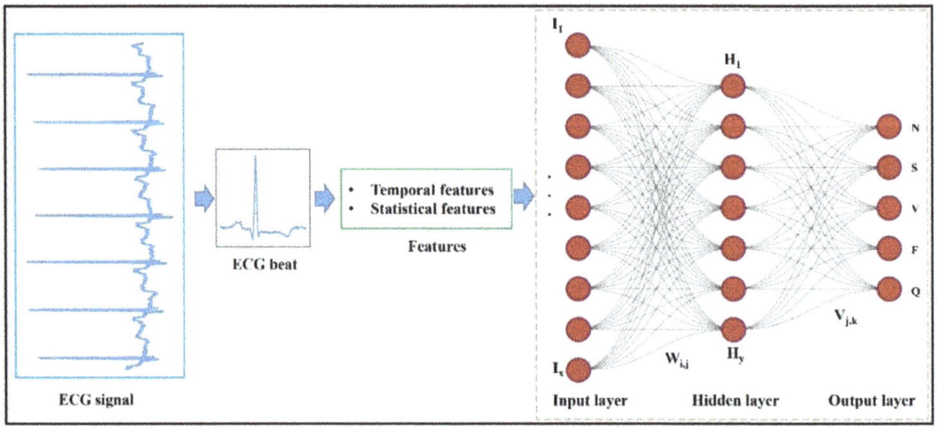

Figure 10.6. The ANN classifier and feature extraction.

The size and design of the network, the quantity and quality of training data, the selection of activation functions, and hyperparameters such as learning rate and regularization strength are a few of the variables that affect an ANN classifier's effectiveness. Enhancing performance and generalizing to unknown data requires meticulous model evaluation through cross validation and hyperparameter modification.

10.5.1 Rectified linear unit functions

ReLUs are popular activation functions in ANN hidden layers. ReLUs add nonlinearity to a model by substituting zero for all negative values and allowing positive values to flow unaltered. ReLU's non-saturation property and simplicity help it to converge more quickly during training than other activation functions, such as sigmoid or hyperbolic tangent (tanh) functions. Deep neural networks can learn more efficiently and effectively by preventing the output from approaching a constant for extreme inputs or the saturation area:

$$\phi_1 = \max(0, F_i). \tag{10.22}$$

10.5.2 Softmax function

The softmax activation function is typically employed in neural network output layers for multiclass classification tasks. It converts the raw output scores (logits) into probability distributions. The following expression mathematically represents K-class categorization:

$$\phi_2 = \frac{e^{F_i}}{\sum_{i=1}^{N} e^{F_i}}. \tag{10.23}$$

10.5.3 Step function

The most basic activation function returns a value of one if the input is greater than or equal to zero; if not, it returns zero. Due to its abrupt nature and inability to support gradient-based optimization, it is rarely employed in current neural networks:

$$\phi_3 = \begin{cases} 1; & 0 \leqslant F_i \\ 0; & \text{elsewhere} \end{cases}. \tag{10.24}$$

10.5.4 Sigmoid function

This function is helpful when difficulties are encountered with binary classification. It provides probabilities, since it normalizes the input values into the range from zero to one. Unfortunately, it has a problem with vanishing gradients, which makes deep network training challenging:

$$\phi_4 = \frac{1}{1 + e^{F_i}}. \tag{10.25}$$

10.5.5 Hyperbolic tangent function

The tanh function flattens the input values into the range from −1 to 1, which is similar to the behavior of the sigmoid function. Under certain conditions, its more comprehensive output range (compared to that of the sigmoid) may accelerate convergence:

$$\phi_5 = \frac{e^{F_i} + e^{-F_i}}{e^{F_i} - e^{-F_i}}. \quad (10.26)$$

10.5.6 Exponential linear unit function

While the exponential linear unit (ELU) function is comparable to the ReLU function, it can assist in solving the vanishing gradient problem by yielding a straight line for negative input values:

$$\phi_6 = \begin{cases} F_i; & 0 \leqslant F_i \\ \alpha(e^{F_i} - 1); & \text{elsewhere} \end{cases}. \quad (10.27)$$

10.5.7 Implementation of ANN

The ANN employed in this work is organized as follows: as illustrated in figure 10.6, it has an input layer with x nodes, a hidden layer with y nodes, and an output layer with five nodes. The number of input variables (denoted by p) changes based on the model's specific design factors. Equation (10.28) governs the computation of the number of nodes, N, in the hidden layer. The architecture of the neural network used in the study is described in this form:

$$N \leqslant \frac{y^{\mathrm{TR}}}{y^{I} + 1} \quad (10.28)$$

In equation (10.28), y denotes the number of nodes in the hidden layer, y^{TR} is the number of samples used for training, and y^{I} is the total number of inputs [52].

The output values are transformed into probabilities by softmax to make sure they add up to one. Every node in the final result indicates the likelihood of the input fitting into a particular class. The network is more confident in its predictions when it employs the exponential function in the softmax to emphasize the outstanding values and suppress smaller ones. Softmax can be particularly helpful when there are several classes and the network needs to assign a probability distribution over all possible classes. It is an essential part of the last layer of neural networks constructed for classification tasks, since it makes the results easy to comprehend. The RELU and softmax functions are each node's two distinct activation functions, based on equations (10.22) and (10.23), respectively. In this work, softmax was used as the activation function for the nodes in the output layer, while RELU was chosen as the activation function for the hidden layer nodes.

The weight matrices $W_{i,j}$ and $V_{j,k}$ reflect the node connections within each layer. The initial values of these weights are chosen randomly, with values selected from a uniform distribution between −1 and 1. These starting weights and biases are modified throughout training to improve the network's performance [53]:

$$H_j = \phi_1\left(\sum_{i=1}^{x} I_i W_{i,j} + b1_j\right) \tag{10.29}$$

$$O_k = \phi_2\left(\sum_{j=1}^{y} H_j V_{j,k} + b2_k\right). \tag{10.30}$$

10.6 Results and discussion

10.6.1 Experimental setup

The AAMI standard ECG beat classification using an ANN classifier combines FOD and HT approaches. The complete implementation uses an STM32F407VE microcontroller for ECG beat classification in real time, as shown in figure 10.7. These parts are combined into a single apparatus for thorough ECG data processing and classification. The 33500B waveform generator, a capable instrument, facilitates data acquisition for this setup. The ability to produce ECG signals allows the system to be tested thoroughly and validated under controlled conditions with various simulated cardiac signals, thus ensuring the reliability and versatility of the device across a spectrum of cardiac conditions.

The essence of this system's signal processing ability comes from the use of FOD. This affects the preprocessing applied to the ECG signal and the extraction of its analytic representation, which are crucial for identifying the instantaneous phase and amplitude. These features are needed because they establish the basis for distinguishing unique characteristics in ECG beats. The use of FOD also emphasizes the signal's features, particularly harsh transitions and peaks that signify cardiac

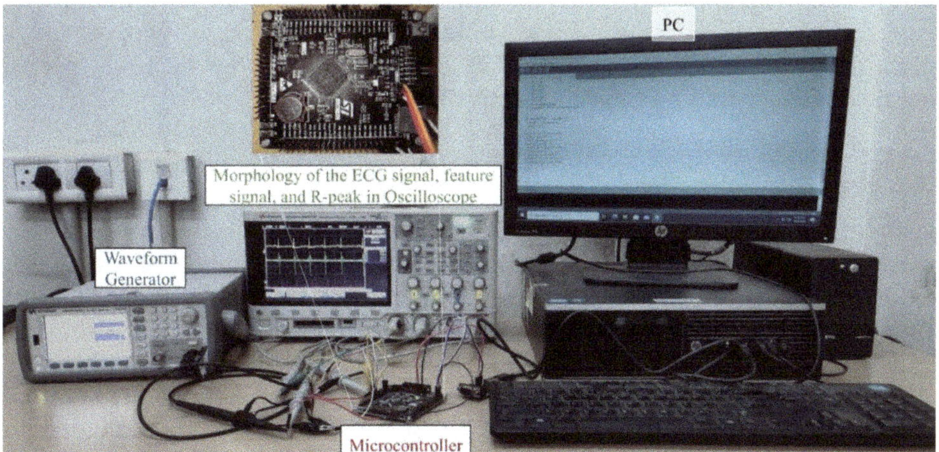

Figure 10.7. Experimental setup for arrhythmia classification.

events. This method surpasses traditional differentiation by enabling more precise manipulation of the frequency components within the signal and enhancing the visibility of features, which are vital for classification. The heart of the classification is the ANN, often known as an ANN classifier. The ANN is perfectly trained to categorize ECG beats by learning from a data set of labeled ECG signals.

This exemplary machine learning is instrumental in distinguishing different beat types. It uses the features extracted during the signal processing stage to achieve high classification accuracy. The signal processing and machine learning operations are implemented on the STM32F407VE microcontroller. Chosen for its strong computational power and efficiency, it also has an ideal, compact form factor; it is perfect for real-time analysis and portable medical applications. It runs the preprocessing, feature extraction, and classification algorithms, showing its ability to handle the complex operations necessary for accurate ECG beat classification.

Following the AAMI standards is a sure-fire way to ensure that a system's classifications are medically relevant and trustworthy. These standards benchmark the system's performance, confirming that its classifications align with clinical expectations and contribute effectively to medical diagnostics. All these advanced technologies and methodologies, and their integration into a single device, represent significant advancements in portable medical diagnostics, offering complete solutions for ECG beat classification in real time. This integration not only meets the needs of healthcare professionals today but also provides the foundation for future innovations.

A systematic framework for classifying ECG results is provided by the AAMI standard classifications of ECG interpretation: N (normal), S (supraventricular), V (ventricular), F (fusion), and Q (unknown), as shown in figure 10.2. A typical ECG trace that displays a regular heart rhythm and shape is represented by the N class. Abnormalities such as atrial fibrillation or superventricular flutter are classified as S class. The V class contains ventricular arrhythmias such as ventricular fibrillation and tachycardia. The F class represents fusion beats resulting from normal and aberrant electrical activity. Finally, patterns not consistently classified into the other classes fall under the Q class. These standardized classifications support efficient communication and decision-making in clinical practice by helping specialists accurately identify and address cardiac problems.

10.6.2 R peak identification

The algorithm for R peak detection works as shown in figure 10.2, and a summary of R peak detection can be seen in table 10.5. This study highlights the use of digital fractional order differentiation (DFOD), which is preferred over traditional differentiation techniques. To accurately identify the true QRS complex within ECG signals and to make it easier to compute A-CLT for preprocessing tasks, this DFOD approach incorporates an adaptive threshold technique. In this context, we propose a new technique based on DFOD, whose performance is thoroughly evaluated using the MITDB database. Figure 10.8 illustrates real-time R peak detection displayed in a digital storage oscilloscope.

Table 10.5. Performance summary for QRS complex identification using the MITDB. Key: T_P—true peaks; F_P—false positives; F_N—false negatives; P_P—positive predictivity; S_e—sensitivity.

ECG record	Total peaks	T_P	F_P	F_N	P_P (in %)	S_e (%)	F1-score (%)
100	2273	2273	0	0	100	100	100
101	1865	1864	4	1	99.78	99.94	99.86
102	2187	2186	1	1	99.95	99.95	99.95
103	2084	2084	1	0	99.95	100	99.97
104	2230	2225	10	5	99.55	99.77	99.66
105	2574	2567	11	7	99.57	99.73	99.65
106	2027	2015	4	12	99.80	99.41	99.60
107	2138	2136	3	2	99.86	99.91	99.88
108	1762	1749	26	13	98.53	99.26	98.89
109	2532	2532	3	0	99.88	100	99.94
111	2124	2123	2	1	99.90	99.95	99.93
112	2539	2539	1	0	99.96	100	99.98
113	1795	1793	1	2	99.94	99.89	99.91
114	1879	1877	1	2	99.95	99.89	99.92
115	1953	1953	0	0	100	100	100
116	2410	2399	4	11	99.83	99.54	99.68
117	1535	1535	0	0	100	100	100
118	2278	2278	6	0	99.74	100	99.86
119	1987	1987	1	0	99.95	100	99.97
121	1863	1863	0	0	100	100	100
122	2477	2476	0	1	100	99.96	99.98
123	1518	1518	1	0	99.93	100	99.97
124	1620	1619	0	1	100	99.94	99.97
200	2601	2600	8	1	99.70	99.96	99.82
201	1963	1961	2	2	99.90	99.90	99.90
202	2136	2134	0	2	100	99.90	99.95
203	2980	2843	16	137	99.44	95.40	97.38
205	2656	2654	0	2	100	99.92	99.96
207	2306	2154	19	152	99.12	93.41	96.18
208	2955	2949	2	6	99.93	99.80	99.86
209	3005	3005	1	0	99.97	100	99.98
210	2650	2646	2	4	99.92	99.85	99.88
212	2748	2748	1	0	99.96	100	99.98
213	3251	3248	0	3	100	99.91	99.95
214	2262	2261	1	1	99.96	99.96	99.95
215	3363	3361	1	2	99.97	99.94	99.95
217	2208	2208	2	0	99.91	100	99.95
219	2155	2154	0	1	100	99.95	99.97
220	2049	2048	1	1	99.95	99.95	99.95
221	2427	2427	0	0	100	100	100
222	2483	2481	4	2	99.84	99.92	99.88

(*Continued*)

Table 10.5. (*Continued*)

ECG record	Total peaks	T_P	F_P	F_N	P_P (in %)	S_e (%)	F1-score (%)
223	2605	2605	1	0	99.96	100	99.98
228	2053	2048	10	5	99.51	99.75	99.63
230	2257	2256	2	1	99.911	99.95	99.93
231	1571	1567	5	4	99.68	99.74	99.71
232	1780	1778	5	2	99.72	99.88	99.80
233	3080	3079	0	1	100	99.97	99.98
234	2753	2753	1	0	99.96	100	99.98
Total	**109 935**	**109 559**	**157**	**376**	**99.85**	**99.66**	**99.75**

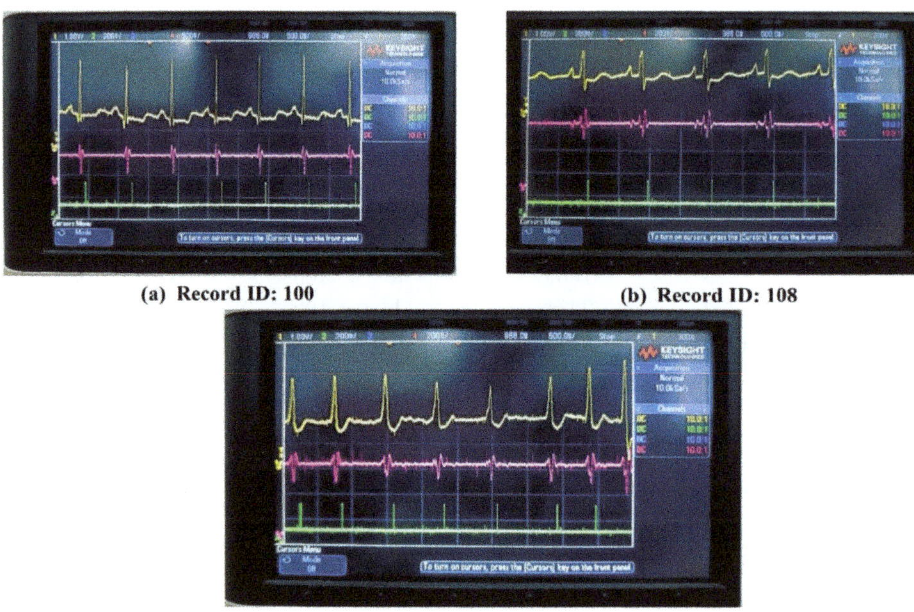

(a) Record ID: 100 **(b) Record ID: 108**

(c) Record ID: 203

Figure 10.8. Real-time ECG beat identification for record IDs 100, 108, and 203.

The research findings show that the suggested technique can correctly identify 109 559 true beats out of an extensive data set of 109 935 beats in total. This validation highlights the stability and reliability of the DFOD-based approach and confirms its effectiveness in consistently detecting true QRS complexes within the complex patterns of ECG signals. Multiple measures must be evaluated to properly evaluate the technique's performance, as table 10.5 extensively illustrates. The total number of ECG beats (TB), the accurate determination of true positive peaks (TP), the occurrence of false negative peaks (FN), the sensitivity (Se), the positive predictivity (PP), and the F-score are just a few of the parameters included in these measures. Upon closer examination of the results, it is evident that a perfect 100% score for positive predictivity is achieved for some recordings. In particular, recordings 115, 117, 121, 122, 124, 202, 205, 213, 219, 221, and 233 stand out as excellent instances, demonstrating the accuracy with which the system can recognize true beats. In addition, records 100, 103, 109, 112, 115, 117, 118, 119, 121, 123, 209, 212, 217, 221, 223, and 234 demonstrate an incredible sensitivity of 100%, confirming the algorithm's ability to identify true peaks reliably.

This thorough analysis of the algorithm's performance metrics offers essential new information about how well and consistently it handles various ECG signals. Moreover, it is necessary to highlight that, as illustrated by specific instances such as records 108, 203, and 207, the suggested DFOD-based algorithm functions well even when applied to complicated ECG recordings. These illustrations prove the technique's capacity to negotiate complex signal patterns successfully. The algorithm performs relatively well; for example, in record 108, it recognizes only 26 incorrect peaks and achieves a positive predictivity rate of 98.53% for R peak identification. It is also important to note that this data set has a maximum of 152 false negative peaks, emphasizing the algorithm's robustness and capacity to manage difficult situations while retaining consistent reliability and precision.

Furthermore, the data in table 10.4 shows that 99.85% of the QRS complexes are accurately identified. The accuracy of this detection is demonstrated by the fact that only 0.14 of the recorded peaks are incorrectly classified as false beats but are nevertheless recognized as true QRS complexes. Although the algorithm's accuracy is commendable, the slight inadequacy in recognizing 0.34 of true QRS complexes should be highlighted. However, it is important to highlight how much this technique contributes to producing outstanding results for particular ECG recordings. In particular, it makes it easier to identify 12 ECG recordings in which false positive (FP) beats are not recognized and 16 records in which false negative (FN) beats are not detected. The accuracy and dependability of the algorithm are further demonstrated by the fact that none of the beats in the five records is incorrectly categorized as a false positive or a false negative. The ECG signal's various characteristics, including many artifacts, must also be emphasized for study. This variability highlights the complexity of the signal analysis and illustrates the algorithm's robustness and adaptability to various changes and difficulties.

10.6.3 ECG beat identification

Following R peak identification, the data set's ECG beat classification is divided into two parts, DS1 and DS2, as shown in table 10.6. DS1 contains 22 thirty-minute recordings, which are employed to train and test the ANN. The other twenty-two records, designated as DS2, are kept for testing. DS2 contains examples of each record type in the MITDB collection. This section ensures that the evaluation framework is strong enough for an in-depth evaluation of the ANN's performance

Table 10.6. Different classes contained in the training and testing data sets.

ECG beat	Total data set	Training data set (DS1)	Testing data set (DS2)
N	46,074	3883	42,191
S	3871	1642	2229
V	6816	2345	4471
F	1413	760	653
Q	62	42	20

	N	S	V	F	Q
N	40243	45	900	924	4
S	172	1726	128	63	160
V	202	102	4037	20	165
F	86	61	17	438	51
Q	1	8	1	1	9

Figure 10.9. Confusion matrix for ECG beat classification.

on various data sets. Careful segmentation like this is essential for establishing confidence in the ANN's performance and capacity to generalize outside the training set, increasing its applicability in a wide range of real-world applications.

Using a tenfold cross validation technique, the classifier chosen for the final model design was extensively evaluated. This approach guaranteed the dependability of the test method. Key indicators, such as true positives (TPs), true negatives (TNs), FPs, and FNs, were rigorously computed during the evaluation procedure. Figure 10.9 represents the confusion matrix for the ECG types. These metrics offer insightful information about the classifier's capacity to categorize data set members correctly.

Cross validation is used to verify the classifier's performance and reduce the possibility of overfitting; it confirms that the model's generalization abilities have been sufficiently evaluated using various data subsets. This comprehensive assessment procedure enhances the classifier's efficacy and establishes an adequate basis for its easy incorporation into the final model, improving its predictive capabilities and applicability.

$$\text{accuracy} = \frac{\text{TP} + \text{TN}}{\text{TP} + \text{FP} + \text{TN} + \text{FN}} \tag{10.31}$$

$$\text{sensitivity} = \frac{\text{TP}}{\text{TP} + \text{FN}} \tag{10.32}$$

$$\text{F1-score}=2 \cdot \frac{\text{precision} \cdot \text{recall}}{\text{precision} + \text{recall}}. \tag{10.33}$$

Table 10.7 represents a complete classifier performance evaluation. A comprehensive assessment of the classifier's predicted performance across a range of tasks is provided in this table. The vertical axis of the confusion matrix format shows the actual activity labels, and the horizontal axis indicates the predicted activity labels. Numerical data indicating the classifier's predictions against the actual truth are contained in each matrix cell. To be more precise, the correct predictions for each assignment are represented by the confusion matrix's diagonal members. These numbers demonstrate the degree to which the classifier identified distinct activities. Conversely, the off-diagonal elements show the false prediction rate for each activity by showing the times when the classifier made inaccurate predictions. Figure 10.9 is a graphic illustration of these metrics, showing incorrect prediction rates. With the help of this representation, one can gain a more profound knowledge of the classifier's performance and its advantages and disadvantages over other activity classifiers.

Advancements in the field of real-time ECG arrhythmia detection made by implementing digital neural networks suggest the potential replacement of conventional ANN classifiers with more effective structures. The efficiency and accuracy of ECG arrhythmia identification in clinical applications can be significantly improved. Digitally implemented neural networks can replace conventional ANN classifiers, improving processing speed and resource efficiency and increasing the viability and accuracy of real-time detection. One can reduce processing overhead and preserve or even enhance detection performance by emphasizing the most critical components of the ECG signal through selective feature extraction, which optimizes computational complexity.

Table 10.7. Performance matrix.

ECG type	Accuracy (%)	Sensitivity (%)	F1-score
N	94.90	95.56	0.97
S	98.33	76.75	0.82
V	96.60	67.96	0.57
F	97.26	67.08	0.41
Q	99.11	45.00	0.04
Average	**97.24**	**70.47**	**0.56**

10.7 Conclusions

R peak detection in ECG signals is effectively achieved using this hardware implementation on the Arduino Mega 2560, yielding outstanding efficiency metrics such as a positive predictivity of 99.85%, a sensitivity of 99.66%, and an F1-score of 99.75%. In addition, the ANN classifier complies with the AAMI standard and achieves a respectable accuracy of 97.24% in detecting ECG beats. These results highlight the effectiveness and dependability of our suggested approach for processing and analyzing ECG signals in real time. We developed a reliable solution that has the potential for application in various clinical and personal health monitoring applications by utilizing the Arduino Mega 2560's processing capability. In the future, further improvements and optimizations can be explored to boost the system's efficiency. However, the results indicate a substantial advancement in developing portable and practical ECG monitoring devices, advancing patient care and healthcare technology.

Acknowledgments

This research has received no external funding.

References and further reading

[1] Attack H 2013 What is the electrocardiogram ECG

[2] Azuaje F, Clifford G D, McSharry P E *et al* 2006 *Advanced Methods and Tools for ECG Data Analysis* **vol 10** (Boston, MA: Artech House) https://us.artechhouse.com/Advanced-Methods-and-Tools-for-ECG-Data-Analysis-P957.aspx

[3] Dai M and Lian S-L 2009 Removal of baseline wander from dynamic electrocardiogram signals *2nd Int. Congress on Image and Signal Processing* (Piscataway, NJ: IEEE) 1–4

[4] Ziarani A K and Konrad A 2002 A nonlinear adaptive method of elimination of power line interference in ecg signals *IEEE Trans. Biomed. Eng.* **49** 540–7

[5] Friesen G M, Jannett T C, Jadallah M A, Yates S L, Quint S R and Nagle H T 1990 A comparison of the noise sensitivity of nine QRS detection algorithms *IEEE Trans. Biomed. Eng.* **37** 85–98

[6] Nayak C, Saha S K, Kar R and Mandal D 2020 Efficient design of zero-phase riesz fractional order digital differentiator using manta-ray foraging optimisation for precise electrocardiogram QRS detection *IEEE Open J. Circuits Syst.* **1** 280–92

[7] Tekeste T, Saleh H, Mohammad B and Ismail M 2018 Ultra-low power QRS detection and ECG compression architecture for IoT healthcare devices *IEEE Trans. Circuits Syst.* I **66** 669–79

[8] Sharma L D and Sunkaria R K 2016 A robust QRS detection using novel pre-processing techniques and kurtosis based enhanced efficiency *Measurement* **87** 194–204

[9] Arif M, Malagore I A and Afsar F A 2012 Detection and localization of myocardial infarction using k-nearest neighbor classifier *J. Med. Syst.* **36** 279–89

[10] Lin H-Y, Liang S-Y, Ho Y-L, Lin Y-H and Ma H-P 2014 Discrete-wavelet-transform-based noise removal and feature extraction for ECG signals *Irbm* **35** 351–61

[11] Liu H, Hu J and Rauterberg M 2009 Music playlist recommendation based on user heartbeat and music preference *2009 Int. Conf. on Computer Technology and Development* (Piscataway, NJ: IEEE) **vol 1** 545–9
[12] Khare S K, Gadre V M and Acharya U R 2023 ECGPsychNet: an optimized hybrid ensemble model for automatic detection of psychiatric disorders using ECG signals *Physiol. Meas.* **44** 115004
[13] Rakshit M and Das S 2017 An efficient wavelet-based automated R-peaks detection method using Hilbert transform *Biocybern. Biomed. Eng.* **37** 566–77
[14] Deepu C J and Lian Y 2014 A joint QRS detection and data compression scheme for wearable sensors *IEEE Trans. Biomed. Eng.* **62** 165–75
[15] Pandit D, Zhang L, Liu C, Chattopadhyay S, Aslam N and Lim C P 2017 A lightweight QRS detector for single lead ECG signals using a max-min difference algorithm *Comput. Methods Programs Biomed.* **144** 61–75
[16] Sahoo S, Biswal P, Das T and Sabut S 2016 De-noising of ECG signal and QRS detection using hilbert transform and adaptive thresholding *Procedia Technol.* **25** 68–75
[17] Manikandan M S and Soman K 2012 A novel method for detecting R-peaks in electrocardiogram (ECG) signal *Biomed. Signal Process. Control* **7** 118–28
[18] Kaur A, Agarwal A, Agarwal R and Kumar S 2019 A novel approach to ECG R-peak detection *Arab. J. Sci. Eng.* **44** 6679–91
[19] Nayak C, Saha S K, Kar R and Mandal D 2019 An optimally designed digital differentiator based preprocessor for R-peak detection in electrocardiogram signal *Biomed. Signal Process. Control* **49** 440–64
[20] Madeiro J P, Cortez P C, Marques J A, Seisdedos C R and Sobrinho C R 2012 An innovative approach of QRS segmentation based on first-derivative, Hilbert and wavelet transforms *Med. Eng. Phys.* **34** 1236–46
[21] Nayak C, Saha S K, Kar R and Mandal D 2019 An efficient and robust digital fractional order differentiator based ECG pre-processor design for QRS detection *IEEE Trans. Biomed. Circuits Syst.* **13** 682–96
[22] Thurner T, Hintermueller C, Blessberger H and Steinwender C 2021 Complex-pan-tompkins-wavelets: cross-channel ECG beat detection and delineation *Biomed. Signal Process. Control* **66** 102450
[23] Rahul J, Sora M and Sharma L D 2021 Dynamic thresholding based efficient QRS complex detection with low computational overhead *Biomed. Signal Process. Control* **67** 102519
[24] Tueche F, Mohamadou Y, Djeukam A, Kouekeu L C N, Seujip R and Tonka M 2021 Embedded algorithm for QRS detection based on signal shape *IEEE Trans. Instrum. Meas.* **70** 1–12
[25] Zidelmal Z, Amirou A, Ould-Abdeslam D, Moukadem A and Dieterlen A 2014 QRS detection using S-transform and Shannon energy *Comput. Methods Programs Biomed.* **116** 1–9
[26] Mukhopadhyay S K and Krishnan S 2020 Robust identification of QRS-complexes in electrocardiogram signals using a combination of interval and trigonometric threshold values *Biomed. Signal Process. Control* **61** 102007
[27] Yakut Ö and Bolat E D 2018 An improved QRS complex detection method having low computational load *Biomed. Signal Process. Control* **42** 230–41
[28] Xiong H, Liang M and Liu J 2021 A real-time QRS detection algorithm based on energy segmentation for exercise electrocardiogram *Circuits Syst. Signal Process.* **40** 4969–85

[29] Zhang F and Lian Y 2009 QRS detection based on multiscale mathematical morphology for wearable ECG devices in body area networks *IEEE Trans. Biomed. Circuits Syst.* **3** 220–8
[30] Chen Z, Luo J, Lin K, Wu J, Zhu T, Xiang X and Meng J 2017 An energy-efficient ECG processor with weak-strong hybrid classifier for arrhythmia detection *IEEE Trans. Circuits Syst. Express Briefs* **65** 948–52
[31] Pławiak P 2018 Novel methodology of cardiac health recognition based on ECG signals and evolutionary-neural system *Expert Syst. Appl.* **92** 334–49
[32] Raj S and Ray K C 2018 A personalized point-of-care platform for real-time ECG monitoring *IEEE Trans. Consum. Electron.* **64** 452–60
[33] Raj S 2020 An efficient IoT-based platform for remote real-time cardiac activity monitoring *IEEE Trans. Consum. Electron.* **66** 106–14
[34] Raj S, Chand G P and Ray K C 2015 Arm-based arrhythmia beat monitoring system *Microprocess. Microsyst.* **39** 504–11
[35] Raj S and Ray K C 2018 Sparse representation of ECG signals for automated recognition of cardiac arrhythmias *Expert Syst. Appl.* **105** 49–61
[36] Thomas M, Das M K and Ari S 2015 Automatic ECG arrhythmia classification using dual tree complex wavelet based features *AEU-Int. J. Electron. Commun.* **69** 715–21
[37] Das M K and Ari S 2014 ECG beats classification using mixture of features *Int. Sch. Res. Notices* **2014** 178436
[38] Marsili I A, Biasiolli L, Masè M, Adami A, Andrighetti A O, Ravelli F and Nollo G 2020 Implementation and validation of real-time algorithms for atrial fibrillation detection on a wearable ECG device *Comput. Biol. Med.* **116** 103540
[39] Martis R J, Acharya U R and Min L C 2013 ECG beat classification using PCA, LDA, ICA and discrete wavelet transform *Biomed. Signal Process. Control* **8** 437–48
[40] Allam J P, Samantray S and Ari S 2020 Spec: a system for patient specific ECG beat classification using deep residual network *Biocybern. Biomed. Eng.* **40** 1446–57
[41] Mar T, Zaunseder S, Martínez J P, Llamedo M and Poll R 2011 Optimization of ECG classification by means of feature selection *IEEE Trans. Biomed. Eng.* **58** 2168–77
[42] Anwar S M, Gul M, Majid M, Alnowami M *et al* 2018 Arrhythmia classification of ECG signals using hybrid features *Comput. Math. Methods Med.* **2018** 1380348
[43] Arif M and Kattan A 2015 Physical activities monitoring using wearable acceleration sensors attached to the body *PLoS One* **10** e0130851
[44] Rosenstein M T, Collins J J and De Luca C J 1993 A practical method for calculating largest lyapunov exponents from small data sets *Physica* D **65** 117–34
[45] Shen Y, Cai Z, Zhang L, Lin B-S, Li J and Liu C 2024 Efficient premature ventricular contraction detection based on network dynamics features *IEEE Trans. Instrum. Meas.* **73** 1–15
[46] Sadhukhan D, Dhar S, Pal S and Mitra M 2019 Automated screening of myocardial infarction based on statistical analysis of photoplethysmo-graphic data *IEEE Trans. Instrum. Meas.* **69** 2881–90
[47] Tripathy R K, Bhattacharyya A and Pachori R B 2019 A novel approach for detection of myocardial infarction from ECG signals of multiple electrodes *IEEE Sens. J.* **19** 4509–17
[48] Chen Z, Xu H, Luo J, Zhu T and Meng J 2018 Low-power perceptron model based ECG processor for premature ventricular contraction detection *Microprocess. Microsyst.* **59** 29–36
[49] Beyramienanlou H 2021 A robust method to reliable cardiac QRS complex detection based on Shannon energy and teager energy operator *Circuits Syst. Signal Process.* **40** 980–92

[50] El Bouny L, Khalil M and Adib A 2020 A Wavelet Denoising and Teager Energy Operator-Based Method for Automatic QRS Complex Detection in ECG Signal *Circuits Syst. Signal Process.* **39** 4943–79

[51] Kamath C 2011 ECG beat classification using features extracted from Teager energy functions in time and frequency domains *IET Signal Proc.* **5** 575–81

[52] Tian W, Liao Z and Zhang J 2017 An optimization of artificial neural network model for predicting chlorophyll dynamics *Ecol. Modell.* **364** 42–52

[53] Zhao Y, Shang Z and Lian Y 2019 A 13.34 μw event-driven patient-specific ann cardiac arrhythmia classifier for wearable ECG sensors *IEEE Trans. Biomed. Circuits Syst.* **14** 186–97

[54] Sharma L D and Sunkaria R K 2018 Inferior myocardial infarction detection using stationary wavelet transform and machine learning approach *Signal Image Video Process.* **12** 199–206

[55] 2011 *ECG Signal Processing, Classification and Interpretation: A Comprehensive Framework of Computational Intelligence* ed A Gacek and W Pedrycz (Berlin: Springer Science & Business Media)

[56] D'Aloia M, Longo A and Rizzi M 2019 Noisy ECG signal analysis for automatic peak detection *Information* **10** 35

[57] Hou Z, Dong Y, Xiang J, Li X and Yang B 2018 A real-time QRS detection method based on phase portraits and box-scoring calculation *IEEE Sens. J.* **18** 3694–702

[58] Chen S-W, Chen H-C and Chan H-L 2006 A real-time QRS detection method based on moving-averaging incorporating with wavelet denoising *Comput. Methods Programs Biomed.* **82** 187–95

Chapter 11

Simulation and review of blood smear image-based leukemia classification using machine learning methods

Gopal Singh Tandel, Nitin Kumar Mishra and Vivek Sharma

Leukemia imposes a substantial global health burden, necessitating precise and prompt detection to optimize treatment outcomes. This study delves into the integration of advanced machine learning (ML) methodologies for the detection and classification of leukemia, leveraging smear blood images. Conventional diagnostic modalities encounter inherent limitations in accurately discerning various leukemia sub-types, underscoring the urgency for sophisticated computational techniques. By harnessing the capabilities of many machine learning methods such as ResNet50, ResNet101, Al,exNet, Inception-V3, EfficientNet, Support Vector Machine (SVM), K-Nearest Neighbors (KNN), Naive Bayes (NB), Decision Tree (DT) and Linear Discrimination (LD). we propose a holistic framework tailored to leukemia detection and classification tasks. Our method encompasses meticulous preprocessing strategies for image enhancement, coupled with robust feature extraction mechanisms designed to effectively encapsulate pertinent information from smear blood images. After conducting extensive experiments on a diverse and representative dataset, we thoroughly evaluate the performance of our proposed method. Various metrics such as accuracy, precision, recall, F-Score, and ROC curves are utilized to comprehensively evaluate the effectiveness of the developed models. When employing an automated feature extraction technique, ResNet101 demonstrated outstanding classification performance with accuracy: 97.02; recall: 96.87; precision: 97.14; F-Score: 97.00, and area under the curve (AUC): 98.64. Conversely, for handcrafted features, SVM achieved the highest classification performance with accuracy: 96.40; recall: 96.49; precision: 96.44; F-Score: 91.69, and AUC: 97.98.

doi:10.1088/978-0-7503-5964-1ch11

11.1 Introduction

Leukemia, characterized by aberrant proliferation and immature growth of blood cells, poses a formidable challenge in the medical landscape, particularly due to its pervasive impact across diverse age groups, with children being significantly affected [1]. This hematological malignancy inflicts considerable damage to crucial components of the circulatory system, including red blood cells, bone marrow, and the immune defense apparatus, thus precipitating profound health ramifications on a global scale. In the United States alone, leukemia comprises a substantial portion, with over 3.5% of new cancer diagnoses attributed to it, and the year 2018 witnessed an alarming tally of more than 60 000 new cases reported. Central to the pathology of leukemia is the infiltration of malignant white blood cells, known as lymphoblasts, which metastasize to vital organs such as the spleen, brain, liver, and kidneys, exacerbating the disease's severity and complicating treatment regimens [2, 3]. The diagnostic landscape of leukemia, navigated by hematologists in cell transplant laboratories, relies heavily on microscopic examination of blood samples. However, the variability in staining techniques and the nuanced presentation of early symptoms, including lymph node enlargement, pallor, fever, and weight loss, often pose challenges to accurate diagnosis, with symptoms sometimes overlapping with those of other medical conditions [4].

While the microscopic evaluation of peripheral blood smears (PBS) serves as a standard diagnostic tool, the gold standard necessitates the invasive procedure of bone marrow sampling for a definitive diagnosis [5]. In response to the limitations and intricacies inherent in conventional diagnostic modalities, there has been a discernible shift towards the adoption of ML and computer-aided diagnostic methods in recent decades [2–5]. These innovative approaches harness the computational power of ML algorithms to meticulously analyze blood smear images, facilitating not only accurate diagnosis but also the nuanced classification of distinct leukemia subtypes. The integration of ML into clinical research represents a paradigm shift in medical diagnostics, empowering practitioners with the ability to leverage vast datasets and intricate data patterns to inform clinical decision-making processes. ML, as a cornerstone of artificial intelligence, embodies a transformative approach, enabling computers to learn from data without explicit programming, thereby revolutionizing the landscape of medical image processing. However, as the volume and complexity of medical data continue to burgeon, the quest for advanced data analysis methodologies capable of robustly handling such datasets becomes increasingly imperative.

Convolutional neural networks (CNNs) have emerged as the preferred ML algorithm for analyzing PBS in leukemia diagnosis [2, 5]. Their exceptional efficiency lies in their ability to autonomously learn hierarchical features directly from raw image data, enabling precise identification of abnormal cells indicative of leukemia. This autonomy significantly enhances the accuracy and speed of leukemia detection, facilitating prompt diagnosis and treatment initiation.

ML techniques have demonstrated significant success in the diagnosis and classification of acute lymphoblastic leukemia (ALL) and acute myeloid leukemia (AML) [2]. These subtypes, known for their diagnostic challenges using traditional methods, have seen notable advancements through ML algorithms such as CNNs and SVMs. By effectively analyzing microscopic images of blood smears, these algorithms contribute to improved accuracy in identifying and distinguishing between ALL and AML, facilitating more targeted and effective treatment strategies [5–8]. The integration of ML methods into healthcare systems offers numerous benefits for leukemia detection and diagnosis. Automated analysis of blood smear images using ML algorithms enhances diagnostic accuracy while streamlining the diagnostic process, reducing turnaround times, and enabling timely interventions. This not only improves patient outcomes but also optimizes resource allocation in healthcare settings. By empowering healthcare professionals with advanced diagnostic tools, ML-driven approaches pave the way for personalized treatment strategies tailored to individual patient needs. The findings from the comprehensive data analysis and quality assessment underscore the pivotal role of ML algorithms, particularly CNNs, in revolutionizing leukemia diagnosis and classification. The adoption of ML-driven approaches promises to usher in a new era of precision medicine, where timely and accurate diagnoses pave the way for improved patient care and outcomes in the realm of hematological malignancies.

The following are the major objective of this study. First, identifying gaps and limitations in existing research underscore the need for further investigation and development of robust ML-based approaches for leukemia detection and classification using smear blood images. Second, current study seeks to address these gaps by leveraging state-of-the-art methodologies, utilizing standardized datasets, and striving for interpretable ML models. Third, there is rigorous simulation of leukemia classification on various deep learning (DL) and ML models. The chapter is structured as follows: introduction to the subject in section 11.1, literature review in section 11.2, materials and methods in section 11.3, results and discussion in section 11.4 and conclusion in section 11.5.

11.2 Literature review

In this review, we summarize the current state-of-the-art methodologies, theories, and findings pertaining to the application of ML in the detection and classification of leukemia using blood smear images. By synthesizing existing research, this section aims to identify gaps or limitations in the literature that motivate the current study and provide insights into avenues for further investigation. Numerous studies have explored the use of ML algorithms for analyzing blood smear images to aid in leukemia diagnosis and classification. Key methodologies employed in these studies include preprocessing techniques for image enhancement, feature extraction methods to capture relevant information from the images, and the implementation of ML classifiers.

The state-of-the-art methods in this field leverage CNNs due to their ability to automatically learn hierarchical features directly from raw image data. CNNs have demonstrated remarkable efficiency in accurately identifying and classifying leukemia cells, contributing to improved diagnostic accuracy and prognostic stratification [8–10]. Additionally, SVMs have been widely utilized for their ability to handle high-dimensional data and effectively discriminate between different leukemia subtypes based on extracted features. A plethora of studies have investigated the utilization of ML techniques for the detection and classification of leukemia using blood smear images. CNNs have emerged as a prominent method due to their ability to automatically learn hierarchical features from raw image data, leading to improved accuracy in leukemia detection and classification. Transfer learning, a technique where pre-trained CNN models are fine-tuned on leukemia-specific datasets, has shown promise in overcoming limitations associated with small datasets and accelerating model convergence. Some of the CNN-based works are summarized below.

This chapter [11] discusses the use of DL, specifically CNNs, in the diagnosis and classification of ALL through bone marrow image analysis. Studies from 2013 to 2023 show DL models achieving up to 100% accuracy in cancer cell classification. Innovative techniques like Cat-Boosting and transfer learning enhance classification accuracy, surpassing traditional methods. Despite challenges, such as dataset diversity, DL demonstrates promising potential for improving ALL diagnostics with high accuracy levels, indicating a positive trajectory in clinical applications. Park *et al* [12] aimed to develop an artificial intelligence model capable of classifying peripheral blood images of various cell types, including those associated with acute leukemia. Using EfficientNet-V1 (B1) and EfficientNet-V2 (B2) models, an ensemble model was created, significantly improving classification accuracy and F1 scores. The ensemble model performed well for 12 cell types, with high accuracy and F1 scores, particularly for myeloblasts and lymphoblasts. The findings suggest the model's potential to aid in the rapid and precise diagnosis of acute leukemia in challenging healthcare settings. Arivuselvam *et al* [13], utilized a CNN-based DL (DCNN) strategy, specifically employing ResNet-34 and DenseNet-121, to improve the quality of low-intensity medical images and classify leukemia. By enhancing image intensity using histogram equalization-based adaptive gamma correction and guided filtering, the DCNN served as a feature extractor to classify leukemia types. The approach achieved high classification accuracy (99.2% and 98.4%) and outperformed various other ML classifiers in terms of specificity, sensitivity, and precision. The findings suggest that the DCNN strategy is effective in enhancing image quality and accurately classifying leukemia types compared to traditional ML methods. Brunning *et al* [14] proposed a study of classification for acute leukemias emphasizing genetic events and immunology alongside morphology for diagnosis and treatment. It follows a hierarchal approach, giving precedence to genetic changes in acute myeloid leukemias and a combination of immunology and genetic changes in acute lymphoblastic leukemias. Acute myeloid leukemias are grouped into four major categories, while acute lymphoblastic leukemias are categorized based on immunologic characteristics. Additionally, precursor B acute lymphoblastic leukemia/lymphoma is further classified into prognostic genetic groups, and biphenotypic leukemia is acknowledged as a type of ambiguous lineage acute leukemia. Vogado *et al* [15] utilized CNN with transfer learning to overcome the need for a large image dataset. By testing three CNN architectures and utilizing SVM classifier, a new methodology achieved high accuracy rates above 99% in correctly classifying diverse image characteristics across different databases, outperforming nine existing methods. Sampathila *et al* [16] proposed a DL algorithm proposed for microscopic images of blood smears detection leukemic cells using a CNN model called ALLNET. Trained on open-source data using a Nvidia Tesla P-100 GPU on Google Collaboratory, the model achieved high accuracy (95.54%) and can aid in early detection during pre-screening tests like complete blood count and peripheral blood tests. Abunadi *et al* [17] focused on developing diagnostic systems for early leukemia detection using image databases. Three systems were proposed: one utilizing artificial neural networks (ANNs) and SVMs with high accuracy, another employing CNN models like AlexNet, GoogleNet, and ResNet-18 achieving 100% accuracy, and a hybrid system combining CNN and SVM technologies, all showing promising results for leukemia detection.

Feature extraction methods such as histogram-based features, texture analysis, and morphological operations have been extensively utilized to capture salient characteristics of leukemia cells, contributing to the development of robust ML models. Ensemble learning techniques, including random forests and gradient boosting machines, have been employed to aggregate predictions from multiple ML models, resulting in improved classification performance and model robustness. Some of the handcrafted feature-based leukemia classification studies are as follows. Das *et al* [18] highlight the limitations of manual methods and propose an automatic method for blast cell counting and leukemia classification using the Gini index-based Fuzzy Naive Bayes (GFNB) classifier. The proposed method shows high accuracy and reliability in detecting leukemia from multi-cell blood smear images. The paper emphasizes the need for efficient leukemia classification methods to prevent fatalities, especially in low-income regions lacking adequate diagnostic resources. The proposed system aims to improve diagnosis speed and accuracy through pre-processing, segmentation, feature extraction, and classification steps. In [19] the authors present a system for automatic detection and classification of white blood cells in microscopic blood smear images, aiming to accelerate the diagnostic process. The system involves locating white blood cells, segmenting them into nucleus and cytoplasm regions, extracting features, and classifying them into basophil, eosinophil, neutrophil, lymphocyte, and monocyte types. The method demonstrates high accuracy in segmentation and classification, with performance comparison between linear and naïve Bayes classifiers showing promising results in terms of segmentation quality and cell classification accuracy. The proposed method showed high consistency and coherence with dice similarity scores of 98.9% and 91.6% for segmented nucleus and cell regions. In the classification phase, correction rates were about 98% for linear models and 94% for naive Bayes models. Liu *et al* [20], An ML model was developed to automatically classify AML-M1 and M2 subtypes in bone marrow smear images using morphological, radiomics, and clinical features. The model, mainly utilizing a random forest method, demonstrated high performance with accuracy, AUC, F1-score, recall, and precision scores close to 1. This suggests the potential of the model as a useful tool for clinicians in accurately categorizing AML-M1 and M2 subtypes. Dese *et al* [2] developed an automated optical image processing system to categorize common types of leukemia using blood smear slides.

The system, employing image segmentation and SVM classification, achieved high accuracy, sensitivity, and specificity rates for leukemia type classification and white blood cell counts. It significantly reduced processing time compared to manual methods and improved diagnosis accuracy. This technology aims to support healthcare workers in resource-limited settings, particularly in sub-Saharan Africa, enhancing screening for blood-related diseases like leukemia. Mandal *et al* [21] have developed an automated system for cancer cell detection in blood cell images using features extraction and ML classifiers. The study compared Gradient Boosting DT and SVM algorithms, with the former showing better performance. Important features such as adjacent nuclei presence and irregularity in nucleus shape were identified as crucial for cancer cell detection. The approach achieved an 85.6% F1 score on validation data and highlighted features that can aid healthcare professionals in diagnosing leukemia patients from stained images.

Despite the advancements in ML-based approaches for leukemia diagnosis, several gaps and limitations exist in the current literature. One notable limitation is the lack of standardized datasets for evaluating the performance of ML algorithms across different studies. Many studies utilize proprietary or small-scale datasets, which may limit the generalizability of their findings. Additionally, there is a need for more comprehensive validation and benchmarking of ML models using large, diverse datasets encompassing various leukemia subtypes and imaging conditions. Furthermore, while ML algorithms show promise in enhancing diagnostic accuracy, there remains a need for interpretable models that provide insights into the features driving classification decisions. The black-box nature of some ML algorithms poses challenges in understanding the underlying biological mechanisms and may hinder their clinical adoption. The gaps and limitations identified in existing research underscore the need for further investigation and development of robust ML- based approaches for leukemia detection and classification. The current study seeks to address these gaps by leveraging state-of-the-art methodologies, utilizing standardized datasets, and striving for interpretable ML models to advance the field of leukemia diagnosis and improve patient outcomes. Through rigorous experimentation and validation, this study aims to contribute novel insights and methodologies to the burgeoning intersection of ML and medical image analysis in the context of leukemia detection and classification.

11.3 Materials and method

Diagnosing leukemia in peripheral blood images relies heavily on the quality of stained slides. As a result, there is a scarcity of large-scale, high-quality standardized datasets. Many studies have resorted to using publicly available datasets for designing and developing ML algorithms. One of the most widely used datasets is ALL-IDB, which has been utilized in numerous articles focusing on the diagnosis and classification of ALL using various ML techniques. Additionally, another published dataset known as Benchmark has been employed in some studies for the development of ML algorithms. While most researchers test their models on homogeneous or private databases, achieving robust detection and classification across datasets with distinct characteristics remains a significant challenge. To address this challenge and ensure the reliability of results, some studies have combined multiple datasets, including local datasets, to develop cross-dataset models. For instance, Sharif utilized three datasets to create a system with high precision and efficiency in diagnosing various leukocytes. The most frequently diagnosed and classified type of leukemia using ML techniques is ALL. Furthermore, some articles have focused on image analysis for leukocyte counting.

11.3.1 Overview of machine vision techniques in PBS image analysis

An analysis of methods employed by reviewed studies [22] reveals two main categories of machine vision techniques used in PBS image analysis: ML and its subset, DL. The former approach involves selective image feature extraction, where mathematical and ML algorithms are used to extract a variety of image features. The goal of feature extraction is to obtain a comprehensive set of image descriptors, allowing for the establishment of relationships between these descriptors. On the other hand, DL algorithms, which have gained prominence in recent years, operate by learning hierarchical representations directly from raw data. Unlike traditional ML methods, DL algorithms can automatically learn features from data without the need for manual feature engineering. This enables them to capture intricate patterns and relationships in PBS images, leading to enhanced diagnostic accuracy in leukemia detection and class. ML algorithms play a crucial role in blood cell segmentation, which is a fundamental step in identifying leukemia in blood smear images. Various ML algorithms have been employed in segmentation techniques, with the aim of identifying the boundary between the nucleus and cytoplasm for further characterization. This characterization includes analyzing nuclear properties, cytoplasmic properties, and the nuclear-to-cytoplasmic ratio, all of which are valuable for leukemia identification. Numerous segmentation algorithms have been proposed in the literature, with traditional ML algorithms based on selected features being the most popular. These algorithms are used in two main types of segmentation: pixel-based image segmentation and region-based segmentation. Some studies have also utilized shape-based segmentation techniques, such as threshold-based, edge-based, and region-based methods. Among the various ML algorithms, clustering algorithms have gained significant acceptance and efficiency in segmentation tasks. Clustering algorithms, such as k-means and fuzzy c-mean, have been utilized for pixel clustering and region growing segmentation. Additionally, the watershed algorithm, which treats pixel values as local topography, has been widely employed for segmentation tasks, particularly in separating components based on morphological features. The application of ML algorithms for segmentation extends beyond traditional methods, with algorithms like SVMs, ANNs, and DTs being frequently used to segment blasts in blood smear images. Segmentation is crucial for leukemia detection and diagnosis, as accurate feature extraction and classification heavily rely on correctly segmented lymphocytes. Figure 11.1 illustrates the diagnostic objectives for various types of leukemia based on PBS image processing. Based on the systematic review conducted on leukemia detection and diagnosis

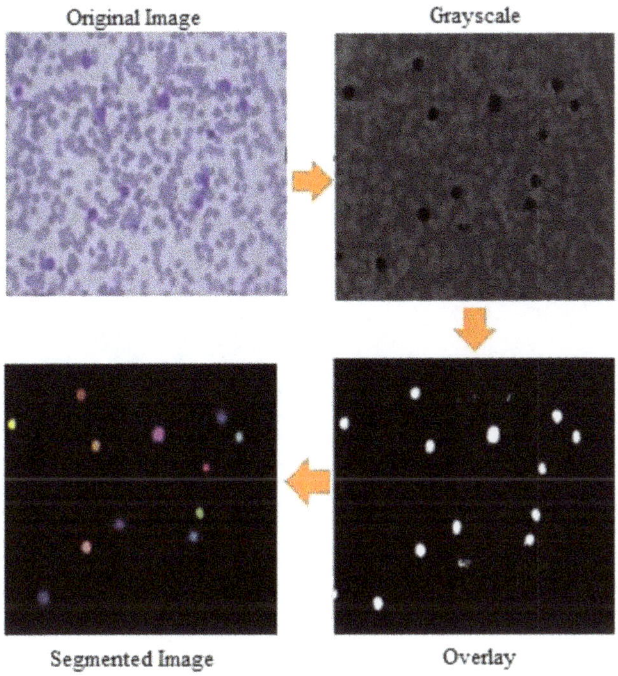

Figure 11.1. PBS image processing.

using ML techniques for PBS image analysis, the following important image features for blood cell images include characteristics such as the presence of adjacent nuclei, irregularity in the shape of the nucleus, texture patterns, cell size, cell density, color intensity, and morphological parameters like roundness, compactness, and eccentricity. These features play a crucial role in automated systems designed for cell classification and disease diagnosis.

Our study used public leukemia data ALL-IDB for simulation. Automated feature extraction methods are compared with handcrafted feature classification methods. It used many features in image analysis that refer to the shape, size, and structure of objects within an image, in addition to the features like nuclei, irregularity in the shape of the nucleus, texture patterns, cell size, cell density, color intensity, and morphological parameters like roundness, compactness, and eccentricity. These features can include parameters such as area, perimeter, aspect ratio, circularity, convexity, solidity, orientation, and texture. In the context of blood cell images, morphological features are essential for distinguishing between different types of cells and aiding in disease diagnosis through automated analysis. The segmented process is exhibited in figure 11.2 and sample segmented images depicted in figure 11.3.

11.3.2 Methodology

We implemented a variety of ML algorithms suitable for image classification tasks on medical datasets. We utilized CNNs as the primary algorithm due to their ability

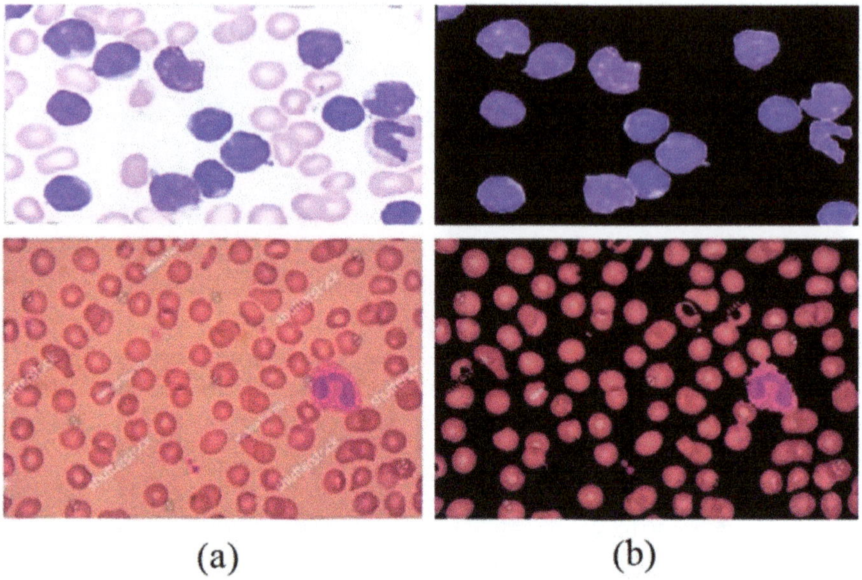

Figure 11.2. Image cell segmentation process. (a) Input image and (b) segmented image.

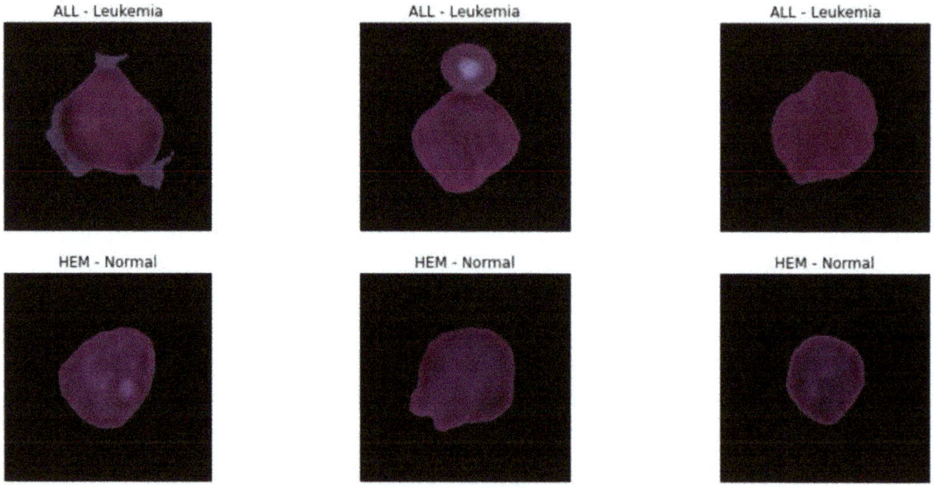

Figure 11.3. Processed image for classification.

to effectively learn hierarchical features from image data and achieve state-of-the-art performance in image classification tasks. We experimented with different CNN architectures, including ResNet50, ResNet101, Al,exNet, Inception-V3, EfficientNet, to identify the most suitable model architecture for leukemia detection and classification. Additionally, we explored the use of traditional ML algorithms such as SVM, KNN, NB, DT and LD for comparison and benchmarking purposes. We divided the dataset into training, validation, and testing sets to facilitate model

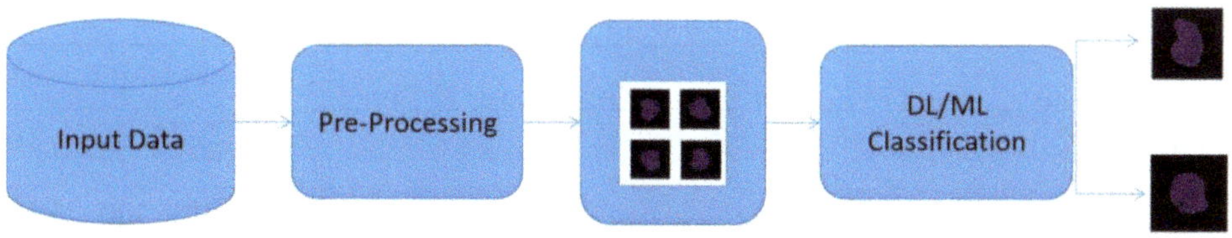

Figure 11.4. Flow chart of methodology.

training and evaluation. We trained ML models on the training data using appropriate loss functions and optimization algorithms. We validated model performance on the validation set to fine-tune hyperparameters and prevent over-fitting. We evaluated the final trained models on the independent testing set using metrics such as accuracy, sensitivity, specificity, and AUC to assess classification performance. We conducted cross-validation experiments to assess the robustness and generalizability of the training models. We performed k-fold cross-validation to validate model performance across different subsets of the dataset and mitigate potential biases introduced by data partitioning. We evaluated model robustness to variations in input data and imaging conditions to ensure reliable performance in real-world clinical settings. We adhered to ethical guidelines and regulations governing the use of medical data and patient information. We ensured compliance with data privacy laws and obtained appropriate consent for the use of blood smear images in research. We protectd patient confidentiality and anonymized sensitive information to prevent the identification of individuals from the dataset (figure 11.4).

11.4 Results

The simulation was performed on the ALL Challenge dataset of ISBI, 2019 [22–25]. The datasets contained cell images of both normal individuals and patients diagnosed with ALL. The C NMC 2019 data included 10 661 images from 73 participants. It included 7272 blast (infected) cell images and 3389 healthy cell images. Images in this dataset were standardized to 450 × 450 × 3 and preprocessed to extract the object of interest (WBC) while excluding all other elements. 80% of the dataset was preserved in the training set, with the remaining 20% kept in the test set. The simulation was evaluated on performance matrix, accuracy, recall, precision, F1-Score and AUC value. Mathematical formulas are depicted in table 11.1. The performance of all the models is compared in table 11.2 and figure 11.5 and shows that highest classification accuracy of 97.02% was seen via ResNet101 using automated feature extraction method. On the other-hand, SVM exhibited maximum classification accuracy of 96.40%.

11.5 Discussion

The utilization of ML techniques in the detection and classification of leukemia using smear blood images has shown promising advancements. This discussion aims to delve into the implications, challenges, and future directions of this innovative

Table 11.1. Performance parameters.

Parameter	Mathematical formula
Accuracy	$\frac{(TP + TN)}{(TP + TN + FP + FN)} \times 100$
Recall	$\frac{(TP)}{(TP + FN)} \times 100$
Precision	$\frac{(TP)}{(TP + FP)} \times 100$
F1-score	$2 \times \frac{(\text{precision} \times \text{recall})}{(\text{precision} \times \text{recall})} \times 100$

Table 11.2. Comparison of performance between ML and DL models.

Method	Model	Accuracy	Recall	Precision	F-Score	Mean (AUC)
Automated features (DL)	ResNet50	96.55	96.39	96.44	96.41	98.65
	ResNet101	**97.02**	**96.87**	**97.14**	**97.00**	**98.64**
	AlexNet	93.28	91.83	92.11	91.97	98.11
	Inception-V3	93.64	93.46	94.12	93.79	98.44
	EfficientNet	87.05	80.80	87.55	84.04	94.38
Handcrafted features (ML)	**SVM**	**96.40**	**96.49**	**96.44**	**91.69**	**97.98**
	KNN	90.77	96.83	93.80	92.87	96.06
	NB	59.06	89.28	74.17	71.69	82.98
	DT	88.55	95.65	92.10	89.34	95.29
	LD	94.24	96.46	95.35	91.69	97.21

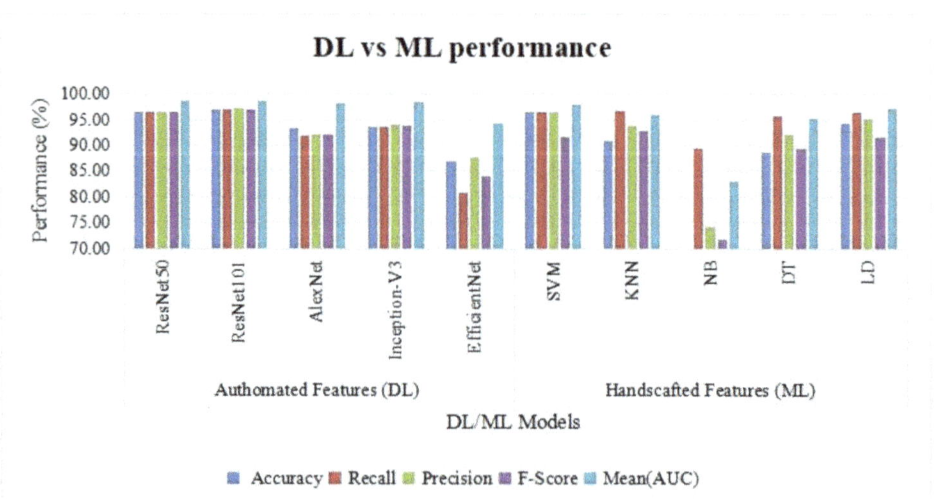

Figure 11.5. Ml versus DL performance comparison for leukemia classification.

approach. Microscopic evaluation of PBS images serves as a primary method for diagnosing leukemia in its early stages. In the simulation process, we compared an automated feature extraction method with handcrafted features. Established CNN models like ResNet50, ResNet101, AlexNet, Inception-V3, and EfficientNet were compared with conventional ML models SVM, KNN, NB, DT, and LD. While conventional CNNs extracted features directly from images, in conventional ML models, various image features were designed, as discussed previously. A mixed performance was observed, with ResNet101 outperforming conventional ML models. Among conventional ML models, SVM displayed the maximum performance.

However, manual examination of these smears can lead to errors in disease typing and non-standardized reports, affecting diagnostic accuracy and efficiency. The tedious and time-consuming nature of manual examination further exacerbates diagnostic challenges, highlighting the need for automated methods unaffected by technician experience or operator fatigue. Given the lack of a comprehensive systematic review on PBS image analysis via ML methods, the authors conducted a review study to explore the applications of ML in leukemia diagnosis and classification based on PBS images. Through a comparative analysis of previous studies [1–5], this research aimed to address key questions surrounding the use of ML in this context. Preprocessing of smear images is essential due to various factors such as illumination conditions, staining variations, and defects in the film, which can introduce visual artifacts and color inconsistencies. Effective preprocessing techniques, including preparation, normalization, and segmentation, are crucial for enhancing the precision of leukemia detection via ML algorithms [6–9]. The selection of relevant features is pivotal in the preliminary processing of blood smears using ML methods. While some studies have focused on color and shape features, others have explored texture metrics and morphological characteristics of blast cells. Manual feature selection, however, poses challenges and may lead to errors. To address this, algorithmic approaches for feature selection are recommended, with hybrid algorithms or swarm intelligence methods offering potential for improved feature extraction and selection. A significant challenge in leukemia diagnosis via ML algorithms is the lack of comprehensive datasets of leukemia smear images, leading to issues such as overfitting. The utilization of small or local datasets hampers algorithm performance and limits the generalizability of results. Augmentation techniques and data processing methods can mitigate this challenge, improving pattern recognition and overall diagnostic accuracy. Despite these challenges, studies employing ML techniques for leukemia diagnosis have demonstrated remarkable results, with high mean accuracy rates exceeding 96%. The expanding applications of ML in disease diagnosis and blood cell imaging, particularly in cell counting and differentiation, underscore the growing significance of these algorithms in healthcare. Looking ahead, the integration of ML-based applications and software, especially DL, holds promise for enhancing diagnostic precision and efficiency in bone marrow transplant laboratories and clinical settings.

ML techniques exhibited promising efficiency in leukemia diagnosis and classification based on PBS images. Across reviewed studies [1–9], ML algorithms consistently demonstrated high accuracy rates in differentiating between leukemia and normal blood cells, highlighting their potential as valuable diagnostic aids. CNNs emerged as the predominant ML algorithm achieving high efficiency in PBS analysis. CNNs showcased superior performance in capturing intricate features and patterns from PBS images, enabling accurate leukemia classification across various subtypes. ML techniques achieved better results in diagnosing and classifying ALL and AML. These leukemia subtypes, known for their diagnostic complexities, benefitted significantly from ML algorithms, particularly CNNs and ensemble learning approaches. Integration of ML methods in healthcare systems promises substantial benefits for leukemia detection and diagnosis. ML-based approaches streamline diagnostic workflows, enhance accuracy, and facilitate timely interventions, ultimately leading to improved patient outcomes and resource optimization.

11.5.1 Implications

The integration of ML algorithms into leukemia detection and classification workflows has revolutionized the field of hematology. ML-based approaches offer the potential for automated and accurate diagnosis, enabling early detection and intervention, which are crucial for improving patient outcomes. By analyzing PBS images, ML algorithms can identify subtle morphological changes in blood cells associated with leukemia, facilitating timely diagnosis and treatment planning. Furthermore, ML algorithms can enhance the efficiency and accuracy of blood cell segmentation, a critical step in leukemia diagnosis. By accurately delineating the boundaries between different cell components, such as the nucleus and cytoplasm, ML-based segmentation techniques enable precise characterization of cell morphology and identification of abnormal cells characteristic of leukemia.

11.5.2 Challenges

Despite the promising implications, several challenges hinder the widespread adoption of ML-based approaches in leukemia detection and classification. One significant challenge is the availability of high-quality annotated datasets for training ML models. The scarcity of standardized datasets with comprehensive annotations poses a bottleneck for algorithm development and validation. Additionally, variability in staining techniques and image quality across different laboratories further complicates algorithm training and generalization. Moreover, the interpretability of ML models remains a concern in clinical settings. Understanding how ML algorithms arrive at their predictions is essential for gaining trust and acceptance among healthcare professionals. The black-box nature of some ML models poses challenges for interpreting results and integrating them into clinical decision-making processes.

11.5.3 Future directions

To address these challenges and unlock the full potential of ML in leukemia detection and classification, several avenues for future research can be explored. Firstly, efforts should be directed towards creating standardized datasets with comprehensive annotations to facilitate algorithm development and evaluation.

Collaborative initiatives involving multiple institutions can help address the variability in data collection and annotation practices. Furthermore, research focusing on explainable AI techniques can enhance the interpretability of ML models in clinical settings. Developing methods to interpret and visualize the decision-making process of ML algorithms can improve trust and transparency, enabling seamless integration into clinical workflows. Additionally, leveraging emerging technologies such as DL and multi-modal imaging can further enhance the accuracy and robustness of ML-based approaches. Integrating data from multiple imaging modalities, such as microscopy and flow cytometry, can provide complementary information for more comprehensive leukemia diagnosis and classification. In conclusion, while ML holds great promise for advancing leukemia detection and classification, addressing challenges related to data availability, interpretability, and technological integration is essential for realizing its full potential in clinical practice. Collaborative efforts and interdisciplinary research initiatives will be key to overcoming these challenges and driving innovation in hematology.

11.6 Conclusion

The integration of ML techniques in the detection and classification of leukemia using smear blood images represents a significant advancement in hematology. Through a systematic review of existing literature, this study has shed light on the potential of ML algorithms to revolutionize leukemia diagnosis and classification. The reliance on manual evaluation of PBS images for leukemia diagnosis poses challenges in terms of accuracy, standardization, and efficiency. ML-based approaches offer a promising solution to these challenges by automating the diagnostic process and minimizing human error. By leveraging ML algorithms, healthcare professionals can achieve precise and timely diagnoses, independent of technician experience or fatigue. Preprocessing of smear images plays a critical role in optimizing the performance of ML algorithms. Techniques such as normalization and segmentation are essential for enhancing the precision of leukemia detection and classification. Additionally, the selection of relevant features is crucial for accurate disease typing, with algorithmic approaches offering more robust solutions compared to manual feature selection methods. However, challenges such as the lack of comprehensive datasets and issues related to overfitting pose significant hurdles to the widespread adoption of ML in leukemia diagnosis. Addressing these challenges requires collaborative efforts to create standardized datasets and develop augmentation techniques to expand the data space for training ML models. Despite these challenges, studies utilizing ML techniques for leukemia diagnosis have demonstrated impressive results, with high accuracy rates exceeding 96%. The growing applications of ML in disease diagnosis and blood cell imaging highlight the increasing significance of these algorithms in healthcare. Looking ahead, the integration of ML-based applications and software, particularly DL approaches, holds promise for enhancing diagnostic precision and efficiency in clinical settings. By embracing ML technologies, healthcare professionals can usher in a new era of leukemia diagnosis characterized by improved accuracy, speed, and accessibility.

References

[1] Ghaderzadeh M, Asadi F, Hosseini A, Bashash D, Abolghasemi H and Roshanpour A 2021 Machine learning in detection and classification of leukemia using smear blood images: a systematic review *Sci. Prog.* **2021** 9933481

[2] Dese K, Raj H, Ayana G, Yemane T, Adissu W, Krishnamoorthy J and Kwa T 2021 Accurate machine-learning-based classification of leukemia from blood smear images *Clin. Lymphoma Myeloma Leuk.* **21** e903–14

[3] Baig R, Rehman A, Almuhaimeed A, Alzahrani A and Rauf H T 2022 Detecting malignant leukemia cells using microscopic blood smear images: a deep learning approach *Appl. Sci.* **12** 6317

[4] Shah A, Naqvi S S, Naveed K, Salem N, Khan M A and Alimgeer K S 2021 Automated diagnosis of leukemia: a comprehensive review *IEEE Access* **9** 132097–124

[5] Hegde R B, Prasad K, Hebbar H, Singh B M K and Sandhya I 2020 Automated decision support system for detection of leukemia from peripheral blood smear images *J. Dig. Imag.* **33** 361–74

[6] Al-Ghraibah A and Al-Ayyad M 2024 Automated detection of leukemia in blood microscopic images using image processing techniques and unique features: cell count and area ratio *Cog. Eng.* **11** 2304484

[7] Salah H T, Muhsen I N, Salama M E, Owaidah T and Hashmi S K 2019 Machine learning applications in the diagnosis of leukemia: current trends and future directions *Int. J. Lab. Hematol.* **41** 717–25

[8] Acharya V, Ravi V, Pham T D and Chakraborty C 2021 Peripheral blood smear analysis using automated computer-aided diagnosis system to identify acute myeloid leukemia *IEEE Trans. Eng. Manage.* **70** 2760–73

[9] Kocatürk C, Candemir C and Kocabaş İ 2022 A Comparative study of automatic detection of acute lymphocytic leukemia with machine learning methods *Dokuz Eylül Üni. Mühendis. Fak. Fen ve Mühendis. Derg.* **24** 1021–32

[10] Mittal A, Dhalla S, Gupta S and Gupta A 2022 Automated analysis of blood smear images for leukemia detection: a comprehensive review *ACM Comput. Surv. (CSUR)* **54** 1–37

[11] Elsayed B, Elhadary M, Elshoeibi R M, Elshoeibi A M, Badr A, Metwally O and Yassin M 2023 Deep learning enhances acute lymphoblastic leukemia diagnosis and classification using bone marrow images *Front. Oncol.* **13** 1330977

[12] Park S, Park Y H, Huh J, Baik S M and Park D J 2024 Deep learning model for differentiating acute myeloid and lymphoblastic leukemia in peripheral blood cell images via myeloblast and lymphoblast classification *Dig. Health* **10** 20552076241258079

[13] Arivuselvam B and Sudha S 2022 Leukemia classification using the deep learning method of CNN *J. X-Ray Sci. Technol.* **30** 567–85

[14] Brunning R D 2003 Classification of acute leukemias *Seminars in Diagnostic Pathology* vol 20 (Philadelphia, PA: WB Saunders) pp 142–53

[15] Vogado L H, Veras R M, Araujo F H, Silva R R and Aires K R 2018 Leukemia diagnosis in blood slides using transfer learning in CNNs and SVM for classification *Eng. Appl. Artif. Intell.* **72** 415–22

[16] Sampathila N, Chadaga K, Goswami N, Chadaga R P, Pandya M, Prabhu S, Bairy M G, Katta S S, Bhat D and Upadya S P 2022 Customized deep learning classifier for detection of acute lymphoblastic leukemia using blood smear images *Healthcare (Basel)* **10** 1812

[17] Abunadi I and Senan E M 2022 Multi-method diagnosis of blood microscopic sample for early detection of acute lymphoblastic leukemia based on deep learning and hybrid techniques *Sensors (Basel)* **22** 1629
[18] Das B K and Dutta H S 2020 GFNB: Gini index-based fuzzy naive bayes and blast cell segmentation for leukemia detection using multi-cell blood smear images *Med. Biol. Eng. Comput.* **58** 2789–803
[19] Prinyakupt J and Pluempitiwiriyawej C 2015 Segmentation of white blood cells and comparison of cell morphology by linear and naïve Bayes classifiers *Biomed. Eng.* **14** 63
[20] Liu K and Hu J 2022 Classification of acute myeloid leukemia M1 and M2 subtypes using machine learning *Comput. Biol. Med.* **147** 105741
[21] Mandal S, Daivajna V and Rajagopalan V 2019 Machine learning based system for automatic detection of leukemia cancer cell *2019 IEEE 16th India Council Int. Conf. (INDICON)* (Piscataway, NJ: IEEE) pp 1–4
[22] Anil kumar K K, Manoj V J and Sagi T M 2020 A survey on image segmentation of blood and bone marrow smear images with emphasis to automated detection of leukemia *Biocyber. Biomed. Eng.* **40** 1406–20
[23] Mourya S, Kant S, Kumar P, Gupta A and Gupta R 2019 ALL challenge dataset of ISBI 2019 (C-NMC 2019) (version 1) [dataset] *The Cancer Imaging Archive*
[24] Gehlot S, Gupta A and Gupta R 2020 SDCT-AuxNet$^{\theta}$: DCT augmented stain deconvolutional CNN with auxiliary classifier for cancer diagnosis *Med. Image Anal.* **61** 101661
[25] Goswami S, Mehta S, Sahrawat D, Gupta A and Gupta R 2020 Heterogeneity loss to handle intersubject and intrasubject variability in cancer *ICLR Workshop on Affordable AI in Healthcare* arXiv:2003.03295
[26] Clark K *et al* 2013 The Cancer Imaging Archive (TCIA): maintaining and operating a public information repository *J. Digit. Imag.* **26** 1045–57

IOP Publishing

Artificial Intelligence
A tool for effective diagnostics
Smith K Khare, Sachin Taran and Ankush D Jamthikar

Chapter 12

Subject-independent emotion classification using galvanic skin response and electroencephalogram data

Tanishqa Tyagi, Anukul Pandey, Sachin Taran and Amit Kumar Dwivedi

Emotion recognition using electroencephalograms (EEGs) and galvanic skin response (GSR) is important for affective computing and human–computer interfacing. This paper presents a novel framework for emotion recognition using EEG and GSR signals. EEG and GSR signals contain useful information for emotion classification. GSR signals are useful in identifying extremely high or low levels of emotional arousal. Emotion recognition is achieved using singular spectrum analysis (SSA). SSA decomposes an EEG signal into multiple sub-bands (SBs), from which a large number of time-domain features are extracted. These features are used as the inputs of various classification algorithms. The performance of various classification algorithms is measured using the leave-one-subject cross validation to ensure that the emotion classification is subject independent. The z-score normalization strategy is used to reduce intersubject variability. The normalization feature results in better classification accuracy. This study used the publicly available LUMED-2 multi-modal data set. The proposed method achieved the best average classification accuracy of 62.2% using GSR and EEG signals for three-class emotion classification, outperforming existing methods using the same data set.

12.1 Introduction

Emotion recognition has been a subject of philosophy and psychology. Emotions significantly affect our daily behavior; they are responsible for strongly influencing our perception, memory, and decision-making. Emotions have been a critical aspect of understanding human behavior [1]. In light of this, the role of emotions in human–computer interfaces has grown significantly. Emotion recognition, which is useful in education, gaming, and marketing, is receiving a lot of attention because it helps to identify the consumer's behavior [2]. Analyzing the face, body language, or

doi:10.1088/978-0-7503-5964-1ch12

speech is useful for emotion recognition; these parameters are defined as the explicit channels humans use for communication and are easily controllable, leading to deliberate deception [3]. So, it is important to look at physiological signals, such as EEGs, functional magnetic resonance imaging (fMRI), and GSRs, which arise from involuntary reactions inside the body [4–6]. Studies documented in the research literature have examined numerous emotion recognition models using both multimodal and unimodal methods [7]. Scholars have found multimodal models which use multiple signal sources for emotion recognition to be more accurate. Body language, voice changes, sweating, and changes in skin temperature can significantly identify emotions [6–8].

In [8], binary classification was done using data sets from DEAP and MAHNOBI-HCI. This study created several hierarchical network architectures, fused the final feature vector, and mined the data for possible information using a hierarchical fusion convolutional model. The authors of [9] used fine-grained emotion classification, in which they classified emotions using a 1D convolutional neural network (CNN) and a simple fast Fourier transform (FFT) for feature extraction. The authors of [10] trained the data set for classification using a capsule neural network and tested the unseen-subject, unseen-record type. Emotion recognition based on EEG data used the flexible analytic wavelet transform (FAWT) for feature extraction. A *k*-nearest neighbors (*k*-NN) classifier used sub-band features for classification. The authors of [11, 12] investigated the identification of emotions using EEG signals from a single electrode, thereby simplifying the brain–computer interaction system. The tunable Q-factor wavelet transform was used for decomposing EEGs into SBs, and the SBs were further used for feature extraction. An extreme learning machine (ELM) was used for the classification of features from SBs. As described in [13], while the GSR can accurately identify the arousal (high or low), an ECG signal is required to ascertain the emotion's positive or negative valence. ECG signals and GSR signals are the two types of signals used to classify emotions, specifically 'happy' and 'sad,' 'happy' and 'neutral,' and 'neutral' and 'sad.'

Multiple physiological signals, such as the GSR and the EEG, combine to classify high or low arousal points [14, 15]. The authors of [16] used SSA to examine EEG signals. Six-level multiresolution wavelet decomposition was performed using 8 dB wavelets, treating the emotion recognition problem as a three-class problem. High frequencies in EEG signals are sensitive to emotional activation, and gamma band activity mediates emotional states.

In [17], sliding-mode singular spectrum analysis (SM-SSA) was used to decompose the signals into reconstructed components (RCs), and two entropy-based features were extracted from the RCs for classification. The adaptive SSA (a-SSA) algorithm was used to extract different EEG rhythms [18]. The alpha rhythms were used for classifying EEG signals into 'eyes-open' and 'eyes-closed' groups. The a-SSA algorithm outperformed both SSA and other wavelet decomposition algorithms, according to observations. The authors of [19] proposed a flexible EEG rhythm for feature extraction, which relied on circular singular spectrum analysis (CiSSA). In [20], researchers discussed multiple methods for emotion recognition based on the EEG rhythm and the timing characteristics of the EEG signal. They used a discrete wavelet transform to extract different rhythms. For classification, they used various window sizes of other rhythm signals as inputs to a long short-term memory network (LSTM). Using rhythm, their model achieved the highest accuracy of 69.1% for the arousal dimension, with a time window of 0.5 s. The authors of [21] presented an experiment that classified EEG signals using SSA to distinguish between alcoholic and non-alcoholic subjects. They used a sliding SSA algorithm to decompose and denoise the brain signals before classifying them with 98% accuracy. The authors of [22] presented an EEG feature extraction technique that combined data space adaptation (DSA) and common spatial patterns (CSPs) to reduce the performance decline in emotional classification due to daily fluctuations and variability in the collected EEG data. The authors of [23] extracted discriminant energy spectral density characteristics from EEG recordings using a principal component covariate adaptive transformation technique based on principal component analysis. In addition, they suggested using a stacked autoencoder-based deep learning network to classify emotions according to their valence and arousal levels. Compared to conventional support vector machine (SVM) and naive Bayes classifiers, this technique increased classification accuracy by 5.55% and 6.53%, respectively. The authors of [24] recorded EEG signals from participants who either produced facial expressions matching positive or negative emotions elicited by image stimuli or suppressed their facial expressions. They discovered that frontal asymmetry is linked to facial emotional expression regulation. The random forest approach used event-related potential and multiscale sample entropy to classify emotions [25]. The combination of a stacked autoencoder and an LSTM-based recurrent neural network classified EEG signals with an accuracy of 79.26%. Using an EEG signal, a three-dimensional CNN recognized emotions with an accuracy of 87.44% for valence and 84.49% for arousal [26]. Because EEG recordings are intricate compound waves with individual variations, feature-generating techniques are divided into the two general categories of time-domain and frequency-domain features. Time-domain features, sometimes referred to as linear features, provide an accurate description of an EEG signal's waveform properties, such as amplitude, mean, variance, skewness, and kurtosis. Frequency-based analysis identifies the fundamental frequencies that comprise the EEG signal. For this analysis, we typically divide the EEG signal into five SBs: delta (1–4 Hz), theta (4–8 Hz), alpha (8–13 Hz), beta (13–30 Hz), and gamma (30–60 Hz). From these five SBs, frequency-domain parameters are then calculated [27]. A high-resolution time-frequency representation of an EEG and its spectral fluctuations over time can be obtained using the quadratic time–frequency distribution (QTFD), as described in [28]. The data indicates that the average accuracy of classification ranges from 73.8% to 86.2%.

Our study used EEG and GSR signals from the LUMED-2 data set for the multiclass emotion detection problem. The local maxima in the GSR signal represent highly stimulated response (arousal) points. The EEG signal for the time interval prior to 5 s was collected and processed. The SSA algorithm broke down the EEG signal into SBs. A machine learning model was trained on reduced features using principal component analysis. To get better cross-subject emotion classification results, the feature matrix was subjected to personal Z-score normalization prior to classification [29].

12.2 Methodology

This section explains the methodology of the proposed work. Three stages are important in the methodology used to solve the emotion recognition problem. The first stage involves preprocessing physiological signals and extracting the optimal frequency ranges for emotion classification. Figure 12.1 displays a basic flowchart of the overall methodology followed. The second stage uses the SSA algorithm for decomposition. Figure 12.1 illustrates the process of creating a feature set for a

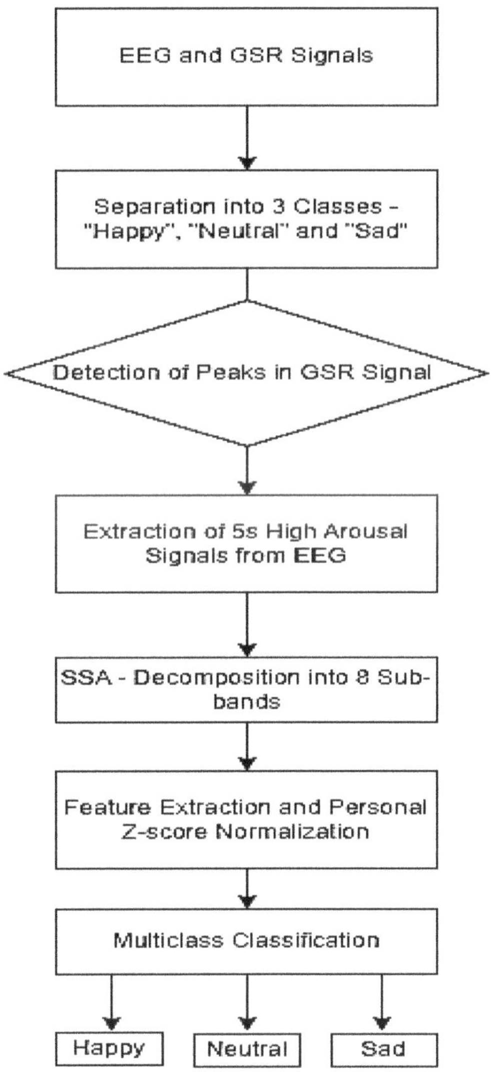

Figure 12.1. Basic flow of the methodology used to form the feature sets of all subjects.

single subject, which subsequently aids in analyzing the model's subject-independent performance. The process is repeated for each subject and then used to calculate the leave-one-subject-out accuracy. The following sections further explain the process.

12.2.1 Preprocessing

First, the physiological signals are divided into the three classes. After a 5 s segment of EEG signal is extracted, the common average reference (CAR) filter approach is used, which is based on local maxima derived from the GSR signal. The CAR filter removes spatial noise from EEG electrodes that interferes with recording [30]. After the filtering has been performed, the signal that represents the individual activity captured by an electrode is unaffected by the regular activities of the nearby electrodes. It can be calculated using the following equation (12.1):

$$X_i(t) = x_i(t) - \frac{1}{N}\sum_{j=1}^{N} x_j(t). \tag{12.1}$$

Here, X_i is the CAR-filtered Nth electrode signal, and the second term represents the average of all electrodes for that point. First, the physiological signals are divided into the three classes. Reference [13] shows that the GSR exhibits an increase in skin conductance in response to a high level of arousal, regardless of the emotion, i.e. happy or sad. In addition, [13] demonstrates that the categorization of high and low arousal situations can rely solely on the GSR signal. The peaks of the GSR signal represent a higher state of arousal, and the region of the EEG signal surrounding these peaks contains crucial information for classification [13]. Figure 12.2 illustrates the use of this information to extract the EEG signal five seconds prior to the local maxima peaks in the GSR signal.

12.2.1.1 Data set

The data set LUMED-2 [14] was recorded at Loughborough University. It consists of recordings of the EEGs, GSRs, and facial video signals of a total of 13 participants, of whom six were women and seven were men. The total length of each physiological signal is 8 min and 50 s, including a rest period of 20 s between each emotionally stimulating video clip. After watching each video, participants were asked to label it as belonging to one of three classes, namely 'happy,' 'sad,' or 'neutral.'

12.2.2 Feature extraction

The EEG signal undergoes SSA decomposition, which reduces it to a set of RCs. The method for deriving these RCs is described below:

We start with x, a single-channel EEG time series defined by the Nth vector $x = (x_1, x_2, \ldots, x_N)^T$; here, T is the transpose, and N is the total number of points in the series. The one-dimensional vector x is converted to a multidimensional trajectory matrix M using a sliding window. M is defined in equation (12.2):

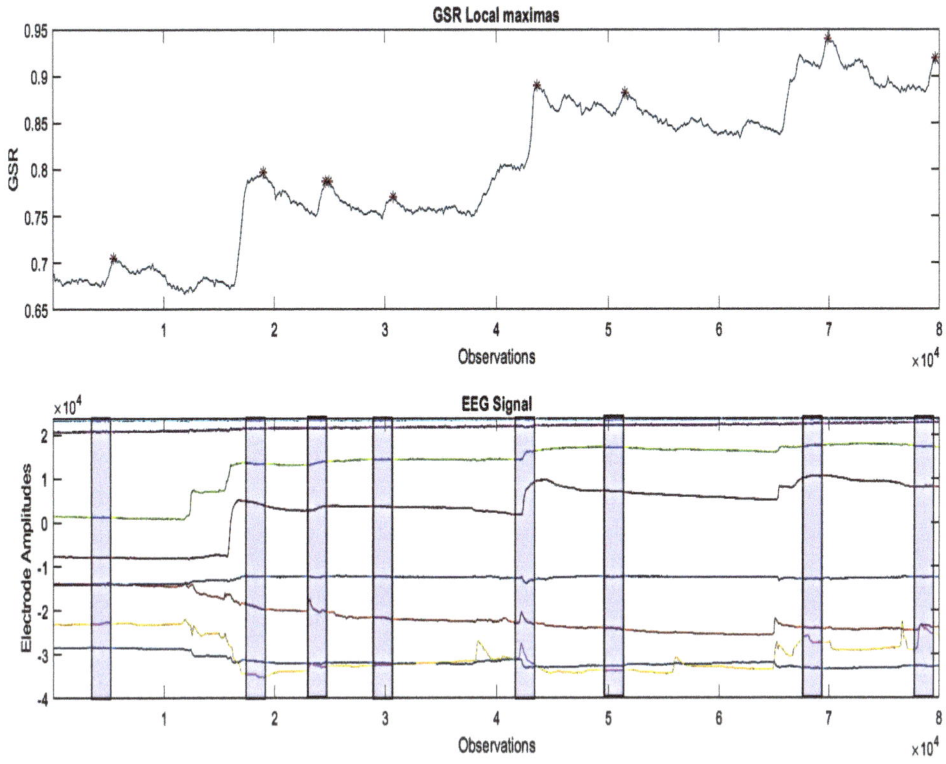

Figure 12.2. GSR local maxima highlighted in red (above) and the corresponding EEG signals obtained 5 s before the maxima were extracted (below).

$$M = (\boldsymbol{X_1}, \boldsymbol{X_2}, \ldots, \boldsymbol{X_K}) = \begin{bmatrix} x_1 & x_2 & \cdots & x_K \\ x_2 & x_3 & \cdots & x_{K+1} \\ \vdots & \vdots & \ddots & \vdots \\ x_L & x_{L+1} & \cdots & x_N \end{bmatrix}. \tag{12.2}$$

Here, L is the embedding dimension, $K = N - L + 1$, and $X_i(1 \leqslant i \leqslant K)$ is the lagged vector. In the next step, the singular value decomposition (SVD) of matrix M is calculated using equation (12.3):

$$M = \sum\nolimits_{i=1}^{L} M_i = \sum\nolimits_{i=1}^{L} \sqrt{\lambda_i} v_i p_i^T \tag{12.3}$$

where M_i denotes the elementary matrix, λ_i denotes the eigenvalues in decreasing order of magnitude, v_i are the corresponding eigenvectors of the covariance matrix defined by $C = MM^T$, and $p_i = M^T v_i / \sqrt{\lambda_i}$ are known as the principal components. For reconstruction, the elementary matrices are split into several groups and summed within each group. The diagonal averaging transforms each matrix into a time series generally called the RCs. $L = 8$ is used because the embedded dimension is defined as $(L \geqslant f_s / f_l)$, where the frequencies are the sampling frequency and the lowest frequency of interest, respectively. The features for this problem are reduced by applying principal component analysis.

It is suggested in [30] that the optimal duration for detecting human emotion is 1 s, hence the SSA is carried out using EEG signals that have a length of 1 s. The raw EEG signals for the classes happy, sad, and neutral, depicted in figures 12.3–12.5, respectively, for eight principal components, are extracted using an embedding dimension of $L = 8$. Using the first principal component obtained by applying SSA [32, 33], features are extracted from 1 s snippets of the component. The seven features extracted are the mean, the standard deviation, the variance, the peak-to-peak value, the power bandwidth, skewness, and kurtosis. The list of features extracted from each of the eight electrodes is given below:

Mean—the mean of a decomposed SSA sub-band is calculated by summing all values in the sub-band and dividing by the number of values. The mean of the sub-band is defined as

$$\text{Mean}(\mu) = \frac{1}{N}\sum_{i=1}^{N} S_i \tag{12.4}$$

where S_i is the sub-band variable of segment i, and N is the total number of samples.

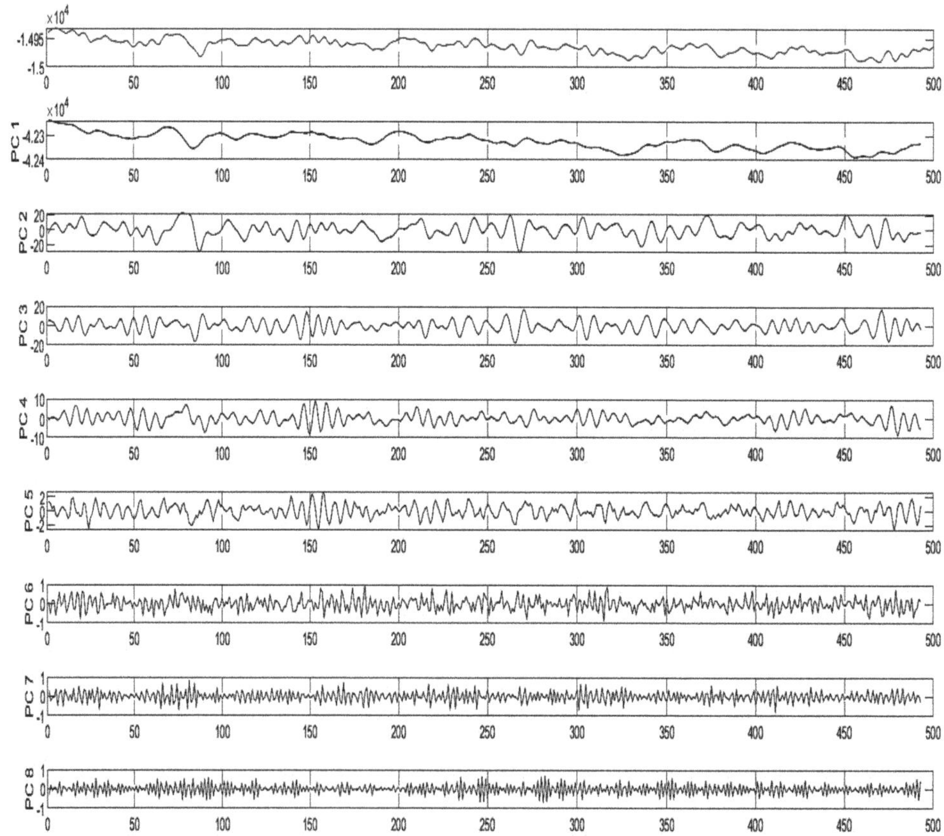

Figure 12.3. Raw EEG signal for the 'happy' class and eight principal components extracted using an embedding dimension of $L = 8$.

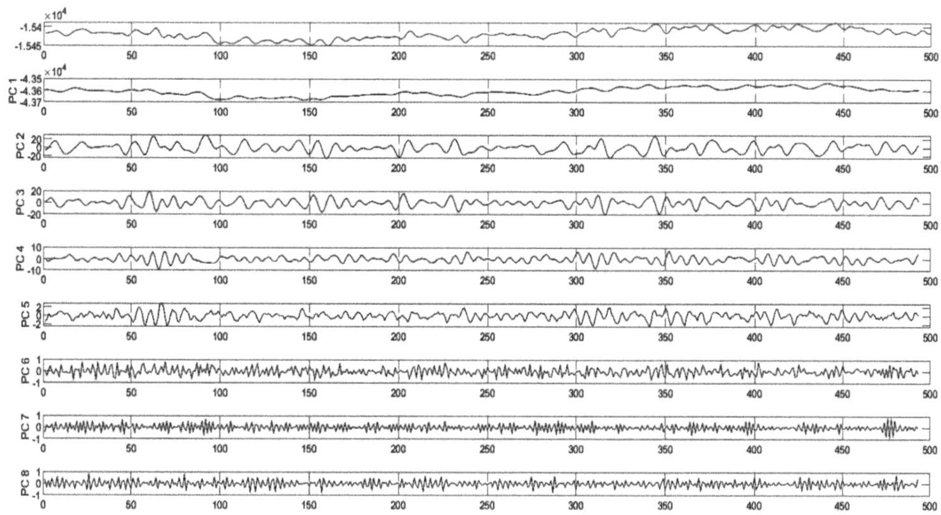

Figure 12.4. Raw EEG signal for the 'sad' class and eight principal components extracted using an embedding dimension of $L = 8$.

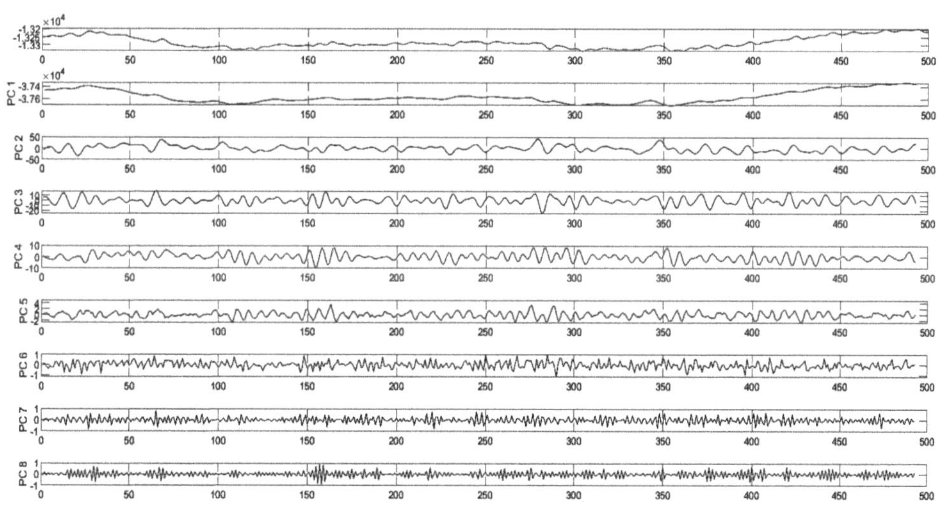

Figure 12.5. Raw EEG signal for the 'neutral' class and eight principal components extracted using an embedding dimension of $L = 8$.

Variance—the variance of each sub-band decomposed using SSA is defined as the average squared deviation from the mean value. The variance is defined as

$$\sigma^2 = \frac{1}{N}\sum_{i=1}^{N}(S_i - \mu) \tag{12.5}$$

where S_i is the segment i of the sub-band, N is the total number of samples in the sub-band, and μ is the mean value.

Standard deviation–this measures the deviation from the mean (on either side). The standard deviation is given by

$$\mathrm{SD} = \sqrt{\frac{1}{N}\sum_{i=1}^{N}(S_i - \mu)} \tag{12.6}$$

where S_i is the segment i of the sub-band, N is the total number of samples in the sub-band, and μ is the mean value.

Peak-to-peak value—the difference between a SSA sub-band's highest and lowest values.

Power bandwidth—the frequency fluctuates by at least 3 dB below the reference level at the lowest point of the spectrum. When using a rectangular window to compute the periodogram power spectrum estimation, the reference level represents the estimated maximum value.

Skewness—skewness measures the asymmetry of the data around the sample mean. When the skewness is negative, the data are more dispersed to the left than to the right of the mean. Data that have a positive skewness extend farther to the right. Skewness is given by

$$s = \frac{E(S - \mu)^3}{\sigma^3} \tag{12.7}$$

where S is the sub-band, μ is the mean, and σ is the standard deviation.

Kurtosis—this is an indicator of a distribution's propensity for outliers. It is given by

$$k = \frac{E(S - \mu)^4}{\sigma^4} \tag{12.8}$$

where S is the sub-band, μ is the mean, and σ is the standard deviation.

12.3 Results and discussion

This section discusses the details of the results obtained for the multiclass classification method. A subject-independent technique based on cross subject cross validation is used to verify the effectiveness of the classification algorithm. In this technique, any randomly selected subject feature vector is used as a testing set, and the model is trained using the features of the remaining subjects. The testing accuracy is measured for each subject, and its average is found to be significantly better than the results shown for the same data set. The data set consists of recordings of the EEGs, GSRs, and facial video signals of a total of 13 participants, of whom six were women and seven were men. The sampling frequency of the EEG and GSR signals is 500 Hz. The EEG data are preprocessed by a filter in the range of 0–75 Hz, and baseline subtraction is applied. The GSR and EEG signals are used for this problem.

Before processing, the data set is segregated class-wise for all 13 subjects. The project is a multiclass problem; it is observed from the data set that four of the

Table 12.1. Time duration for each class, shown by subject.

Subject	Duration in minutes		
	Class 1	Class 2	Class 3
Subject 1	4.38	2.70	1.52
Subject 2	0.00	2.28	5.72
Subject 3	0.00	2.70	5.83
Subject 4	4.20	2.84	1.80
Subject 5	0.00	2.70	5.99
Subject 6	4.38	2.69	1.49
Subject 7	4.48	2.69	1.51
Subject 8	4.38	2.69	1.65
Subject 9	4.33	2.26	1.51
Subject 10	4.38	2.70	1.51
Subject 11	4.21	2.69	0.00
Subject 12	4.05	2.69	1.51
Subject 13	4.38	2.69	1.51

subjects have labeled data for only two classes. Therefore, these subjects are not taken into account during the experiment. The durations of the EEG signals for each subject are given per class in table 12.1. The preprocessing steps utilize the CAR filter and extract high-arousal snippets using GSR peaks. The EEG signals are subjected to decomposition using the SSA algorithm. SSA is applied to EEG segments 1 s long, and feature extraction is performed using the extracted SBs. The feature matrix consists of seven features extracted from each of the eight SBs obtained by the SSA algorithm and also from each of the eight electrodes, making 448 features in total.

The discriminative abilities of the features can be seen in figures 12.6–12.8, which show the histogram distributions of the top seven features from the first sub-band of the first electrode. The features have visibly different histogram graphs for each of the three classes.

In our study, we observed that the personal *Z*-score (PZ) feature processing method can discriminate emotions better than the original data set, according to leave-one-subject-out cross validation. This is the case because this method can reduce the individual differences between different subjects when recording EEG signals. These individual differences result in low accuracy, as seen in the first three columns of table 12.2. Therefore, every subject's feature set is normalized using the *z*-score, as defined in equation (12.9), before we perform the leave-one-subject-out accuracy calculation.

$$Z_{\text{score}}(f) = \frac{f - \mu}{\sigma} \tag{12.9}$$

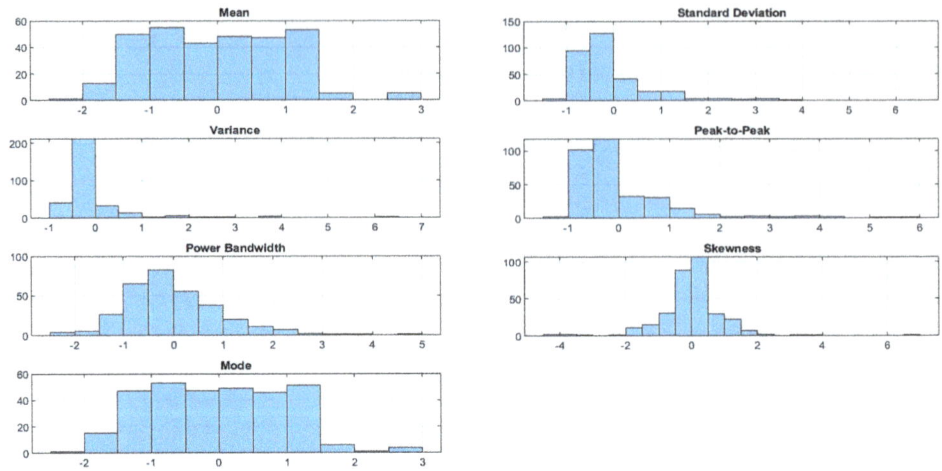

Figure 12.6. Histogram representation of feature values of the first sub-band from the first electrode for the 'sad' class.

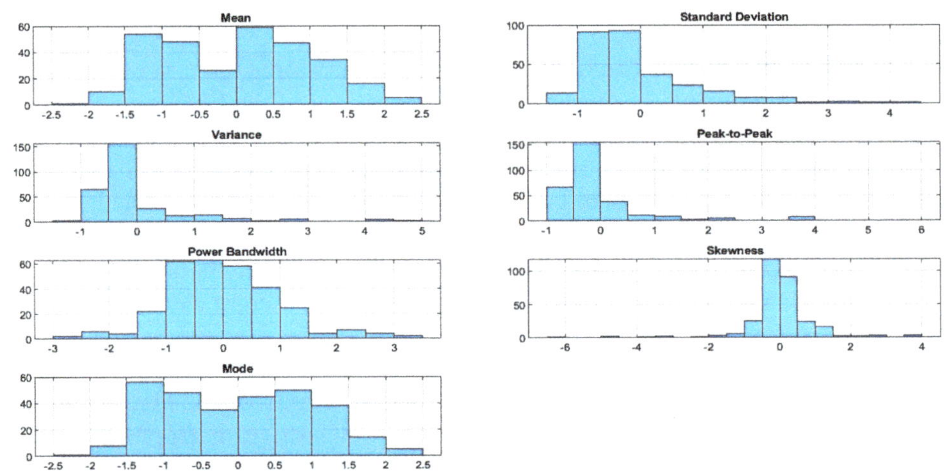

Figure 12.7. Histogram representation of feature values of the first sub-band from the first electrode for the 'happy' class.

Here, μ is the mean of one feature vector, and σ is the standard deviation. After z-score normalization, each feature or column of a feature set is normally distributed with mean = 0 and std = 1. As a result, a significant improvement of 58.8% is observed in the fine trees classifier, as shown in table 12.2.

Table 12.3 shows a leave-one-subject-out accuracy comparison between our proposed method and the only other study [31] that has worked on the LUMED-2 data set. It should be noted that the accuracy considered in this study is obtained from physiological signals only.

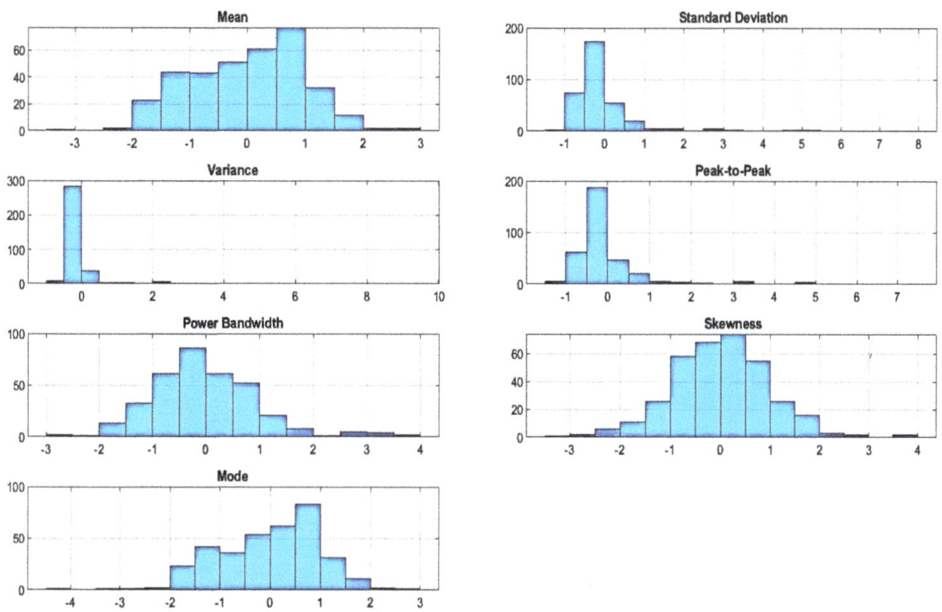

Figure 12.8. Histogram representation of feature values of the first sub-band from the first electrode for the 'neutral' class.

Table 12.2. Leave-one-subject-out accuracy improvement after normalization with the PZ.

	Without PZ normalization			With PZ normalization		
One-subject-out	Fine trees	LDA	SVM	Fine trees	LDA	SVM
Subject 1	4.3	1.7	60.3	77	75	75
Subject 4	58.3	25.5	65.8	76	55.7	55.7
Subject 6	28.5	45.1	25	59.7	61.8	60
Subject 7	54.7	46.5	59.4	70.6	53	51
Subject 8	43	26.9	53.9	64.8	50.8	40
Subject 9	64.3	58.6	58.6	67.1	64	60
Subject 10	53.9	15.7	35.6	43.5	40.7	40.5
Subject 12	37.3	53	49.2	41.6	43	40
Subject 13	8.7	11.1	56.3	59.5	50.6	49
Average	39.166 67	31.566 67	51.566 67	62.2	54.95	52.355 56

This can overcome the privacy concerns reported in [34] related to the usage of facial data by human–computer interaction (HCI) systems based on emotion recognition technologies. This chapter reports higher subject-independent accuracy for a three-class problem than [31] while reducing the number of modalities used for

Table 12.3. Comparison of leave-one-subject-out accuracies (%).

Subject	Accuracies for physiological signals from [31]	Proposed method
Subject 1	63	77
Subject 4	61.1	76
Subject 6	40.1	59.7
Subject 7	45.7	70.6
Subject 8	53.3	64.8
Subject 9	54.2	67.1
Subject 10	39.3	43.5
Subject 12	52.2	41.6
Subject 13	49.1	59.5
Average	50.88	62.2

the classification model. Other published studies have reported much higher accuracies because they considered a subject-dependent model for emotion classification.

12.4 Conclusions

The physiological changes in the human body provide accurate emotional predictions. Changes in skin conductance, which can be measured by GSR, are a notable consequence of any heightened emotional state. This study identifies local maxima in EEG signals. SSA is used to decompose the EEG signals. A classification algorithm is then used to classify reduced statistical features using the principal components. We normalize feature sets using a PZ and compare the results with the non-normalized data to improve subject-independent accuracy. The normalized feature sets provide improved classification accuracy. The use of either EEG or physiological signals from the LUMED-2 data set yields a mean leave-one-subject-out accuracy of 52%. The mean accuracy for three-class emotion classification increases to 62.2% with multimodal GSR and EEG signals. The proposed method provides better accuracy than that of the other study that used the same data set.

References

[1] Izard C E 2009 Emotion theory and research: highlights, unanswered questions, and emerging issues *Annu. Rev. Psychol.* **60** 1–25

[2] Mehta D, Siddiqui M F H and Javaid A Y 2019 Recognition of emotion intensities using machine learning algorithms: a comparative study *Sensors* **19** 1897

[3] Cowie R *et al* 2001 Emotion recognition in human-computer interaction *IEEE Signal Process. Mag.* **18** 32–80

[4] Hattingh C J *et al* 2013 Functional magnetic resonance imaging during emotion recognition in social anxiety disorder: an activation likelihood meta-analysis *Front. Hum. Neurosci.* **6** 347

[5] Ranganathan H, Chakraborty S and Panchanathan S 2016 Multimodal emotion recognition using deep learning architectures in *2016 IEEE Winter Conf. on Applications of Computer Vision (WACV)* (Lake Placid, NY: IEEE) pp 1–9

[6] Zheng W-L, Liu W, Lu Y, Lu B-L and Cichocki A 2019 EmotionMeter: a multimodal framework for recognizing human emotions *IEEE Trans. Cybern.* **49** 1110–22

[7] Bahreini K, Nadolski R and Westera W 2016 Data fusion for real-time multimodal emotion recognition through webcams and microphones in e-learning *Int. J. Hum.–Comput. Int.* **32** 415–30

[8] Cimtay Y and Ekmekcioglu E 2020 Investigating the use of pretrained convolutional neural network on cross-subject and cross-dataset EEG emotion recognition *Sensors* **20** 2034

[9] Li M, Xu H, Liu X and Lu S 2018 Emotion recognition from multichannel EEG signals using K-nearest neighbor classification *THC* **26** 509–19

[10] Zhang Y, Cheng C and Zhang Y 2021 Multimodal emotion recognition using a hierarchical fusion convolutional neural network *IEEE Access* **9** 7943–51

[11] Hasan M, Rokhshana-Nishat-Anzum , Yasmin S and Pias T S 2021 Fine-grained emotion recognition from EEG signal using fast fourier transformation and CNN in *2021 Joint 10th Int. Conf. on Informatics, Electronics & Vision (ICIEV) and 2021 5th Int. Conf. on Imaging, Vision & Pattern Recognition (icIVPR)* (Kitakyushu, Japan: IEEE) pp 1–9

[12] Jana G C, Sabath A and Agrawal A 2022 Capsule neural networks on spatio-temporal EEG frames for cross-subject emotion recognition *Biomed. Signal Process. Control* **72** 103361

[13] Bajaj V, Taran S and Sengur A 2018 Emotion classification using flexible analytic wavelet transform for electroencephalogram signals *Health Inf. Sci. Syst.* **6** 12

[14] Krishna A H, Sri A B, Priyanka K Y V S, Taran S and Bajaj V 2019 Emotion classification using EEG signals based on tunable-*Q* wavelet transform *IET Sci. Meas. Technol.* **13** 375–80

[15] Tarnowski P, Kolodziej M, Majkowski A and Rak R J 2018 Combined analysis of GSR and EEG signals for emotion recognition *2018 Int. Interdisciplinary PhD Workshop (IIPhDW)* (Swinoujście: IEEE) pp 137–41

[16] Das P, Khasnobish A and Tibarewala D N 2016 Emotion recognition employing ECG and GSR signals as markers of ANS *2016 Conf. on Advances in Signal Processing (CASP)* (Pune, India: IEEE) pp 37–42

[17] Li M and Lu B-L 2009 Emotion classification based on gamma-band EEG *2009 Annual Int. Conf. of the IEEE Engineering in Medicine and Biology Society* (Minneapolis, MN: IEEE) pp 1223–6

[18] Aydin S, Demirtaş S, Ateş K and Tunga M A 2016 Emotion recognition with eigen features of frequency band activities embedded in induced brain oscillations mediated by affective pictures *Int. J. Neur. Syst.* **26** 1650013

[19] Sharma L D and Bhattacharyya A 2021 A computerized approach for automatic human emotion recognition using sliding mode singular spectrum analysis *IEEE Sens.* J **21** 26931–40

[20] Hu H, Guo S, Liu R and Wang P 2017 An adaptive singular spectrum analysis method for extracting brain rhythms of electroencephalography *PeerJ* **5** e3474

[21] Agarwal S and Zubair M 2021 Classification of alcoholic and non-alcoholic EEG signals based on sliding-SSA and independent component analysis *IEEE Sens.* J **21** 26198–206

[22] Chen J X, Zhang P W, Mao Z J, Huang Y F, Jiang D M and Zhang Y N 2019 Accurate EEG-based emotion recognition on combined features using deep convolutional neural networks *IEEE Access* **7** 44317–28

[23] Jirayucharoensak S, Pan-Ngum S and Israsena P 2014 EEG-based emotion recognition using deep learning network with principal component based covariate shift adaptation *Sci. World J.* **2014** 1–10

[24] Takehara H, Ishihara S and Iwaki T 2020 Comparison between facilitating and suppressing facial emotional expressions using frontal EEG asymmetry *Front. Behav. Neurosci.* **14** 554147

[25] Zheng X, Zhang M, Li T, Ji C and Hu B 2021 A novel consciousness emotion recognition method using ERP components and MMSE *J. Neural Eng.* **18** 046001

[26] Schirrmeister R T *et al* 2017 Deep learning with convolutional neural networks for EEG decoding and visualization *Hum. Brain Mapp.* **38** 5391–420

[27] Suhaimi N S, Mountstephens J and Teo J 2020 EEG-based emotion recognition: a state-of-the-art review of current trends and opportunities *Comput. Intell. Neurosci.* **2020** 1–19

[28] Alazrai R, Homoud R, Alwanni H and Daoud M 2018 EEG-based emotion recognition using quadratic time-frequency distribution *Sensors* **18** 2739

[29] Chen H *et al* 2021 Personal-Zscore: Eliminating Individual Difference for EEG-based Cross-Subject Emotion Recognition *IEEE Trans. Affect. Comput.* 1

[30] Jatupaiboon N, Pan-ngum S and Israsena P 2013 Real-time EEG-based happiness detection system *Sci. World J.* **2013** 1–12

[31] Cimtay Y, Ekmekcioglu E and Caglar-Ozhan S 2020 Cross-subject multimodal emotion recognition based on hybrid fusion *IEEE Access* **8** 168865–78

[32] Vautard R and Ghil M 1989 Singular spectrum analysis in nonlinear dynamics, with applications to paleoclimatic time series *Physica* D **35** 395–424

[33] Yu X, Chum P and Sim K-B 2014 Analysis the effect of PCA for feature reduction in non-stationary EEG based motor imagery of BCI system *Optik* **125** 1498–502

[34] McStay A 2020 Emotional AI, soft biometrics and the surveillance of emotional life: an unusual consensus on privacy *Big Data Soc.* **7** 205395172090438

Chapter 13

Speech emotion recognition using empirical wavelet transform and cubic support vector machine

Mehrab Hosain, Anukul Pandey, Sachin Taran, Ravi, Asmar Hafeez and Nikhil

The human voice is an essential tool for conveying emotions; therefore, this chapter proposes a novel speech emotion recognition (SER) framework based on a combination of empirical wavelet transform (EWT) and cubic support vector machine (CSVM). The system is designed for multiclass SER and uses a combination of auditory spectrograms, cepstral coefficients, spectral descriptors, periodicity, and harmonicity for feature extraction. The extracted features are used as CSVM classifier inputs, and the classifier is trained to recognize the speaker's emotional state. The proposed system is evaluated using the Toronto Emotional Speech Set (TESS) data set, which has seven emotion classes labeled 'angry,' 'sad,' 'fear,' 'neutral,' 'disgust,' 'pleasant surprise,' and 'happy.' Our proposed system achieves an experimental accuracy of 99.2%, outperforming other state-of-the-art systems. This study demonstrates the effectiveness of the CSVM classifier in multiclass SER and provides a promising solution for SER.

13.1 Introduction

SER is a vital area for research into human emotions, due to its numerous applications in areas such as communication technologies, human–computer interaction, and psychology. SER is a growing field that has attracted researchers in recent years due to its wide range of uses in several fields, including entertainment, speech treatment, and human–computer interfacing [1–4]. SER refers to the process of automatically classifying the emotional state of a speaker based on the acoustic features of speech signals. The ultimate objective of SER is to provide a framework that can identify the emotions of a speaker with high accuracy and robustness. In recent years, various techniques have been proposed for SER, including machine learning algorithms, feature extraction methods, and signal processing techniques.

doi:10.1088/978-0-7503-5964-1ch13

The machine learning algorithms most frequently employed for SER include artificial neural networks (ANNs), the k-nearest neighbors algorithm, support vector machines (SVMs), and decision trees [5, 6]. The feature extraction methods used include auditory spectrograms, cepstral coefficients, spectral descriptors, and prosodic features [7–9]. Signal processing techniques such as EWT have been used for feature extraction and signal decomposition [10].

Emotion recognition, particularly recognition carried out using speech and electroencephalogram (EEG) signals, has gained significant attention in the last few years due to its application in human–computer interactions. In [11], a sophisticated architecture leveraging decomposition techniques is discussed that improves the accuracy of emotion recognition across all languages. Similarly, the author of [12] introduces a nonlinear feature extraction method combined with variational mode decomposition (VMD) and the Teager–Kaiser energy operator (TKEO), which significantly enhances the precision of emotion detection using speech signals. This approach is very effective at separating intrinsic mode functions and capturing emotional nuances in speech.

In the context of emotion recognition, the authors of [13] develop a novel two-stage filtering method that can perform correlation and instantaneous frequency analysis. This improves emotion classification using EEG data. This approach is very useful for its effectiveness in analyzing single-channel EEGs, simplifying hardware requirements and making the technology more useful for practical applications. In addition, work on emotion classification using flexible analytic wavelet transform [15] and tunable-Q wavelet transform [14] again demonstrates a commitment to refining signal processing techniques for speech emotion detection. All these contributions collectively highlight the innovative strategies being used to develop accurate and applicable SER modalities.

In this study, we propose a SER system that combines the advantages of CSVM and EWT [10, 16]. The system is designed to perform multiclass SER. It uses a combination of features from auditory spectrograms, cepstral coefficients, and spectral descriptors of speech signals. The extracted features are then used as the input of a CSVM classifier, which is trained to categorize the emotional state of its input speech signals. The main objective of this chapter is to demonstrate the effectiveness of the CSVM classifier in a multiclass SER environment [17]. Our experimental findings demonstrate that this proposed SER method performs better than all current state-of-the-art related machine learning algorithms, such as SVMs and ANNs, in terms of accuracy and robustness [18]. In addition, our results demonstrate that the combination of EWT and CSVM provides a powerful framework for multiclass SER that can be applied to various domains.

13.2 Related work

SER is an increasingly prominent field of research, and many different algorithms and methods have been presented in an effort to increase its accuracy. ANNs, convolutional neural networks (CNNs), SVMs, and deep belief networks (DBNs) are some of the common methods that have been utilized in SVM-based sequential event reconstruction. In recent years, researchers have placed strong emphasis on the utilization of numerous feature extraction strategies in an attempt to increase the accuracy of SER systems. The authors of [19] studied the classification of audio files using traditional classifiers on three data sets: combined, Ryerson Audio-Visual Database of Emotional Speech and Song (RAVDESS), and TESS. To extract speech features, they utilized three techniques: mel-frequency cepstral coefficients (MFCCs), chromagrams, and mel spectrograms (MelSpecs), resulting in 180 features. The authors compared the accuracy of different classifiers and found that the gradient boosting classifier outperformed the other classifiers, achieving the highest accuracy of 84.96% for the mixed data set. Another study described the continuous development of a deep-learning-based system for recognizing speech emotions using acoustic data from spectrograms, chromagrams, and MFCCs [20]. Their proposed framework was capable of recognizing emotions and achieved an accuracy of 89% on combined data sets using data augmentation techniques.

To prevent overload and improve the performance of SER systems, a feature selection strategy is needed to choose vital features rather than increasing their number. Yao *et al* presented a speech emotion classification model that combined a deep neural network, a CNN, and a recurrent neural network (RNN). Their model recognized four common emotion classes: happy, sad, angry, and neutral [21]. ReddyBandela and Kumar presented an unsupervised feature selection approach that increased the classification accuracy of a SER system without increasing processing time. They used a combination of gammatone cepstral coefficients (GTCCs), interspeech paralinguistic features, and power-normalized cepstral coefficients (PNCCs) and applied dense non-negative matrix factorization (NMF) to remove noise in a noisy environment [22]. This study proposes a multi-input deep neural network for SER that simultaneously learns MelSpec and Geneva minimalistic acoustic parameter set (GeMAPS) audio features. The model achieved higher accuracy than those of existing methods and could effectively recognize emotions, particularly 'happy.' A focal loss function was introduced to address imbalanced data [23]. The lack of standardized dataset testing restricts SER model to compare with state-of-the-art methods and generalizability of SER systems to practical applications. Another research gap is the need for more robust and accurate feature extraction methods for speech analysis [24].

13.3 Methodology

The process of emotion recognition using CSVM and EWT is as follows:

Data loading:

1. The first step is to load the TESS data set, which contains speech samples with different emotions.
2. Signal Decomposition: the next step is to decompose the speech signal into sub-signals using EWT.
3. Feature Extraction: after signal decomposition, 84 features are extracted from 18 unique features utilizing feature extraction techniques such as auditory spectrograms, cepstral coefficients, spectral descriptors, and prosodic features.

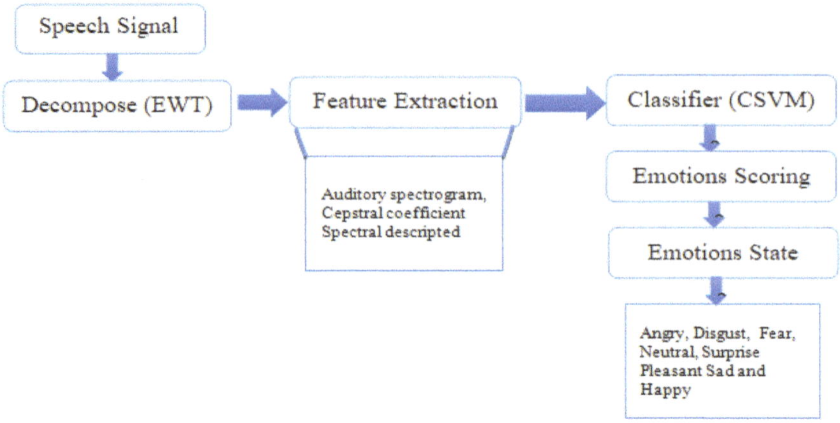

Figure 13.1. SER flow diagram.

4. Classifier Training: the computed spectral features are then utilized as input to a SVM classifier, which is trained to classify the emotional state of the input speech signal.
5. Emotional Scoring: based on the extracted features, the SVM classifier is then utilized to predict the speaker's emotional state, and an emotional score is produced.
6. Emotional State Recognition: finally, the emotional scoring system is used to identify the speaker's emotional state.

   This study demonstrates the effectiveness of using a CSVM classifier for multiclass SER and provides a promising solution for this research field. A flow diagram of the proposed framework is presented in figure 13.1. Detailed descriptions of each step are presented in the following sections.

13.3.1 Empirical wavelet transform

EWT, developed by Jerome Gilles in 2013, is an adaptive wavelet filter bank for signal decomposition [10]. Like EMD, EWT seeks to decompose a signal into AM and FM components. EWT is a simple, straightforward, and adjustable algorithm with a robust mathematical foundation. EWT presents a way to create a wavelet family adjustable to the processed speech signal. This is analogous to developing a set of band-pass filters when viewed through the window of Fourier analysis. Construct a bank of N wavelet filters using well-chosen Fourier supports (N band-pass filters and one low-pass filter that correspond to the estimate and specific components). This is done by picking suitable modes in the signal spectrum. To accomplish adaptability, assume that the filter supports are dependent on the spectrum of the analyzed signal. Indeed, an IMF's spectrum is compact, in addition to being oriented around a certain frequency. The subdivision scheme in classical wavelet transforms is fixed, whereas in EWT it is determined empirically.

To start, local maximum and minimum filters are applied to the frequency spectrum in order to discover and sort extreme values. Second, a peak sequence is formed by the highest m neighboring local maxima. Then, between two consecutive

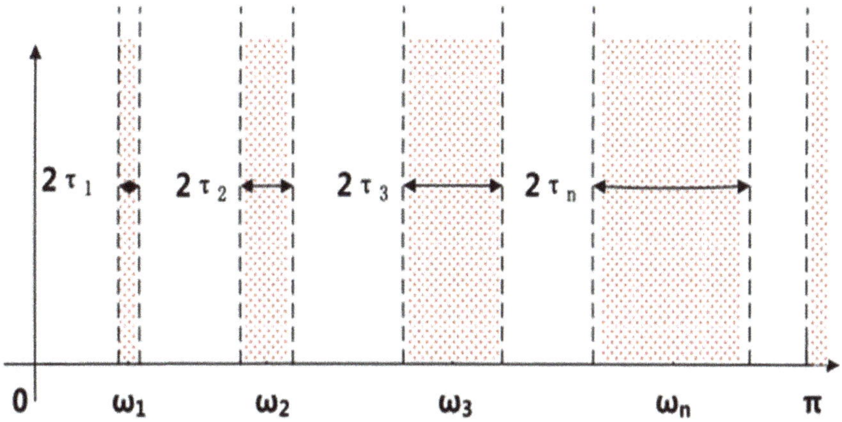

Figure 13.2. Fourier spectrum segmenting.

peak values, the lowest local minima were obtained and used as the components of the boundary. As illustrated in figure 13.2, the Fourier spectrum has a frequency range of 0–π [25]. At the same time, the Fourier spectrum is split into N different components using the detected boundary, which is denoted by ω_n ($n = 0,1,\ldots,N$, $\omega_0 = 0$, and $\omega_N = \pi$). Centered around every ω_n, we define a transition zone (the hatched area in figure 13.1) whose width is $2\tau n$ ($\tau n = \gamma\, \omega_n, 0 < \gamma < 1$).

Now, using the same approach that we used to define the traditional wavelet transform [26, 27], this study we further specifies the EWT as $\mathcal{W}_f^{\varepsilon}(n, t)$. The inner products with the empirical wavelets determine the detail coefficients; they are defined by (13.1) and (13.2), as follows:

$$\begin{aligned} \mathcal{W}_f^{\varepsilon}(n, t) &= \langle f, \psi_n \rangle = \int f(\tau)\overline{\psi_n(\tau - t)}d\tau \\ &= (\hat{f}(\omega)\overline{\hat{\psi}_n(\omega)})^{\vee}. \end{aligned} \tag{13.1}$$

The estimation coefficients (we use the convention $\mathcal{W}_f^{\varepsilon}(0, t)$ to denote them) are obtained by internal multiplication of the scaling function

$$\begin{aligned} \mathcal{W}_f^{\varepsilon}(0, t) &= \langle f, \phi_1 \rangle = \int f(\tau)\overline{\phi_1(\tau - t)}d\tau \\ &= (\hat{f}(\omega)\overline{\hat{\phi}_1(\omega)})^{\vee} \end{aligned} \tag{13.2}$$

where the variables $\hat{\psi}_n(\omega)$ and $\hat{\phi}_1(\omega)$ are defined by (13.3) and (13.4), respectively. The reconstruction is obtained as follows:

$$\begin{aligned} f(t) &= \mathcal{W}_f^{\varepsilon}(0, t) \times \phi_1(t) + \sum_{n=1}^{N} \mathcal{W}_f^{\varepsilon}(n, t) \times \psi_n(t) \\ &= \left(\hat{\mathcal{W}}_f^{\varepsilon}(0, \omega)\hat{\phi}_1(\omega) + \sum_{n=1}^{N} \hat{\mathcal{W}}_f^{\varepsilon}(n, \omega)\hat{\psi}_n(\omega) \right)^{\vee}. \end{aligned} \tag{13.3}$$

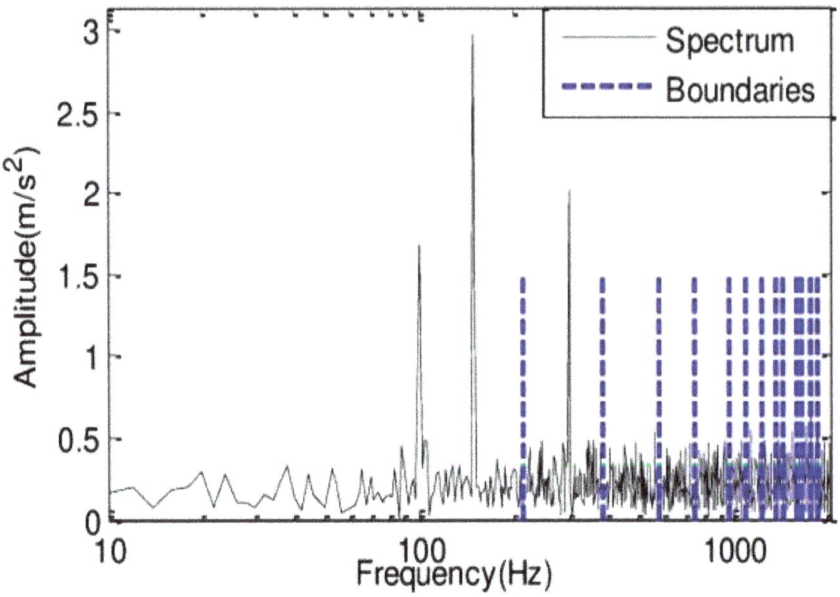

Figure 13.3. Representation of spectrum segmentation in scale space.

In accordance with this formalism, the empirical mode f_k is given by (13.4)

$$\begin{aligned} f_0(t) &= \mathcal{W}_f^{\varepsilon}(0, t) \times \phi_1(t) \\ f_k(t) &= \mathcal{W}_f^{\varepsilon}(k, t) \times \psi_k(t) \end{aligned} \tag{13.4}$$

where k is the number of modes.

In the spectrum, the signal can be seen to have three vertical lines. In a perfect world, EWT would divide all three frequencies without using any invalid or extraneous components. In order to divide up the spectrum, a scale-space representation approach is utilized, such as that shown in figure 13.3.

13.3.2 Feature extraction

In feature extraction, meaningful and distinctive qualities are obtained from the raw speech signal. The extracted features selected are those that can be utilized to identify different emotional states in speech emotion detection. These characteristics are selected from the speech signal. The voice signal is parsed in order to extract these features, which are then used to train machine learning models that are able to identify emotions based on the features.

In order for speech emotion identification to be successful, suitable features must be chosen. This is because the extracted features must be able to accurately represent the significant emotional information contained within the speech signal. In SER, a variety of feature extraction strategies, including MFCC, linear predictive coding (LPC), and prosodic features, have been utilized [28–30].

13.3.3 Auditory spectrograms

The primary application of auditory spectrograms is in speech processing, where they are utilized to analyze the spectral content of speech signals [31]. In speech analysis, auditory spectrograms can be used to extract phonetic features, such as formants (resonant frequencies determining vowel sounds), by computing the following equation:

$$S(f,\ t) = |X(f,\ t)|^2 \tag{13.5}$$

where $X(f, t)$ is the short-time Fourier transform of the speech signal, and $S(f, t)$ denotes the spectrogram.

13.3.4 Auditory cepstral coefficients

Auditory cepstral coefficients (ACCs) are a type of feature extraction method for speech signals that is often used in speech processing and speech recognition applications. ACCs are based on a model of the auditory system and are designed to work like the human ear. ACCs have been shown to be good at recognizing speech, and they have been used in many different ways [32].

(a) Gammatone cepstral coefficients (GTCCs): the GTCC method involves the extraction of GTCCs, delta, and log energy. The data is divided into overlapping parts using the following equation (13.6):

$$\text{gtcc} = \text{GammatoneFilterBank}(X) \times \text{CepstralTransform} \tag{13.6}$$

where X represents the input speech signal, GammatoneFilterBank denotes the gammatone filter bank applied to X, and CepstralTransform denotes the cepstral transformation applied to the filtered signal.

(b) MFCCs: the MFCC method is a very popular method for the extraction of speech features, and ongoing research is aimed at improving its performance. The delta-delta MFCC is an MFCC implementation that improves speaker verification. It can be computed using the following equation (13.7):

$$\text{mfcc} = \text{MelFilter Bank}(X) \times \text{CepstralTransform} \tag{13.7}$$

where X represents the input speech signal, MelFilterBank represents the mel-frequency filter bank applied to X, and CepstralTransform represents the cepstral transformation applied to the filtered signal.

13.3.5 Periodicity and harmonicity

Periodicity and harmony play important roles in speech signal processing, since they facilitate the determination of a voice's sound and pitch. Periodicity describes the regularity of the pitch period, and harmonicity describes the number of fundamental frequency harmonics in the signal. These traits have been used for recognizing speech, identifying the speaker, and determining how someone feels [33].

(a) **Harmonic ratio:** the harmonic ratio is used to describe the degree of harmonicity present in a signal and is computed using equation (13.8):

$$\text{hr} = \frac{\text{Power}(f_0)}{\text{TotalPower}} \tag{13.8}$$

where f_0 represents the fundamental frequency and TotalPower represents the total power in an audio frame.

(b) **Pitch:** pitch is the physical characteristic of sound that corresponds to timbre, volume, and rhythm. It can be said to be the property of the auditory perception of speech that organizes sounds on a musical scale. Mathematically, pitch can be represented by equation (13.9):

$$\text{pitch} = \frac{1}{T} \tag{13.9}$$

where T is the time for one complete cycle.

13.3.6 Spectral descriptor

In speech processing, spectral descriptors are utilized in order to carry out an analysis of the signal's spectral properties. Spectral descriptors include all the signal's characteristics and are not limited to the distribution of energy across frequency bands. They have been utilized in the processes of speaker recognition, speech recognition, and emotion recognition because they contain details about the signal's frequency content [34].

(a) **Spectral centroid**: the spectral centroid (SC) is computed by taking the weighted average of the frequency components in the spectrum, using the magnitude of each frequency component as the weight, as given by equation (13.10):

$$\text{CS} = \frac{\Sigma(f \times |X(f)|)}{\Sigma(|X(f)|)} \tag{13.10}$$

where $X(f)$ is the magnitude of the frequency component, f is the frequency, and the sum is taken over all frequency components.

(b) **Spectral crest**: the spectral crest (CR) is the ratio of the peak value of the spectrum to the average value of the spectrum. It is defined in equation (13.11):

$$\text{CR} = \frac{\max(|X(f)|)}{\Sigma(|X(f)|)} \times h \tag{13.11}$$

where h is the number of frequency components.

(c) **Spectral decrease:** spectral decrease (SD) measures the amount of energy lost in the lower-frequency regions of the spectrum. It is calculated using equation (13.12):

$$\text{SD} = \Sigma(|X(f)|) - \Sigma(|X(f)|) \quad \text{for} \quad f < \text{Fc} \tag{13.12}$$

where Fc is a cutoff frequency.

(d) **Spectral entropy:** spectral entropy (*H*) is computed by taking the average of the logarithm of the magnitude of the frequency components in the spectrum. It is defined as follows (equation 13.13):

$$H = -\frac{\Sigma(|X(f)| \times \log(|X(f)|))}{\Sigma(|X(f)|)}. \tag{13.13}$$

(e) **Spectral flatness:** spectral flatness (SF) is defined as the ratio of the geometric mean of the magnitude of the frequency components in the spectrum to the arithmetic mean of the magnitude of the frequency components *X(f)* in the spectrum. It is calculated using equation (13.14):

$$\mathrm{SF} = \frac{\left(\Pi(|X(f)|)^{\frac{1}{N}}\right)}{\frac{\Sigma(|X(f)|)}{N}}. \tag{13.14}$$

(f) **Spectral flux:** spectral flux is computed by taking the difference between the magnitude of the frequency components in the current and previous spectrums (see equation 13.15):

$$\mathrm{SF} = \Sigma(|X(f, t) - X(f, t-1)|) \tag{13.15}$$

where *X(f,t)* is the magnitude of the frequency component at time *t*.

(g) **Spectral kurtosis:** spectral kurtosis (SK) measures the flatness or non-Gaussian nature of the spectrum near its centroid. It is defined in equation (13.16):

$$\mathrm{SK} = \frac{\Sigma((f - C)^4 \times |X(f)|)}{\Sigma(|X(f)|)^2}. \tag{13.16}$$

(h) **Spectral roll-off point:** the spectral roll-off point (SRP) is defined as the frequency of the bin that contains a certain percentage of the total energy of the signal. It is defined in equation (13.17):

$$\mathrm{SRP} = f \text{ where } \Sigma(|X(f)|) \text{ for } f <= \mathrm{SRP} \,/\, \Sigma(|X(f)|) >= P \tag{13.17}$$

where *P* is the percentage of the total energy.

(i) **Spectral skewness:** spectral skewness (SS) measures the extent of symmetry around the centroid. It is defined in equation (13.18):

$$\mathrm{SS} = \frac{\Sigma((f - C)^3 \times |X(f)|)}{\Sigma(|X(f)|)^{\frac{3}{2}}}. \tag{13.18}$$

(j) **Spectral slope:** the spectral slope (SSl) measures the rate of change of the magnitude of the speech signal frequency components in the spectrum. It is defined in equation (13.19):

$$\mathrm{SSl} = \frac{\Sigma(f \times (|X(f)| - C))}{\Sigma(|X(f)|)}. \tag{13.19}$$

13.3.7 Classification algorithms: cubic support vector machine

CSVM is a variant of the SVM machine learning algorithm that is utilized for classification and regression analysis. The main difference between CSVM and other SVMs is that CSVM uses a cubic kernel function instead of a linear or radial basis function kernel. The kernel function is utilized to map the input data into a higher-dimensional space, where a hyperplane can be used to separate the classes [16, 35].

The mathematical expression for the cubic kernel function in CSVM is given by (13.20):

$$k(x, y) = (1 + \langle x, y \rangle)^3 \tag{13.20}$$

where x and y are the vectors of the input and $\langle x, y \rangle$ represents the dot product of x and y. The cubic kernel function enables the CSVM to capture nonlinear relationships between the input data and the target variable, making it more flexible and suitable for complex data sets. CSVM also provides better generalization performance compared to other SVM models and has the potential to handle large data sets. In the context of SER, CSVM has been shown to produce promising results and has the potential to improve the performance of emotion recognition systems. Overall, CSVM is a powerful tool for machine learning applications, especially for complex and nonlinear data sets.

13.4 Data set

The TESS is a very valuable resource for researchers and practitioners in the SER field. This data set is designed to provide a diverse, large set of speech recordings that are free of plagiarism, ensuring that the results generated from this data are reliable and accurate. The TESS data set consists of over 2400 speech samples recorded by actors in a controlled laboratory environment. The TESS Audio Collection features the sounds of two female actors expressing a range of emotions, namely angry, fear, happy, pleasant surprise, disgust, sad, and neutral. This compilation provides a comprehensive representation of various emotional states.

The TESS data set is also notable for its high-quality recordings, which are critical for achieving accurate results in SER. The actors were carefully selected for their ability to accurately convey emotions, and the recordings were made using state-of-the-art equipment to ensure that the audio quality was consistent and reliable.

13.5 Results and discussion

The proposed architecture utilizes EWT to decompose each speech signal into sub-bands. These sub-bands provide simplified representations of the speech signals and make the signals predictable. After that, a set of features is extracted, as discussed in section 13.2. To improve the performance, static measures of the extracted features are also calculated and utilized as features. Finally, we perform a machine learning analysis of a data set consisting of 2800 samples using several different algorithms. Our results, as shown in table 13.1, indicate that the cubic SVM algorithm achieved the highest accuracy, with a score of 99.2%. Other algorithms, such as the neural network, decision tree, and naive Bayes algorithms, also produced relatively high accuracies, reaching scores close to those of cubic SVM except for medium tree, whose accuracy was 82.2%. Table 13.2 lists the per-class results for emotion validation.

The high accuracy achieved by the cubic SVM algorithm suggests that the data set may have a nonlinear relationship between the input features and the target variable. The reason for this is that the cubic SVM algorithm is designed to handle linear as well as nonlinear data, as it uses a kernel function to transform the input data into a higher-dimensional space where a linear decision boundary can be found. In contrast, the neural network, decision tree, and naive Bayes algorithms are all based on linear models, and may not be as effective at handling nonlinear data.

Table 13.1. Comparison of the performance of various ML algorithms in processing the TESS data set.

Classifier name	Accuracy (%)
Cubic SVM	99.2
Quadratic SVM	99.1
Medium Gaussian SVM	99.1
Linear discriminant	98.7
Linear SVM	98.6
Wide neural network	98.3
Bagged trees	98.2
Medium *k*-NN	99.2
Kernel naive Bayes	91.5
Medium tree	82

Table 13.2. Validation classification performance achieved by cubic SVM, per class.

Emotion class	Score (%)
Angry	100
Disgust	100
Fear	95.5
Happy	99.5
Neutral	100
Pleasant surprise	99.5
Sad	100

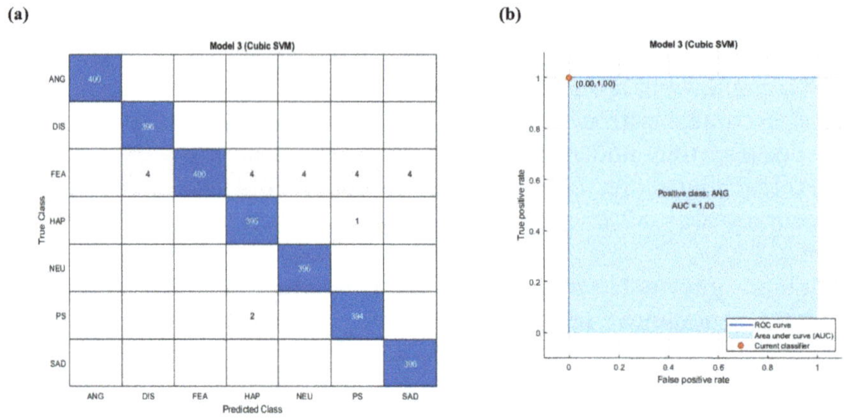

Figure 13.4. (a) Confusion matrices and (b) ROC curve.

In addition, it is worth noting that while the accuracy of the other algorithms is lower than that of cubic SVM, they still produce relatively high scores. This indicates that they may also be useful for this particular data set, especially if interpretability or computational efficiency is an important factor. Figure 13.4 shows the confusion matrices and receiver operating characteristic (ROC) curve. Further analysis, such as feature selection and hyperparameter tuning, may be needed to optimize the performance of these algorithms. The proposed architecture proved highly efficient for the angry, disgust, and sad emotion classes as well as the neutral class.

Advantages:

- Unlike traditional wavelet transforms, which use predefined wavelet functions, EWT adapts to the specific characteristics of the signal being analyzed. This allows for more precise and relevant decomposition of the signal based on its intrinsic properties.
- The empirical approach allows EWT to handle a wide range of signals, including nonstationary and complex signals, more effectively than traditional methods.
- By adapting to the signal's actual structure, EWT can provide better performance in the presence of noise.
- This approach enhances social media content analysis through SER, providing valuable insights into the speech signal.

Disadvantages:

- Validating emotion data sets can be challenging, leading to inaccurate emotion recognition.
- Although EWT can be efficient, the empirical determination of wavelet filters and the preceding EMD process can be computationally intensive, especially for large data sets or signals of high complexity.

- Supporting emotion recognition in multiple languages can be difficult.
- Some software only accepts text data, limiting the effectiveness of image, pattern, video, and audio input.

13.6 Conclusions

This study demonstrated the effectiveness of using EWT, statistical and spectral descriptors, periodicity, and harmonicity as feature extraction methods in recognizing speech emotions. The results showed that the CSVM algorithm achieved a high accuracy rate of 99.2% in recognizing emotions, including the angry, sad, fear, disgust, pleasant surprise, and happy classes, as well as the neutral class. This research contributes to the field of speech recognition and analysis and has the potential to be applied in various areas such as psychology, sociology, and linguistics. The findings of this study provide valuable insights into the relationship between speech and emotions and can be used to further explore this topic. In addition, the proposed system is designed for multiclass SER, and further research is needed to extend the system to handle more classes. Furthermore, the system is designed for English speech, and it would be interesting to assess the performance of the system in analyzing other languages.

Data availability statement

This study used the publicly available data set available at: https://doi.org/10.5683/SP2/E8H2MF.

Conflict of interest statement

The authors declare that there are no conflicts of interest.

References

[1] Wani T M *et al* 2021 A comprehensive review of speech emotion recognition systems *IEEE Access* **9** 47795–814

[2] Schuller B W 2018 Speech emotion recognition: two decades in a nutshell, benchmarks, and ongoing trends *Commun. ACM* **61** 90–9

[3] Lieskovská E *et al* 2021 A review on speech emotion recognition using deep learning and attention mechanism *Electronics* **10** 1163

[4] Khalil R A *et al* 2019 Speech emotion recognition using deep learning techniques: a review *IEEE Access* **7** 117327–45

[5] Harar P, Burget R and Dutta M K 2017 Speech emotion recognition with deep learning *2017 4th Int. Conf. Signal Process. Integr. Netw. SPIN (IEEE, Noida, Delhi-NCR, India)* (Piscataway, NJ: IEEE) 137–40

[6] Gupta V, Juyal S and Hu Y-C 2022 Understanding human emotions through speech spectrograms using deep neural network *J. Supercomput.* **78** 6944–73

[7] Kim C and Stern R M 2016 Power-normalized cepstral coefficients (PNCC) for robust speech recognition *IEEE/ACM Trans. Audio Speech Lang. Process.* **24** 1315–29

[8] Delić V *et al* 2019 Speech technology progress based on new machine learning paradigm *Comput. Intell. Neurosci.* **2019** 4368036

[9] Zhao Z *et al* 2023 A multi-feature sets fusion strategy with similar samples removal for snore sound classification *National Conf. on Man-Machine Speech Communication* (Singapore: Springer Nature)

[10] Gilles J 2013 Empirical wavelet transform *IEEE Trans. Signal Process.* **61** 3999–4010

[11] Ravi S T 2024 A novel decomposition-based architecture for multilingual speech emotion recognition *Neural Comput. Appl.* **36** 9347–59

[12] Ravi S T 2023 A nonlinear feature extraction approach for speech emotion recognition using VMD and TKEO *Appl. Acoust.* **214** 109667

[13] Sachin T and Bajaj V 2019 Emotion recognition from single-channel EEG signals using a two-stage correlation and instantaneous frequency-based filtering method *Comput. Methods Programs Biomed.* **173** 157–65

[14] Krishna A H, Sri A B, Sai Priyanka K Y V, Taran S and Bajaj V 2019 Emotion classification using EEG signals based on tunable-Q wavelet transform *IET Sci. Meas. Technol.* **13** 375–80

[15] Varun B, Taran S and Sengur. A 2018 Emotion classification using flexible analytic wavelet transform for electroencephalogram signals *Health Inf. Sci. Syst.* **6** 12

[16] Jain U, Nathani K, Ruban N, Joseph Raj A N, Zhuang Z and Mahesh V G V 2018 Cubic SVM classifier based feature extraction and emotion detection from speech signals *2018 Int. Conf. Sens. Netw. Signal Process. SNSP (IEEE, Xi'an, China)* 386–91

[17] Zhang W, Meng X, Li Z, Lu Q and Tan S 2015 Emotion Recognition in Speech Using Multi-classification SVM *2015 IEEE 12th Intl Conf Ubiquitous Intell. Comput. 2015 IEEE 12th Intl Conf Auton. Trust. Comput. 2015 IEEE 15th Intl Conf Scalable Comput. Commun. Its Assoc. Workshop UIC-ATC-ScalCom (UIC/ATC/ScalCom 2015) (IEEE, Beijing)* (Piscataway, NJ: IEEE) 1181–6

[18] Ottoni L T C, Ottoni A L C and Cerqueira J de J F 2023 A deep learning approach for speech emotion recognition optimization using meta-learning *Electronics* **12** 4859

[19] Asiya U A and Kiran V K 2021 Speech Emotion Recognition-A Deep Learning Approach *2021 Fifth International Conference on I-SMAC (IoT in Social, Mobile, Analytics and Cloud) (I-SMAC) (IEEE, Palladam, India)* (Piscataway, NJ: IEEE) pp 867–71

[20] Özseven T 2019 A novel feature selection method for speech emotion recognition *Appl. Acoust.* **146** 320–6

[21] Yao Z *et al* 2020 Speech emotion recognition using fusion of three multi-task learning-based classifiers: HSF-DNN, MS-CNN and LLD-RNN *Speech Commun.* **120** 11–9

[22] Bandela S R and Kishore Kumar T 2021 Unsupervised feature selection and NMF de-noising for robust speech emotion recognition *Appl. Acoust.* **172** 107645

[23] Toyoshima I *et al* 2023 Multi-input speech emotion recognition model using mel spectrogram and GeMAPS *Sensors* **23** 1743

[24] Pandey S K, Shekhawat H S and Prasanna S R M 2019 Deep learning techniques for speech emotion recognition: a review *2019 29th Int. Conf. Radioelektronika (RADIOELEKTRONIKA)* (Piscataway, NJ: IEEE)

[25] Daubechies I 1992 *Ten Lectures on Wavelets* (Philadelphia, PA: Society for Industrial and Applied Mathematics)

[26] Perrier V, Philipovitch T and Basdevant C 1995 Wavelet spectra compared to Fourier spectra *J. Math. Phys.* **36** 1506–19

[27] Gilles J and Heal K 2014 A parameterless scale-space approach to find meaningful modes in histograms—application to image and spectrum segmentation *Int. J. Wavelets Multiresolution Inf. Process.* **12** 1450044

[28] Muda L, Begam M and Elamvazuthi I 2010 Voice recognition algorithms using mel frequency cepstral coefficient (MFCC) and dynamic time warping (DTW) techniques *arXiv preprint* arXiv:1003.4083

[29] Marwala T 2023 *Artificial Intelligence, Game Theory and Mechanism Design in Politics* (Singapore: Springer Nature)

[30] Poria S *et al* 2017 A review of affective computing: from unimodal analysis to multimodal fusion *Inf. Fusion* **37** 98–125

[31] 1992 *The Auditory Processing of Speech* ed M E Schouten (Berlin: de Gruyter Mouton)

[32] Ali Z *et al* 2016 Automatic voice pathology detection with running speech by using estimation of auditory spectrum and cepstral coefficients based on the all-pole model *J. Voice* **30** 757–e7

[33] Su L, Chuang T-Y and Yang Y-H 2016 Exploiting frequency, periodicity and harmonicity using advanced time-frequency concentration techniques for multipitch estimation of choir and symphony *ISMIR 2016 7-11 August 2016, New York City (USA)* (Canada: International Society for Music Information Retrieval) 393–9

[34] Dair Z, Donovan R and O'Reilly R 2021 Linguistic and gender variation in speech emotion recognition using spectral features *arXiv preprint* arXiv:2112.09596

[35] Piliouras N *et al* 2004 Development of the cubic least squares mapping linear-kernel support vector machine classifier for improving the characterization of breast lesions on ultrasound *Comput. Med. Imaging Graph.* **28** 247–55

Chapter 14

Spectral and spatial analysis of EEG signals for imagined speech recognition

Ashwin Kamble and Pradnya Ghare

Brain–computer interface (BCI) systems aim to offer a communication channel for both individuals in good health and those living with neurological conditions. The intentions of users are communicated through imagined speech. This study explores the spatial and spectral attributes relevant to imagined speech identification. Our research relies on a publicly accessible data set containing data from 15 subjects and three categories: long words (INDEPENDENT and COOPERATE), short words (IN, OUT, and UP), and vowels (A, I, and U). This chapter examines the spectral characteristics used to classify imagined words in binary and multiclass settings across six frequency bands (FBs), along with spatial features from seven different brain areas (BAs). In addition, the factors influencing the decoding performance are analyzed for both binary classification and multiclass classification. The high-frequency (HF) band shows superior performance to that of the low-frequency bands, achieving a classification accuracy of 94.57% for long words, 94.53% for short–long words, 93.38% for short words, and 94.69% for vowels. Furthermore, the whole BA, Broca's area, Wernicke's area, and the auditory and sensorimotor cortexes, were found to be useful for decoding imagined speech. Moreover, our exploration of the scalability of multiclass decoding of imagined words involved incrementally increasing the number of classes from two to eight, revealing a decrease in decoding performance as the number of classes increased. These findings offer insights that may enhance decoding accuracy in practical BCI applications.

14.1 Introduction

BCIs are being developed to help people with locked-in syndrome or paralysis to directly communicate with their external surroundings [1, 2]. Researchers are developing BCI systems so that both patients and healthy individuals can communicate through their imagination. The conventional paradigms, such as event-related

doi:10.1088/978-0-7503-5964-1ch14

potentials and motor imagery offer enhancement in communication but are restricted by the required stimuli and number of classes for practical communication [3, 4]. Moreover, these paradigms have been shown to be inefficient in terms of BCI (i.e., users who are unable to assert control when using a specific BCI framework), implying the need for a simpler paradigm [5]. For BCI communication to be effective, the user must be able to interact with the devices readily and intuitively. As a result, an intuitive framework that is simple to use and communicates user intent immediately is required [6].

Imagined speech is referred to as the imagination of words or things that a person wants to communicate without any articulation. Imagined speech recognition, also known as silent speech interface, is an emerging technology that aims to decode the neural signals associated with the cognitive process of speech production without any overt articulation or vocalization. This technology holds immense potential for individuals with speech impairments or those operating in environments where audible communication is not feasible.

The imagined speech is captured from the electroencephalogram (EEG) signals, which have evolved as the most common choice of researchers because of their non-invasive nature. Using EEG signals to recognize imagined speech directly from the brain could be helpful for direct BCI control with less training time [3]. In recent years, several attempts have been made to classify the EEG signals generated for imagined speech. These attempts were mainly focused on the classification of imagined vowels, imagined syllables, or a few imagined words [6–14]. The words chosen in the imagined speech application may increase decoding performance.

For a human being, natural communication takes place through speech. The imagined speech application has the advantage of having an unlimited number of words, and each word represents a class. Unlike the other ways of communication, such as motor imagery, where the number of classes is restricted by the number of motor movements, imagined speech has constant discrimination between the words despite the number of words increasing in the classification problem. These properties of imagined speech demonstrate its usefulness for BCI applications with more words.

Previous studies have shown the reliability of the EEG signals in imagined speech applications but fail to attain actual communication along with the restrictions on a number of classes [15]. In recent studies, researchers have focused on spectral and spatial features of the EEG signals for imagined speech [16]. An extensive investigation of the time-frequency content of EEG signals captured for imagined speech applications is required. Hence, this chapter presents the analysis of EEG signals for imagined speech application for various frequency bands, such as Delta, Theta, Alpha, Mu, Beta, and Gamma, and different areas of the brain with Hjorth parameters and entropy features. The global architecture of the proposed system is shown in figure 14.1.

The remainder of the chapter is arranged as follows: section 14.2 describes the dataset acquisition, spectral and spatial analysis, variational mode decomposition, and feature extraction processes in the proposed model. Section 14.3 describes the experimental protocol. Section 14.4 presents the experimental results, and a

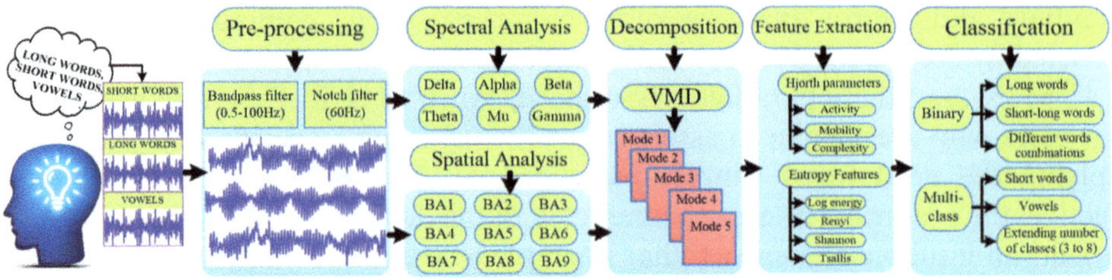

Figure 14.1. The global architecture of the proposed model.

Table 14.1. Number of participants for each category of dataset [2].

Protocol	Prompts	Total participants	IDs of the participants
Long words	'independent' and 'cooperate'	6	S2, S3, S6, S7, S9, and S11
Short–long words	'in' and 'cooperate'	6	S1, S5, S8, S9, S10, and S14
Short words	'in', 'out', and 'up'	6	S1, S3, S5, S6, S8, and S12
Vowels	'/a/', '/i/', and '/u/'	8	S4, S5, S8, S9, S11, S12, S13, and S15

discussion is provided in section 14.5. Finally, section 14.6 provides the conclusion of the paper.

14.2 Materials and methods

14.2.1 Data acquisition

The data used in this study were collected at the Human Oriented Robotics and Controls (HORC) lab at Arizona State University and are publically available [2]. For the dataset acquisition, 15 healthy subjects (4 female and 11 male, aged 22–32 years, mean age 27 years) were recruited. A 64-channel BrainProducts ActiCHamp amplifier system was used to record the data with a sampling rate of 1000 Hz and later down-sampled to 256 Hz. Out of the total 64 electrodes, 60 electrodes (2–9, 11–32, and 34–63) were used for the analysis, while the remaining four (1, 10, 33, and 64), which contributed to the EOG data, were excluded. Although 15 subjects participated in the study, only the data of a subset of them were available for the analysis of each category. Table 14.1 shows the details of the subset of subjects that are available for each category. Further details regarding the dataset can be found in [2].

14.2.2 Data pre-processing

We retrieved 4 seconds of data from each trial of short words and vowels, out of which 3 seconds corresponded to speech imagination and the remaining 1 second was used to capture any residual mental activity after the visual signal had vanished.

We retrieved 4.5 sof data from each trial of long words and short–long words. EEG data were pre-processed using the EEGLAB toolbox in MATLAB 2021. A fifth-order Butterworth filter with a passband of 0.5 to 100 Hz was used to suppress the noise and artifacts [2]. In addition, a 60 Hz notch filter was used to remove the power line noise. Finally, common average referencing was performed for re-referencing [3].

14.2.2.1 Spectral analysis

Spectral analysis plays a crucial role in decoding imagined speech from EEG signals. EEG signals are typically analyzed in the frequency domain, as different cognitive processes are associated with distinct patterns of neural oscillations across various frequency bands. The EEG frequency spectrum is commonly divided into several frequency bands (FBs), each associated with different brain states and cognitive functions [9, 17–20]. The following frequency bands are particularly relevant in the context of imagined speech recognition:

Delta band (0.5–4 Hz): The delta band is characterized by slow oscillations and is typically associated with deep sleep stages. While not directly related to imagined speech, delta activity may provide insights into the overall brain state during the task.

Theta band (4–8 Hz): The theta band has been linked to memory processes, attention, and cognitive control. Some studies have suggested that theta oscillations in frontal and temporal regions may be modulated during imagined speech tasks, reflecting the involvement of memory retrieval and linguistic processing.

Alpha band (8–13 Hz): The alpha band is generally associated with relaxed wakefulness and inhibitory processes. During imagined speech, changes in alpha power have been observed in regions like the auditory cortex, potentially reflecting the suppression of auditory processing during internal speech production.

Beta band (12–30 Hz): Beta oscillations are often related to motor processes and cognitive functions such as decision-making and attention. Modulations in beta power have been reported in areas like Broca's area and the motor cortex during imagined speech tasks, suggesting their involvement in the planning and execution of speech production.

Gamma band (30–100 Hz): The gamma band is associated with higher-order cognitive processes, such as perception, attention, and memory. Increased gamma activity has been observed in regions like the auditory cortex and Wernicke's area during imagined speech, potentially reflecting the processing of speech-related information.

All the 60-channel data were used for the spectral analysis. The dataset was pre-processed from 0.5 to 100 Hz using a fifth-order Butterworth bandpass filter. This frequency range consists of several frequency bands, each having significant information in each band. These FBs are shown in table 14.2. A fifth-order Butterworth bandpass filter was used to filter the EEG data into six FBs. This is performed to evaluate the effect of the imagination of speech in different FBs. Binary and multiclass classifications were performed for each area.

Table 14.2. Brief description of the groups and frequency bands used for analysis.

Groups	Description
Frequency band (FB)	FB1 (0.5–4 Hz, Delta), FB2 (4–8 Hz, Theta), FB3 (8–12 Hz, Mu), FB4 (8–13 Hz, Alpha), FB5 (13–30 Hz, Beta), and FB6 (30–100 Hz, Gamma).
High-frequency group(HFG)	HFG1 (30–50 Hz), HFG2 (30–80 Hz), HFG3 (30–100 Hz), HFG4 (50–80 Hz), HFG5 (50–100 Hz), HFG6 (80–100 Hz)
Brain areas (BA)	BA1 (Visual cortex), BA2 (Motor cortex), BA3 (Auditory cortex), BA4 (Pre-frontal cortex), BA5 (Sensory cortex), BA6 (Broca's and Wernicke's area), and BA7 (whole brain)

14.2.2.2 Spatial analysis

EEG has emerged as a promising modality for capturing the underlying neural activities during imagined speech, making spatial analysis of brain areas, such as visual cortex, auditory cortex, pre-frontal cortex, Broca's and Wernicke's area, a crucial aspect of research in this domain. While the visual cortex is primarily involved in processing visual information, recent studies have suggested its potential involvement in imagined speech recognition [21]. The visual cortex may contribute to the mental imagery aspect of speech production, as individuals often visualize the words or concepts they intend to express silently. However, the precise role and extent of involvement of the visual cortex in imagined speech recognition is an area that warrants further exploration.

The auditory cortex, located in the temporal lobe, is responsible for processing auditory information, including speech perception [22]. During imagined speech, the auditory cortex is believed to be involved in the internal monitoring and feedback mechanisms associated with the covert production of speech. Researchers have observed increased activity in the auditory cortex during imagined speech tasks, suggesting its potential role in the generation and monitoring of the intended speech output.

The prefrontal cortex, situated in the anterior part of the frontal lobe, is known to play a crucial role in cognitive control, working memory, and decision-making processes [23]. In the context of imagined speech recognition, the prefrontal cortex is thought to be involved in the planning, organization, and execution of the cognitive processes associated with speech production. It may also contribute to the inhibition of overt articulation during imagined speech tasks.

Broca's area, located in the inferior frontal gyrus of the frontal lobe, is a crucial region for speech production and language processing [24]. During imagined speech, Broca's area is believed to be responsible for the planning, sequencing, and execution of the motor programs associated with the intended speech output. Researchers have observed increased activity in Broca's area during imagined speech tasks, suggesting its central role in the cognitive processes underlying silent speech production.

Wernicke's area, situated in the posterior part of the superior temporal gyrus, is primarily associated with language comprehension and processing [25]. In the context of imagined speech recognition, Wernicke's area is thought to be involved in the semantic and linguistic aspects of speech production. It may contribute to the generation and retrieval of the intended speech content, as well as the monitoring and feedback mechanisms associated with the production of imagined speech.

The effect of imagination on speech was evaluated by considering the different areas of the brain (BA), such as the visual cortex (BA1: PO3, PO4, POZ, PO7, PO8, O1, O2, OZ), motor cortex (BA2: F1, F2, F3, F4, FZ, FC1, FC2, FC3, FC4, CZ), auditory cortex (BA3: T7, T8, FT7, FT8, TP7, TP8), pre-frontal cortex (BA4: FP1, FP2, AF3, AF4, F5, F7), sensory cortex (BA5: C1, C2, C3, C4, CZ, CP1, CP2, CP3, CP4, CPZ), Broca's and Wernicke's area (BA6: AF3, F3, F5, FC3, FC5, T7, C5, TP7, CP5, and P5), and the whole brain (BA7: all 60 channels) [10, 26]. The binary and multiclass classification was performed for each area.

14.2.3 Variational mode decomposition

Variational mode decomposition (VMD) adaptively determines the relevant bands with simultaneous estimation of associated modes, this helps to balance the errors between them [27]. It has garnered a lot of attention in the signal-processing field, and it has been shown to outperform other adaptive signal decomposition algorithms [1]. VMD uses a constrained variational optimization problem to extract the fixed number of modes (K) from the input signal.

VMD assumes that each mode has a compact bandwidth in its Fourier spectrum. The optimization problem in VMD can be briefly described as:

- Taking Hilbert transforms of real signal to get a single-sideband analytic signal.
- Complex harmonic mixing entails multiplying the frequency spectrum of each mode by an exponential function tuned to the estimated center frequency of the respective mode.
- Determine the bandwidth using the modulated signal's H1-norm Gaussian smoothness, which is the squared L2-norm of the gradient.

The constraint optimization is converted to an unconstrained one by using the Lagrangian multiplier and quadratic penalty factor α. The resulting constrained variational problem is then given by:

$$\min \{u_k\}, \{w_k\}$$

$$\left\{\sum_k \left\| \partial_t\left[\left(\delta(t) + \frac{j}{\pi t}\right) \times u_k(t)\right] e^{-j\omega_k t} \right\|_2^2\right\} \quad s.\ t. \quad \sum_k u_k = f$$

where u_k is the kth mode of the signal and ω_k is the respective center frequency, f is the signal to be decomposed, and δ is the Dirac function.

$\mathcal{L}(\{u_k\}, \{\omega_k\}, \lambda)$:

$$= \alpha \Sigma_k \left\| \partial_t \left[\left(\delta(t) + \frac{j}{\pi t} \right) * u_k(t) \right] e^{-j\omega_k t} \right\|_2^2 + \left\| f(t) - \Sigma_k u_k(t) \right\|_2^2 + \left\langle \lambda(t), f(t) - \Sigma_k u_k(t) \ldots \right\rangle$$

The decomposition of the original signal $f(t)$ using VMD results in several time-domain modes ($u_k(t)$). Even though using VMD for long-term EEG signals has drawbacks due to non-stationarity, this study chose VMD because the time series data was short and the focus was on classification rather than accurate mode decomposition and reconstruction.

14.2.4 Feature extraction

Statistical features such as Hjorth parameters (Hjorth complexity (HC), Hjorth activity (HC), and Hjorth mobility (HM)), difference absolute standard deviation value (DASDV), and entropy features (Shannon entropy (SE), Renyi entropy (RE), Tsallis entropy (TE), and log energy entropy (LEE)) are extracted from each mode of the decomposed signal [28–33]. These features represent the hidden characteristics of the signal. The mathematical expression and a short description of these above-mentioned features are provided in table 14.3.

14.2.5 Classifiers

A features matrix obtained from the above-mentioned features is given to the three different machine learning (ML) algorithms, namely ensemble bagged tree (EBT), k-nearest neighbor (KNN), and random forest (RF). In the context of EEG-based imagined speech recognition, these ML algorithms are the most widely used in ML applications [1, 34].

Table 14.3. Features with their mathematical expression.

Sr No	Feature	Mathematical expression
1	Hjorth activity (HA)	$\text{HA} = \sigma^2(x(t))$
2	Hjorth mobility (HM)	$\text{HM} = \sqrt{\frac{\text{var}(\frac{dx(t)}{dt})}{\text{var}(x(t))}}$
3	Hjorth complexity (HC)	$\text{HC} = \frac{\text{mobility}(\frac{dx(t)}{dt})}{\text{mobility}(x(t))}$
4	Difference absolute standard deviation value (DASDV)	$\text{DASDV} = \sqrt{\frac{1}{N-1}\Sigma_{i=1}^{n}(x(i+1) - x(i))^2}$
5	Log energy entropy (LEE)	$\text{LEE} = -(\Sigma_{i=1}^{N}(\log_2(P_i(x)))^2)$
6	Renyi entropy (RE)	$\text{RE}_\gamma = \frac{1}{1-\gamma}(\log \Sigma_{i=1}^{N} P_i(x)^\gamma)$
7	Shannon entropy (SE)	$\text{SE} = -\Sigma_{i=0}^{N} pi(\hat{u}).\ \log\ (pi(\hat{u}))$
8	Tsallis entropy (TE)	$\text{TE} = \frac{1 - \Sigma_{i=1}^{N} P_i(x)^\gamma}{1-\gamma}$

EBT, also known as Bootstrap Aggregating (Bagging), is an ML ensemble method that combines multiple decision tree models to improve predictive accuracy and reduce overfitting [35]. The bagging algorithm operates by creating multiple bootstrap samples from the original training data and training individual decision trees on each bootstrap sample. During prediction, the outputs of all the individual trees are combined, typically through majority voting for classification tasks or by averaging for regression tasks.

The KNN algorithm is a non-parametric, instance-based learning method widely used for classification and regression tasks [36]. The KNN algorithm operates by determining the k nearest neighbors in the feature space to a new, unlabeled instance based on a distance metric (e.g., Euclidean distance). The class label of the new instance is then assigned based on the majority vote of its k nearest neighbors in the training data. The choice of k and the distance metric can significantly impact the performance of the KNN algorithm.

RF is another ensemble learning algorithm that constructs multiple decision trees during training and combines their outputs for prediction [37]. However, unlike bagged trees, it introduces additional randomness by randomly selecting a subset of features at each node split during the tree-building process. This random feature selection helps to reduce the correlation among individual trees in the ensemble, leading to improved generalization performance and robustness to overfitting.

14.2.6 Performance evaluation

Three different ML algorithms, namely EBT, KNN, and RF, were used to perform binary and multiclass classification. Different performance parameters such as accuracy (ACC), F1-score, precision (PREC), recall (REC), Cohen's kappa (κ), and area-under-the-curve (AUC) are used to analyze the performance of the ML algorithms.

A Confusion matrix is an $N \times N$ matrix used to evaluate the performance of a classification algorithm, where N represents the number of classes. The confusion matrix compares the actual values with those predicted by the classification algorithm. A general structure of the confusion matrix can be found in figure 14.2. In figure 14.2, true positive (TP) represents the values that are correctly classified as positive, whereas true negative (TN) represents the values that are correctly classified as negative. The false positive (FP) represents the values that are falsely classified as positive but are actually negative, whereas the false negative (FN) represents the values that are falsely classified as negative but are actually positive. The performance evaluation metrics are calculated using the following mathematical formulation.

$$\text{Accuracy} = \frac{\text{TP} + \text{TN}}{\text{TP} + \text{TN} + \text{FP} + \text{FN}}$$

$$F_1 \text{ Score} = \frac{\text{TP}}{\text{TP} + \frac{1}{2}(\text{FP} + \text{FN})}$$

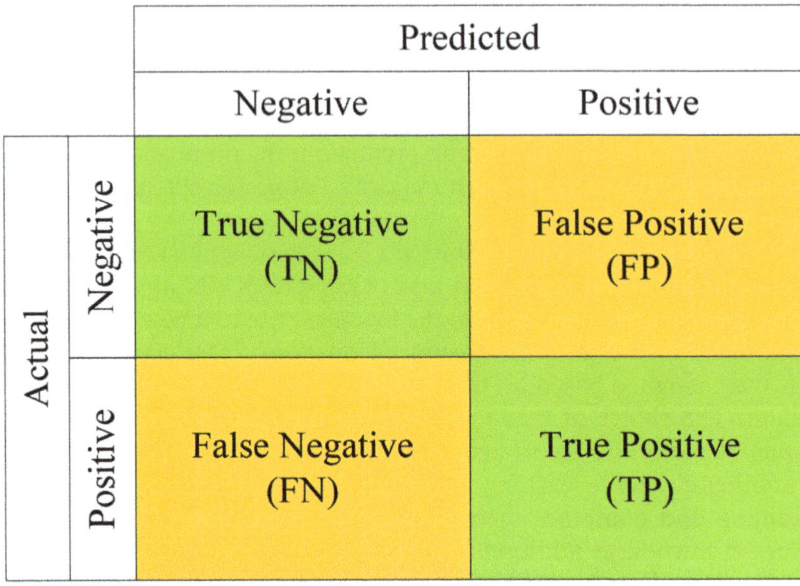

Figure 14.2. General structure of confusion matrix.

$$\text{PREC} = \frac{\text{TP}}{\text{TP} + \text{FP}}$$

$$\text{SEN} = \text{REC} = \frac{\text{TP}}{\text{TP} + \text{FN}}$$

$$\text{SPEC} = \frac{\text{TN}}{\text{TN} + \text{FP}}$$

14.3 Experimental protocol

This section describes the experimental protocol for pre-processing, spectral analysis, spatial analysis, choosing the best ML algorithm, and increasing the number of classes. Figure 14.3 depicts the stages of the proposed model.

14.3.1 Pre-processing

The EEG dataset was pre-processed to remove artifacts. The pre-processed EEG data were divided into six different frequency bands for spectral analysis. For spatial analysis, the EEG data from different areas of the brain are considered. The EEG data was then decomposed into five modes (default in MATLAB 2021) using VMD.

14.3.1.1 Spectral analysis

The most powerful frequency bands containing significant information were analyzed, and the EEG signals were divided into six FBs. It was observed that

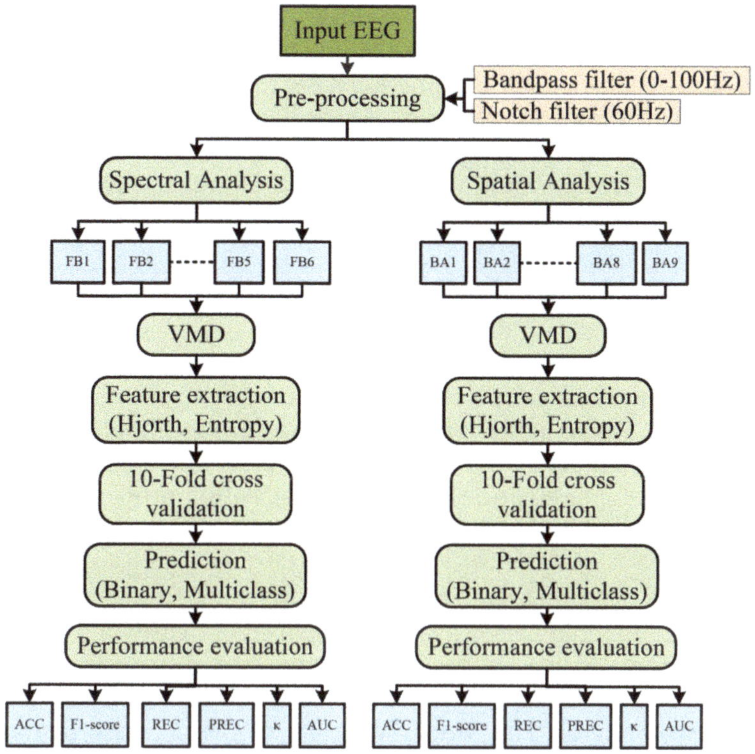

Figure 14.3. Stages of the proposed model.

the performance of the FB6 (Gamma) band was best compared to that of other bands. Thus, the FB6 (Gamma) was again divided into six different bands for the analysis, and we called these bands high-frequency groups (HFG). A fifth-order Butterworth bandpass filter was used to filter the EEG data into six HFGs. These HFGs are HFG1 (30–50 Hz), HFG2 (30–80 Hz), HFG3 (30–100 Hz), HFG4 (50–80 Hz), HFG5 (50–100 Hz), and HFG6 (80–100 Hz) as shown in table 14.2.

14.3.1.2 Spatial analysis

Each brain area is known to be responsible for specific brain functions. So, the effect of different parts of the brain on imagined speech is studied by dividing the data into different brain areas. Seven different brain areas were identified, and three different ML algorithms were used to analyze how imagined speech affects each brain area. The 0.5–100 Hz frequency band was used for this analysis because it has all of the frequencies used for EEG analysis.

14.3.2 Selection of an ML algorithm

A tenfold cross-validation approach was used for all the ML algorithms. This divides the training data into ten equal, non-overlapping independent parts. Out of the ten non-overlapping independent parts, nine were used for training the model, and the remaining one was used for validation. The process is repeated ten times, and the mean measurements of all ten values are utilized as the final cross-validation accuracy of the ML algorithms. Additionally, for ten-by-ten-fold nested validation, the classification process was repeated ten times to ensure the robustness of the classification results. The complete workflow of the proposed model is depicted in figure 14.3. The ML algorithm with the best performance parameter values is selected for the further process.

14.3.3 Expanding the number of classes

Although the binary and multiclass classifications were performed for all four categories, the multiclass classification was restricted to three class problems. Hence, the idea of expanding the number of classes was explored by considering each word as a separate class. Different combinations of words are utilized, adding one word (class) to each combination, and the number of classes is expanded from two to eight. The number of combinations for each classification problem is calculated as:

$$nC_k = \frac{n!}{(n-k)!k!}$$

Where n and k are the number of available (eight in our case) and selected classes, respectively. As the number of classes increases, the drop rate in classification accuracy for each added class is calculated and compared to the drop rate for accuracy at chance levels. The drop rate refers to the decrease in the $(n+1)$th accuracy as compared to the nth accuracy and is defined as

$$d_n = 1 - \frac{a_{n+1}}{a_n}$$

Where n denotes the number of classes increasing sequentially. The chance level accuracy is obtained when one is divided by the number of classes.

14.4 Results

14.4.1 Classification using spectral features

Binary and multiclass classification for all four categories was tested on six FBs using three different ML algorithms, as shown in table 14.4. Table 14.4 shows the significant difference in the classification accuracies for all six FBs using three ML algorithms. Out of the six FBs, FB6 showed the highest classification accuracy of $93.92 \pm 1.69\%$, $91.93 \pm 1.29\%$, $91.80 \pm 0.87\%$, and $91.71 \pm 0.63\%$ for long words, short–long words, short words, and vowels, respectively, and FB1 showed the lowest classification accuracy for all the categories. Out of the three ML algorithms, EBT presented the highest classification accuracy for both binary and multiclass categories.

In addition to the FBs, the binary and multiclass classification for all four categories was tested on six HFGs using three ML algorithms, as shown in table 14.5. Table 14.5 shows the significant difference in the classification accuracies for all six HFGs using three ML algorithms. Out of the six HFGs, the HFG3 has

Table 14.4. Classification accuracy (%) of different classifiers in FBs.

		Frequency bands					
Category	Classifier	FB1	FB2	FB3	FB4	FB5	FB6
Long words	EBT	62.73 ± 1.96	70.61 ± 13.9	74.07 ± 13.36	76.11 ± 2.60	81.38 ± 4.55	**93.92 ± 1.69**
	KNN	55.15 ± 0.93	61.03 ± 2.63	65.48 ± 14.99	69.55 ± 2.06	74.22 ± 6.21	**84.91 ± 2.85**
	RF	59.27 ± 2.59	69.56 ± 2.64	70.96 ± 1.91	73.88 ± 2.65	80.19 ± 2.12	**87.09 ± 1.76**
Short–long words	EBT	64.27 ± 1.62	66.44 ± 3.76	70.54 ± 2.35	74.57 ± 2.49	81.85 ± 2.72	**91.93 ± 1.29**
	KNN	57.73 ± 1.45	59.84 ± 5.93	64.89 ± 6.67	72.41 ± 4.55	77.01 ± 4.51	**85.85 ± 4.12**
	RF	64.41 ± 1.20	67.48 ± 4.84	69.03 ± 4.47	80.83 ± 3.93	82.43 ± 3.28	**88.18 ± 1.50**
Short words	EBT	61.09 ± 2.43	70.97 ± 2.55	71.24 ± 3.27	74.16 ± 1.27	81.24 ± 2.59	**91.80 ± 0.87**
	KNN	57.39 ± 1.73	62.11 ± 2.63	67.79 ± 1.37	68.64 ± 6.91	76.39 ± 6.08	**82.13 ± 1.23**
	RF	59.13 ± 2.86	61.78 ± 1.37	66.10 ± 12.24	75.92 ± 5.33	76.39 ± 6.08	**89.29 ± 1.44**
Vowels	EBT	63.77 ± 3.39	66.60 ± 3.97	72.44 ± 8.80	75.58 ± 1.75	79.99 ± 3.18	**91.71 ± 0.63**
	KNN	56.87 ± 3.07	60.01 ± 4.78	67.74 ± 2.07	72.48 ± 1.68	75.88 ± 2.90	**83.25 ± 1.75**
	RF	58.43 ± 3.90	60.06 ± 9.43	67.66 ± 10.06	75.32 ± 1.87	81.49 ± 2.82	**88.33 ± 2.31**

Table 14.5. Classification accuracy (%) of different classifiers in HFGs.

		High-frequency groups					
Category	Classifier	HFG1(6)	HFG2(3)	HFG3(1)	HFG4(4)	HFG5(2)	HFG6(5)
Long words	EBT	82.19 ± 3.47	87.09 ± 1.76	**93.92 ± 1.69**	85.78 ± 2.82	**90.15 ± 1.84**	84.55 ± 3.17
	KNN	77.78 ± 2.12	81.24 ± 2.73	**84.91 ± 2.85**	80.11 ± 9.02	**82.19 ± 3.47**	79.95 ± 3.05
	RF	81.00 ± 3.74	86.35 ± 1.99	**87.09 ± 1.76**	84.87 ± 2.56	**86.75 ± 1.82**	83.40 ± 1.87
Short–long words	EBT	79.37 ± 2.17	86.61 ± 3.04	**91.93 ± 1.29**	83.43 ± 6.50	**88.09 ± 4.54**	80.43 ± 4.65
	KNN	76.02 ± 1.51	80.76 ± 2.48	**85.85 ± 4.12**	79.59 ± 5.80	**81.85 ± 4.51**	78.39 ± 4.62
	RF	82.87 ± 1.55	86.56 ± 1.45	**88.18 ± 1.50**	82.77 ± 5.22	**87.92 ± 1.65**	82.05 ± 6.50
Short words	EBT	81.24 ± 2.59	86.09 ± 1.82	**91.80 ± 0.87**	83.60 ± 1.43	**89.13 ± 1.66**	82.13 ± 1.23
	KNN	76.78 ± 1.40	79.12 ± 3.38	**82.13 ± 1.23**	78.68 ± 4.65	**81.24 ± 2.59**	75.48 ± 2.60
	RF	78.06 ± 4.78	81.53 ± 1.54	**89.29 ± 1.44**	80.89 ± 2.46	**83.48 ± 1.19**	78.68 ± 4.65
Vowels	EBT	80.00 ± 3.59	86.74 ± 1.52	**91.71 ± 0.63**	85.68 ± 5.10	**88.64 ± 2.23**	84.17 ± 5.12
	KNN	75.11 ± 2.14	80.35 ± 1.63	**83.25 ± 1.75**	80.42 ± 2.70	**81.60 ± 2.65**	76.38 ± 6.84
	RF	81.56 ± 2.06	85.68 ± 5.10	**88.33 ± 2.31**	84.541 ± 1.60	**87.08 ± 1.94**	81.82 ± 5.67

shown the highest classification accuracy of 93.92 ± 1.69%, 91.93 ± 1.29%, 91.80 ± 0.87%, and 91.71 ± 0.63% for long words, short–long words, short words, and vowels, respectively, followed by the HFG5 which obtained the classification accuracies as 90.15 ± 1.84%, 88.09 ± 4.54%, 89.13 ± 1.66%, and 88.64 ± 2.23% for long words, short–long words, short words, and vowels, respectively. Out of the three ML algorithms, EBT presented the highest classification accuracy for both binary and multiclass categories.

14.4.2 Classification using spatial features

Binary and multiclass classification for all four categories was tested on seven BAs using three ML algorithms, as shown in table 14.6. Table 14.6 shows the significant difference in the classification accuracies for all the seven BAs using three ML algorithms. Out of the seven BAs, the BA9 (whole brain) showed the highest classification accuracy of 89.97 ± 2.46%, 90.39 ± 3.57%, 88.30 ± 3.45%, and 85.33 ± 4.22% for long words, short–long words, short words, and vowels, respectively, followed by BA6 (Broca's and Wernicke's area), BA5 (sensory cortex) and BA2 (motor cortex), and BA3 showed the lowest classification accuracy for all the categories. Out of the three ML algorithms, EBT presented the highest classification accuracy for both binary and multiclass categories.

14.4.3 Performance evaluation

Table 14.7 compares the performance parameters for long words, short–long words, short words, and vowel categories for EBT, KNN, and RF algorithms. As shown in table 14.7, for binary classification, the overall ACC, F1-score, PREC, REC, κ, and AUC for the long word category using EBT are 93.92 ± 1.69%, 93.92, 93.92, 93.92, 87.85, and 0.97. Similarly, for the short–long words category, the overall ACC, F1-score, PREC, REC, κ, and AUC using EBT are 91.93 ± 1.29%, 91.92, 91.93, 91.93, 83.86, and 0.91. As shown in figure 14.3, for multiclass classification, the overall ACC, F1-score, PREC, REC, κ, and AUC for the short words category using EBT are 91.80 ± 0.87%, 91.81, 91.82, 91.81, 87.70, and 0.89. Similarly, for the short-vowels category, the overall ACC, F1-score, PREC, REC, κ, and AUC using EBT are 91.71 ± 0.63%, 91.69, 91.71, 91.70, 87.54, and 0.86. The EBT algorithm outperforms the other ML algorithms.

Figure 14.4 shows the ROC plots for binary ((A) long and (B) short–long words) and multiclass ((C) short words, (D) vowels) classification. The EBT algorithm reported the highest AUC of 0.97, 0.94, 0.89, and 0.86 for long words, short–long words, short words, and vowels, respectively. Figure 14.4 shows that the bagging algorithm is the best choice for an imagined speech recognition application.

14.4.4 Selection of ML algorithm

The binary and multiclass classification was performed using three EBT, KNN, and RF ML algorithms. It was observed from tables 14.4–14.7 that the EBT algorithms are providing better classification accuracies for both binary (long words and short–long words) and multiclass (short words and vowels) categories, as well as for the

Table 14.6. Classification accuracy (%) of different classifiers in Bas.

Category	Classifier	Brain areas						
		BA1	BA2	BA3	BA4	BA5	BA6	BA7
Long words	EBT	80.69 ± 4.03	**83.15 ± 4.75**	78.64 ± 4.35	80.25 ± 3.05	**83.84 ± 2.35**	**83.77 ± 2.31**	**89.97 ± 2.46**
	KNN	75.48 ± 3.41	**78.41 ± 2.80**	75.42 ± 3.90	76.65 ± 3.98	**79.69 ± 4.81**	**79.00 ± 2.32**	**83.93 ± 4.08**
	RF	77.92 ± 2.10	**79.62 ± 4.29**	76.44 ± 4.83	77.12 ± 3.24	**80.90 ± 3.93**	**80.61 ± 2.19**	**85.88 ± 2.28**
Short–long words	EBT	79.14 ± 2.52	**84.45 ± 2.56**	78.12 ± 2.62	77.77 ± 4.52	**84.59 ± 3.43**	**85.30 ± 3.21**	**90.39 ± 3.57**
	KNN	77.01 ± 4.12	**79.54 ± 2.86**	73.41 ± 4.16	75.64 ± 4.49	**79.75 ± 3.91**	**79.43 ± 3.34**	**84.06 ± 3.59**
	RF	76.88 ± 3.42	**79.20 ± 2.27**	73.27 ± 2.70	73.45 ± 2.76	**81.62 ± 3.63**	**80.77 ± 3.09**	**88.25 ± 4.58**
Short words	EBT	78.06 ± 2.45	**79.66 ± 3.72**	78.00 ± 2.35	77.40 ± 3.84	**81.53 ± 3.94**	**82.18 ± 4.29**	**88.30 ± 3.45**
	KNN	69.04 ± 3.82	**74.89 ± 4.05**	68.93 ± 3.02	69.54 ± 3.74	**71.69 ± 3.63**	**80.97 ± 3.88**	**82.22 ± 3.18**
	RF	78.02 ± 3.82	**80.76 ± 3.63**	74.04 ± 3.35	79.63 ± 3.62	**80.65 ± 4.16**	**81.23 ± 4.31**	**85.26 ± 4.01**
Vowels	EBT	76.42 ± 2.57	**77.63 ± 3.27**	75.85 ± 3.37	74.16 ± 4.60	**77.24 ± 3.56**	**77.72 ± 4.79**	**85.33 ± 4.22**
	KNN	75.86 ± 3.98	**77.30 ± 3.93**	74.24 ± 4.21	73.48 ± 2.79	**77.39 ± 4.98**	**77.44 ± 4.91**	**80.03 ± 3.56**
	RF	75.96 ± 4.31	**77.85 ± 3.94**	75.30 ± 2.72	74.65 ± 2.95	**78.19 ± 2.65**	**78.85 ± 2.57**	**83.99 ± 3.04**

Table 14.7. Performance parameters.

Category	Classifier	Performance parameters					
		ACC (%)	F1-score	PREC	REC	κ	AUC
Long words	EBT	93.92 ± 1.69	93.92	93.92	93.92	87.85	0.97
	KNN	84.91 ± 2.85	84.91	84.91	84.91	69.83	0.91
	RF	87.09 ± 1.76	87.09	87.09	87.09	74.18	0.92
Short–long words	EBT	91.93 ± 1.29	91.92	91.93	91.93	83.86	0.94
	KNN	85.85 ± 4.12	85.85	85.86	85.85	71.71	0.84
	RF	88.18 ± 1.50	88.18	88.17	88.18	76.37	0.91
Short words	EBT	91.80 ± 0.87	91.81	91.82	91.80	87.70	0.86
	KNN	82.13 ± 1.23	82.12	82.11	82.13	73.19	0.81
	RF	89.29 ± 1.44	89.29	89.33	89.29	83.93	0.81
Vowels	EBT	91.71 ± 0.63	91.69	9.71	91.70	87.54	0.86
	KNN	83.25 ± 1.75	83.26	83.17	83.18	7.76	0.81
	RF	88.33 ± 2.31	88.33	88.26	88.19	82.49	0.81

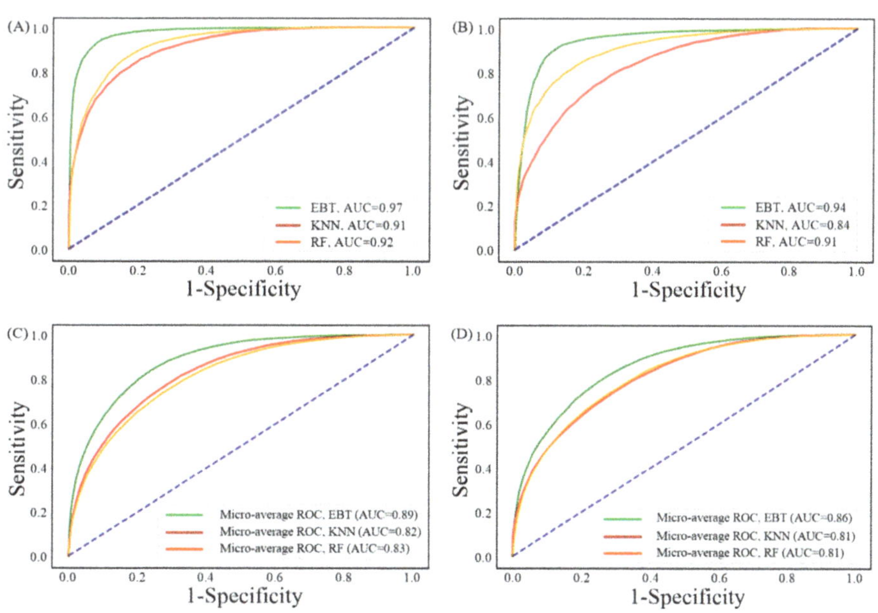

Figure 14.4. ROC curves comparing ML algorithms for binary ((A) long and (B) short–long words) and multiclass ((C) short words, (D) vowels) classification.

other performance parameters. Hence, EBT was selected as the best ML algorithm and was used for further analysis.

14.4.5 Expanding the number of classes

The drop in the classification accuracy with the increase in the number of classes along with the chance level accuracy is shown in figure 14.5. There were 28 binary, 56 three-class, 70 four-class, 56 five-class, 28 six-class, eight seven-class, and one eight-class combination available for classification. As shown in the bar plots in figure 14.5, the classification accuracy decreases as we increase the number of classes. The average binary classification accuracy was 90.64 ± 2.27%, while the eight-class classification accuracy was 77.45 ± 1.81%. The drop in the classification accuracy from binary to eight was compared with the drop in the chance level and is depicted in table 14.8.

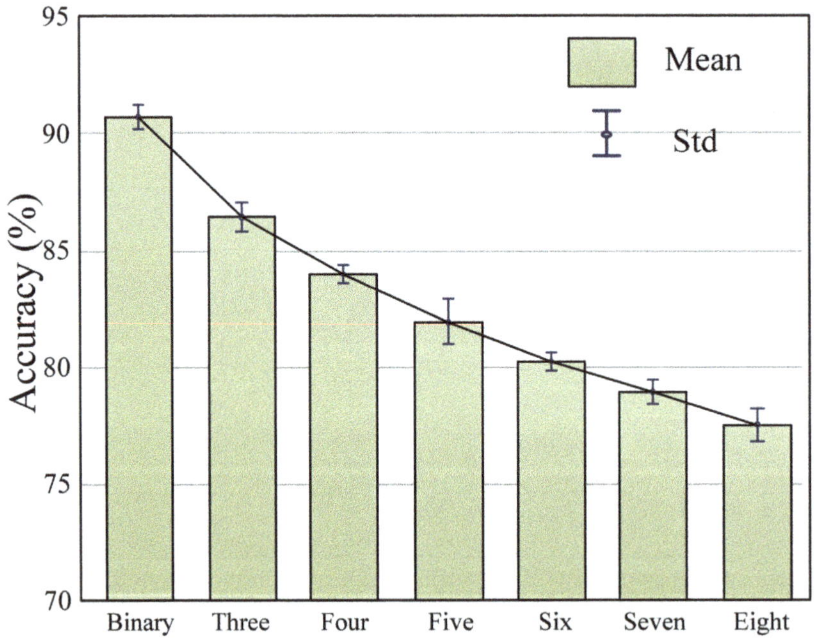

Figure 14.5. Binary and multiclass classification accuracy (%) with drop rate.

Table 14.8. Drop-rate (%) in classification and chance level according to number of classes.

Number of classes	2–3	3–4	4–5	5–6	6–7	7–8
Drop rate	4.66	2.88	2.51	2.05	1.61	1.79
Chance level	33.33	25.00	20.00	16.66	14.28	12.5

14.5 Discussion

EEG-based BCI for imagined speech recognition has applications for both healthy and disabled people, such as those with speech production and speaking disabilities, neuromuscular illness, and other diseases [14, 15, 40]. In addition, this will enhance the quality of rehabilitation and neurology. This chapter focuses on the significant characteristics of EEG signals for imagined speech applications, such as spectral and spatial features, the effect of word choice, and the scalability of multiclass classification. When compared to any other spectral characteristic throughout the whole brain, the high-frequency (HF) band has shown considerable improvement in the classification of imagined speech. Both Broca's and Wernicke's regions, as well as the temporal cortex, performed well in identifying both imagined speech and visual images.

14.5.1 Superior performance in the frequency band

The EEG signals of the imagined speech are divided into six FBs, and the decoding performance of the proposed system was observed for all six FBs. It has been observed that the HF band, especially FB6 (gamma), has shown a remarkable enhancement in decoding performance. It is known that the HF activity shown by the gamma band can help with natural language processing [10]. To explore the decoding performance again, the gamma band was again divided into six HF bands, called HFGs, and the performance was evaluated for six different HFGs (HFG1-HFG6). It was observed that HFG3 had shown the best performance among the other HFGs. Additionally, all the HFGs showed better performance compared to the low-frequency groups (FB1-FB5).

Furthermore, the HF band is evident during cross-modal memory and sensory processing of objects and sounds [41]. The mental arousal of the pre-given stimulus is involved in the imagined speech, and the memory recall process may be represented in the HF band [6]. Although the 0.5–100 Hz group encompasses the HF range, selecting only this range resulted in substantially better performance. It might have been difficult to distinguish between highly active thoughts and sleep when there was a delta or theta band associated with it [42].

14.5.2 Superior performance in the brain area

The decoding performance of the proposed system is observed for different areas of the brain. The EEG signals were categorized into different groups, comprising data from different areas of the brain. It has been observed that the BA7 (whole brain) has the highest classification performance among the seven BAs. This finding indicates that relevant information within the HF band is distributed across the entire brain. While each brain region is generally associated with distinct functions, studies have shown that Broca's and Wernicke's areas, as well as the sensorimotor area, are involved in language and speech production [3, 10]. Language processing occurs in conjunction with brain processes such as sensorimotor, premotor, auditory, and motor cortical regions [43, 44]. Furthermore, the auditory cue of the imagined speech may have stimulated the auditory cortex. Therefore the result confirms the earlier studies. Therefore, in addition to the 60-channel group, Broca's and Wernicke's areas (BA6), the auditory cortex (BA2), and the sensory cortex (BA5) have demonstrated noteworthy performance in the classification of imagined speech.

14.5.3 Best ML algorithm for binary and multiclass classification

This study designed an ML-based system to predict the imagined word from the EEG signal. EBT, KNN, and RF algorithms are used to classify the EEG signals, and the performance of the three algorithms is compared using six different performance evaluation metrics. The study results show that the EBT algorithm showed better performance, followed by RF and KNN algorithms in both binary and multiclass classification. Ensemble learning combines multiple learning models, which improves performance over individual models. Bagging extends ensemble learning by not only relying on the results of multiple models but also allowing each model to train on a different random subset of the original dataset with replacement. Each model obtains a different score. Finally, all the scores are combined and the majority of the votes are taken to get the final score. The same scoring method is used to obtain each score.

14.5.4 Robustness in expanding the number of classes

This chapter presents the results from binary classification to eight-class classification, and the results are satisfactory in terms of classification accuracy. The results show the possibility of expanding the number of classes for imagined speech applications. The chance level accuracy changes (decreases) as we expand the number of classes from two to eight. The results show that the accuracy of the classifications is better than the accuracy at the chance level. The imagined speech can be viewed as a strong paradigm to increase the number of classes for BCI applications, since that multiclass classification in emotion recognition [45] and motor imagery detection [46] showed a rapid drop in the classification accuracy with an increase in the number of classes. In this chapter, the effects of features in an imagined speech application were looked at using a simple classification method. However, deep learning methods that take into account these significant aspects might improve decoding performance and give even more freedom.

14.5.5 Benchmarking with previous studies

Table 14.9 compares the results obtained using the proposed technique to those obtained using current methods on the same dataset. Nguyen *et al* [2] employed CSP-based features and relevance vector machine (RVM) to obtain classification accuracies of 45.1 ± 8.7%, 46.6 ± 8.6%, and 76.2 ± 8.9% for vowels, short words, and short–long words, respectively. With tangent Space wand Artificial Neural Network + Bagging classifiers, Singh *et al* [38] obtained average classification accuracies of 58.66%, 60.40, 75%, and 71% for vowels, short words, short–long words, and long words, respectively. Kamble *et al* [1] employed VMD and ensemble algorithms to obtain average accuracy of 66.16%, 71.54%, 73.57% and 73.74%, for

Table 14.9. Comparative results (accuracy (%) values) with previous results.

(a) Comparing for Vowels

Author	Method	Subjects							
		S4	S5	S8	S9	S11	S12	S13	S15
Nguyen *et al* [2]	Tangent + RVM	47.0 ± 4.6	48.0 ± 7.2	51.0 ± 6.7	47.0 ± 5.5	53.0 ± 4.0	51.0 ± 6.3	46.7 ± 8.2	48.0 ± 7.2
	Tangent + ELM	41.0 ± 13.3	44.6 ± 11.2	45.3 ± 8.9	46.0 ± 5.1	43.3 ± 7.9	48.6 ± 8.9	45.7 ± 7.2	46.7 ± 7.5
Singh *et al* [38]	TS + ANN + Bagging	—	—	62	62	54	54	58	62
Kamble *et al* [1]	VMD + EBT	75.83	51.6	51.98	74.24	67.88	52.82	86.04	66.54
Singh *et al* [39]	TS + ANN	—	—	62.0 ± 4.68	61.66 ± 6.46	54.0 ± 4.16	53.78 ± 4.84	58.44 ± 3.52	61.55 ± 3.69
Proposed	Entropy + VMD	**87.11 ± 4.20**	**89.48 ± 4.01**	**91.52 ± 3.41**	**93.33 ± 2.89**	**88.18 ± 2.20**	**90.78 ± 2.09**	**88.17 ± 3.53**	**93.85 ± 1.744**

(b) Comparing for short words

Author	Method	S1	S3	S5	S6	S8	S12
Nguyen *et al* [2]	Tangent + RVM	48.0 ± 6.1	49.7 ± 5.5	46.3 ± 8.2	54.0 ± 9.1	47.7 ± 9.8	54.7 ± 6.9
	Tangent + ELM	44.6 ± 10.3	45.3 ± 7.4	43.4 ± 7.7	46.3 ± 8.1	45.0 ± 8.5	55.0 ± 9.8
Singh *et al* [38]	TS + ANN + Bagging	57	55	60	—	64	65
Kamble *et al* [1]	VMD + EBT	71.82	56.77	49.91	68.53	61.17	74.26
Singh *et al* [39]	TS + ANN	57.44 ± 4.55	55.0 ± 5.28	59.77 ± 4.91	—	63.88 ± 6.25	65.66 ± 5.99
Proposed	Entropy + VMD	**89.67 ± 3.55**	**87.10 ± 1.51**	**89.12 ± 1.49**	**87.51 ± 5.90**	**88.89 ± 5.14**	**90.04 ± 1.95**

(c) Comparing for short versus long words

Author	Method	S1	S5	S8	S9	S10	S14
Nguyen *et al* [2]	Tangent + RVM	70.3 ± 5.5	71.5 ± 5.0	81.9 ± 6.5	88.0 ± 6.4	79.3 ± 7.7	89.3 ± 3.5
	Tangent + ELM	73.5 ± 8.2	70.0 ± 6.2	80.6 ± 13.2	72.5 ± 12.2	75.5 ± 6.8	85.5 ± 6.8
Singh *et al* [38]	TS + ANN + Bagging	77	71	77	85	78	83
Kamble *et al* [1]	VMD + EBT	74.08	64.48	74.38	74.14	73.19	81.18
Singh *et al* [39]	TS + ANN	76.5 ± 2.83	71.33 ± 5.66	77.08 ± 4.26	85.0 ± 4.73	77.83 ± 5.16	83.33 ± 3.57
Proposed	Entropy + VMD	**86.10 ± 2.11**	**88.06 ± 2.24**	**86.33 ± 2.34**	**89.22 ± 2.18**	**91.49 ± 1.96**	**93.35 ± 1.75**

(d) Comparing for long words

Author	Method	S2	S3	S6	S7	S9	S11
Singh *et al* [38]	TS + ANN + Bagging	75	—	68	75	66	66
Kamble *et al* [1]	VMD + EBT	63.63	71.73	69.96	69.35	84.59	83.18
Singh *et al* [39]	TS + ANN	74.66 ± 4.76	—	69.33 ± 3.53	75.33 ± 6.35	64.33 ± 5.12	63.5 ± 5.39
Proposed	Entropy + VMD	**87.25 ± 3.57**	**90.24 ± 3.16**	**92.73 ± 2.76**	**94.64 ± 2.33**	**89.22 ± 4.53**	**91.63 ± 1.76**

vowels, short words, short–long words, and long words, respectively. In another experiment, Singh *et al* [39] attained average classification accuracies of 57.86 ± 5.03%, 60.35 ± 5.39%, 78.51 ± 4.36%, and 69.43 ± 5.03% for vowels, short words, short–long words, and long words, respectively. The proposed method has an average classification accuracy of 90.95 ± 3.01%%, 89.08 ± 2.09%%, 88.72 ± 3.25% %, and 90.30 ± 3.00%% for long words, short–long words, short words, and vowels, respectively. The proposed method's performance was examined using tenfold cross-validation, which is widely used and was employed by [1, 2, 38] in their study. Table 14.9 results indicate that the proposed approach outperformed the existing ML algorithms for imagined speech recognition.

14.5.6 Limitations and future work

Even though the results from the proposed model are superior to those of the previous study, we believe that a dataset with more words is required for the investigation. A more detailed analysis is required to fully comprehend the impact of word length. In addition, although the dataset was collected from a native English speaker, it is difficult to control the subject's internal language, making us completely dependent on the performance of the subject while recording the dataset. Different words have different lengths, which may contribute to recognizing the words. Therefore, recording the data for the exact length of each word is more important in an imagined speech recognition application. Furthermore, different sessions can have different recordings of the same word with the same subject. So, the experimental design may not be able to control changes between sessions. For further validation of our observations, it may be worthwhile to study session-to-session issues in the future. Furthermore, there is a great potential for robust decoding and adding more classes, both of which could be done by using deep learning approaches that are already available.

14.6 Conclusion

The imagined speech is a form of communication that can immediately communicate the user's intentions to the outside world. Users can be both healthy people and those suffering from brain disabilities. This chapter proves the applicability of EEG signals for the imagined speech application using Hjorth parameters and entropy features. The study of innate features of the imagined speech signals plays a critical role in improving the performance of the imagined speech recognition system and, in the future, approaching 'reading the mind'.

References

[1] Kamble A, Ghare P and Kumar V 2022 Machine-learning-enabled adaptive signal decomposition for a brain-computer interface using EEG *Biomed. Signal Process. Control* **74** 103526

[2] Nguyen C H, Karavas G K and Artemiadis P 2017 Inferring imagined speech using EEG signals: a new approach using Riemannian manifold features *J. Neural Eng.* **15** 016002

[3] Pei X-M *et al* 2011 Decoding vowels and consonants in spoken and imagined words using electrocorticographic signals in humans *J. Neural Eng.* **8** 046028

[4] Chen Y *et al* 2016 A high-security EEG-based login system with RSVP stimuli and dry electrodes *IEEE Trans. Inf. Forensics Secur.* **11** 2635–47

[5] Lee M-H *et al* 2019 EEG dataset and OpenBMI toolbox for three BCI paradigms: an investigation into BCI illiteracy *GigaScience* **8** giz002

[6] Lee S-H *et al* 2019 Towards an EEG-based intuitive BCI communication system using imagined speech and visual imagery *2019 IEEE Int. Conf. on Systems, Man and Cybernetics (SMC)* (Piscataway, NJ: IEEE)

[7] Min B *et al* 2016 Vowel imagery decoding toward silent speech BCI using extreme learning machine with electroencephalogram *BioMed Res. Int.* **2016** 2618265

[8] Idrees B M and Farooq O 2016 Vowel classification using wavelet decomposition during speech imagery *2016 3rd Int. Conf. on Signal Processing and Integrated Networks (SPIN)* (Piscataway, NJ: IEEE) pp 636–40

[9] Deng S *et al* 2010 EEG classification of imagined syllable rhythm using Hilbert spectrum methods *J. Neural Eng.* **7** 046006

[10] Qureshi M N I *et al* 2018 Multiclass classification of word imagination speech with hybrid connectivity features *IEEE Trans. Biomed. Eng.* **65** 2168–77

[11] Hashim N, Ali A and Mohd-Isa W-N 2018 Word-based classification of imagined speech using EEG *Computational Science and Technology 4th ICCST 2017 (Kuala Lumpur, Malaysia, 29–30 November 2017)* (Singapore: Springer) pp 195–204

[12] González-Castañeda E F *et al* 2017 Sonification and textification: proposing methods for classifying unspoken words from EEG signals *Biomed. Signal Process. Control* **37** 82–91

[13] Lee S H, Lee M and Lee S W 2020 Neural decoding of imagined speech and visual imagery as intuitive paradigms for BCI communication *IEEE Trans. Neural Syst. Rehabil. Eng.* **28** 2647–59

[14] Martin S *et al* 2016 Word pair classification during imagined speech using direct brain recordings *Sci. Rep.* **6** 1–12

[15] Saha P, Abdul-Mageed M and Fels S 2019 Speak your mind! Towards imagined speech recognition with hierarchical deep learning *arXiv preprint arXiv:1904.05746*

[16] Kosmyna N, Lindgren J T and Lécuyer A 2018 Attending to visual stimuli versus performing visual imagery as a control strategy for EEG-based brain-computer interfaces *Sci. Rep.* **8** 13222

[17] Akhoun I, McKay C and El-Deredy W 2015 Electrically evoked compound action potentials artefact rejection by independent component analysis: procedure automation *J. Neurosci. Methods* **239** 85–93

[18] Alsharif O *et al* 2015 Long short term memory neural network for keyboard gesture decoding *2015 IEEE Int. Conf. on Acoustics, Speech and Signal Processing (ICASSP)* (Piscataway, NJ: IEEE)

[19] De Asis-Cruz J *et al* 2021 Functional connectivity-derived optimal gestational-age cut points for fetal brain network maturity *Brain Sci.* **11** 921

[20] Martin S *et al* 2014 Decoding spectrotemporal features of overt and covert speech from the human cortex *Front. Neuroeng.* **7** 14

[21] Berry A S, Sarter M and Lustig C 2017 Distinct frontoparietal networks underlying attentional effort and cognitive control *J. Cogn. Neurosci.* **29** 1212–25

[22] Harms H *et al* 2000 Acute treatment of hypertension increases infarct sizes in spontaneously hypertensive rats *Neuroreport* **11** 355–9
[23] Lazar N A *et al* 2002 Combining brains: a survey of methods for statistical pooling of information *Neuroimage* **16** 538–50
[24] Shuster L I and Lemieux S K 2005 An fMRI investigation of covertly and overtly produced mono-and multisyllabic words *Brain Lang* **93** 20–31
[25] Chmielewski W X *et al* 2018 Effects of multisensory stimuli on inhibitory control in adolescent ADHD: it is the content of information that matters *NeuroImage Clin* **19** 527–37
[26] Ashwin Kamble P H G and Kumar V 2021 Classifying phonological categories and imagined words from EEG signal *Biomedical Signal Processing for Healthcare Applications 1* (Boca Raton, FL: CRC Press) p 29
[27] Dragomiretskiy K and Zosso D 2014 Variational mode decomposition *IEEE Trans. Signal Process.* **62** 531–44
[28] Khare S K and Bajaj V 2020 Optimized tunable Q wavelet transform based drowsiness detection from electroencephalogram signals *IRBM* **43** 13–21
[29] Phinyomark A, Phukpattaranont P and Limsakul C 2012 Feature reduction and selection for EMG signal classification *Expert Syst. Appl.* **39** 7420–31
[30] Aydın S, Saraoğlu H M and Kara S 2009 Log energy entropy-based EEG classification with multilayer neural networks in seizure *Ann. Biomed. Eng.* **37** 2626–30
[31] Khare S K and Bajaj V 2020 An evolutionary optimized variational mode decomposition for emotion recognition *IEEE Sens. J.* **21** 2035–42
[32] Khare S K and Bajaj V 2020 A facile and flexible motor imagery classification using electroencephalogram signals *Comput. Methods Programs Biomed.* **197** 105722
[33] Khare S K and Bajaj V 2020 Entropy-based drowsiness detection using adaptive variational mode decomposition *IEEE Sens. J.* **21** 6421–8
[34] Kamble K S and Sengupta J 2021 Ensemble machine learning-based affective computing for emotion recognition using dual-decomposed EEG signals *IEEE Sens. J.* **22** 2496–507
[35] Bühlmann P 2012 Bagging, boosting and ensemble methods *Handbook of Computational Statistics* (Berlin: Springer)
[36] Adeniyi D A, Wei Z and Yongquan Y 2016 Automated web usage data mining and recommendation system using K-nearest neighbor (KNN) classification method *Appl. Comput. Inform.* **12** 90–108
[37] Ho T K 1995 Random decision forests *Proc. of 3rd Int. Conf. on Document Analysis and Recognition* (Piscataway, NJ: IEEE) pp 278–82
[38] Singh A and Gumaste A 2020 Interpreting imagined speech waves with machine learning techniques arXiv:2010.03360
[39] Singh A and Gumaste A 2021 Decoding imagined speech and computer control using brain waves *J. Neurosci. Methods* **358** 109196
[40] Matsumoto M and Hori J 2014 Classification of silent speech using support vector machine and relevance vector machine *Appl. Soft Comput.* **20** 95–102
[41] Kisley M A and Cornwell Z M 2006 Gamma and beta neural activity evoked during a sensory gating paradigm: effects of auditory, somatosensory and cross-modal stimulation *Clin. Neurophysiol.* **117** 2549–63
[42] Lee M *et al* 2017 Network properties in transitions of consciousness during propofol-induced sedation *Sci. Rep.* **7** 1–13

[43] Pulvermüller F and Fadiga L 2010 Active perception: sensorimotor circuits as a cortical basis for language *Nat. Rev. Neurosci.* **11** 351–60
[44] Guenther F H, Ghosh S S and Tourville J A 2006 Neural modeling and imaging of the cortical interactions underlying syllable production *Brain Lang* **96** 280–301
[45] Liu Y-J *et al* 2017 Real-time movie-induced discrete emotion recognition from EEG signals *IEEE Trans. Affect. Comput.* **9** 550–62
[46] Sun A, Fan B and Jia C 2011 Motor imagery EEG-based online control system for upper artificial limb *Proc. 2011 Int. Conf. on Transportation, Mechanical, and Electrical Engineering (TMEE)* (Piscataway, NJ: IEEE)

IOP Publishing

Artificial Intelligence

A tool for effective diagnostics

Smith K Khare, Sachin Taran and Ankush D Jamthikar

Chapter 15

Classifying human attention states in EEG-based brain–computer interfacing using singular spectrum analysis

Ankit Baisoya, Ujjwal Kumar Upadhyay, Vansh Singh, Sachin Taran and Vikram Singh Kardam

Brain–computer interface (BCI) technology assists impaired persons in communicating with the outside world. The effective categorization of various motor imagery (MI) activities can improve the dependability of BCI systems. Recent technological breakthroughs have resulted in innovative operational environments in which human roles are limited to passive observation. While pushing the boundaries of efficiency and lifestyle, such settings also pose risks due to humans' incapacity to retain mental focus during passive control activities. In this study, the classification of focused and drowsy states is performed using singular spectrum analysis (SSA)-based features and a suitable machine learning algorithm. The proposed approach achieves a classification accuracy of 81.1% using the medium Gaussian support vector machine (SVM) classifier.

15.1 Introduction

Brain–computer interface (BCI) research has continued to uncover novel strategies for assisting patients with their conditions [1]. In the last few years, BCIs have expanded far beyond communication and control devices for severely handicapped users. They are already gaining popularity among those who suffer from a wide range of illnesses. BCIs are apparatuses that directly scan the user's brain activity and use it in a real-time, closed-loop system with feedback. Unlike other interfaces, BCIs do not require the user to move; rather, information from the brain is transformed into signals or orders rather than relying on the body's conventional output channels. As a result, BCIs can be particularly useful for people with significant motor impairments who cannot communicate using most (if not all)

doi:10.1088/978-0-7503-5964-1ch15

conventional communication methods [1, 2]. BCIs have applications in various domains and can be used for [1–4] monitoring various aspects of health, such as sleep stages and mood. BCIs can also monitor the cognitive states of pilots, air traffic controllers, and plant workers, such as their workload, weariness, and alertness.

15.2 Literature survey

An MI task involves using the brain to visualize cognitive processes corresponding to a specific task. Differently abled people can use BCI systems based on MI tasks to interact with their environments [5]. The use of electroencephalogram (EEG) data to classify MI tasks has become the preferred choice for the following reasons: (i) the noninvasive nature of EEG-based procedures [6, 7], (ii) the ability to use EEG data for the detection of sleep phases and epileptic seizures, (iii) the strong association of EEG data with mental activity and human brain physiology [8–10], and (iv) the fact that EEG signals make real-time BCI applications such as muscle communication more viable [11].

In BCI systems, solutions that employ feature extraction and classification to differentiate MI tasks are the most successful [11]. A spatial filter is employed to minimize the number of electrodes required and the variations in the spatial filter's projected signal. Such variations are then utilized as input characteristics for a classification algorithm that uses linear discriminant analysis (LDA) [12]. Regarding discernment of MI tasks, [13] presents a complex feature extraction and classification technique implemented using an iterative spatial–spectral pattern-learning algorithm. In [14], the Bayesian technique is employed for feature extraction, and a spectrally weighted decision rule is used for classification. In another study, an enhanced model of the usual spatial subspace decomposition is used for feature extraction, and an SVM is evaluated for classification [15]. In [16], clustering is adopted for feature extraction, while a least-squares support vector machine (LS-SVM) is selected for classification. To categorize MI tasks, the authors of [17] use short-time Fourier transform (STFT) and multivariate decomposition to examine EEG data and calculate the spectrum-related properties in EEG signals [17].

Utilizing advanced wavelet decomposition methods such as rational dilation wavelet transform, EEG signals have been examined in a variety of clinical and non-clinical settings. In addition, these advanced wavelet decomposition techniques have been proven useful in the field of MI [18]. Advanced wavelet transforms, such as the dual complex wavelet transform and the flexible analytic wavelet transform (which employs an iterative filter bank structure) have also been created [19]. The best-first search and pruning process is carried out by the breadth-first tree algorithm until a stopping requirement is satisfied, such as reaching a predetermined depth or when additional splitting does not significantly enhance the evaluation metric. Numerous EEG-based studies of the classification of mental states have employed the breadth-first tree [20]. Features have been extracted from EEG signals using the analysis of adaptive Hermite decomposition for the purpose of detecting drowsy states [21]. The ideal time segment must be chosen, since EEG signals are nonstationary and time varying. In addition, empirical mode decomposition (EMD) has been used to identify a variety of disorders, including mental states [22]. To differentiate between MI activities, features extracted using the tunable Q wavelet transform (TQWT) have been fed into an LS-SVM [23]. Nevertheless, the complexity of BCI systems rises as the number of electrodes increases. Although certain BCIs can perform more accurate recognition, their system architectures are complex [4]. The most popular methods involve the use of STFT, which produces spectral images that can be classified using deep learning techniques [2]. One method that avoids the need to choose a wavelet function is the TQWT. The analysis and investigation of physiological and pathological applications of EEG data have made extensive use of TQWT [24]. To distinguish between an alert and drowsy state using EEGs, EMD has been combined with adaptive Hermite decomposition (AHD) and an extreme learning machine (ELM) [25] for automatic drowsiness detection. For the purpose of detecting drowsiness, clustering variational mode decomposition (CVMD) has been used to investigate the nonstationary behavior of EEGs [26]. This chapter presents the singular spectrum analysis (SSA) method and discusses the use of suitable classification algorithms to distinguish between focused and drowsy human attention states.

15.3 Method

15.3.1 Data set

We employed an EPOC headset, an EEG measuring device that collects 12 channels of real-time EEG data. The equipment was set to use a sampling rate of 128 Hz, frequencies between 0.2 and 43 Hz, and a voltage resolution of 0.51 V. The data set consisted of a total of 25 h of EEG recordings gathered from five subjects doing a low-intensity control task where the subject utilized the 'Microsoft Train Simulator' program to control a computer-simulated train for 35 to 55 min over a mostly featureless course [27, 28]. Three mental states were monitored in the recorded data set. This work used EEG recordings corresponding to focused and drowsy states.

15.3.2 Singular spectrum analysis

In time-series analysis, SSA is a nonparametric spectral estimation approach. The main objective of SSA is the decomposition of time series into several independent components or sub-series, each with its own significance [29]. These independent components are decipherable and can be used for various analyses.

Figure 15.1 depicts the general architecture of SSA-like methods. Principal component analysis (PCA) in the vector space of time-series delay coordinates forms the basis of SSA. A major axis of a series of M-dimensional matrices is generated by extending a series of vectors that are M-dimensional in nature in PCA with regard to an orthonormal premise: $(E^k, 1 \leqslant k \leqslant M)$

$$X_{ij} = \sum_{k=1}^{M} a_i^k E_j^k, \quad 1 \leqslant j \leqslant M. \tag{15.1}$$

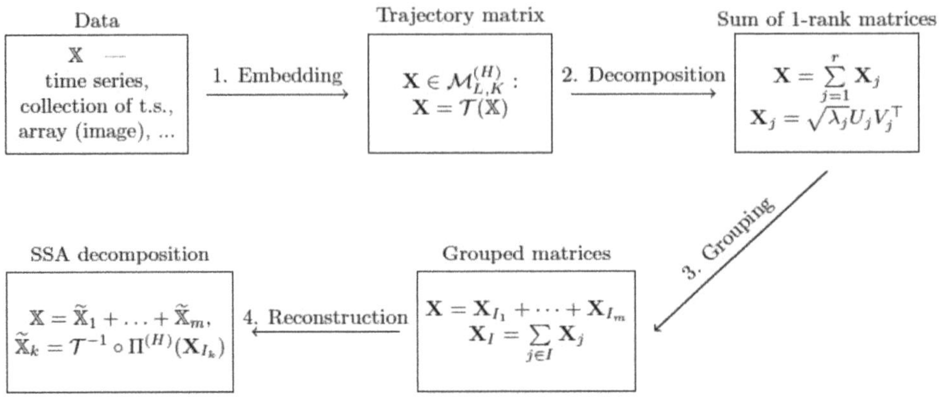

Figure 15.1. The general architecture of SSA-like methods [30].

The projection coefficients a_i^k are the principal components (PCs), and the empirical orthogonal functions (EOFs) E_k are the basis vectors. The sequence of cross-covariance matrices (E_i) is the eigenvectors known as E_k vectors. If the values of a scalar series are represented by (X_i, 1 I N), then the analogous extension for single-channel SSA is

$$X_{i+j} = \sum_{k=1}^{M} a_i^k E_j^k, \quad 1 \leqslant j \leqslant M. \tag{15.2}$$

By transforming the single time sequence X_i into the multivariate time series $X_j = (x_{j+1}, x_{j+2}, \ldots x_{j+M})$, the parallel embedding is created. There is no official distinction between the two expressions. Unlike traditional PCA, where M is the fixed dimension of the input vectors, M is the user-selected window length or embedding dimension. The eigenvectors of the Toeplitz matrix represent the vectors E_k of x. Each row i of this matrix corresponds to the covariance of x at lag $i-j$, with T_x containing the jth column. Singular value decomposition (SVD) is a set of methods in numerical linear algebra with a wide range of applications; we prefer to keep things separate by distinguishing it from SSA, which is a time-series analysis technique.

With initial L-dimensional data vectors for multi-channel SSA $X_{l,\,i}$, $1 \leqslant 1 \leqslant L$, $1 \leqslant i \leqslant N$, the resulting equation is

$$X_{l,\,i+j} = \sum_{k=l}^{L \times M} a_i^k E_{l,\ j}^k, \quad 1 \leqslant l \leqslant L, \quad 1 \leqslant j \leqslant M. \tag{15.3}$$

15.3.3 Feature extraction

(a) **Skewness**

Skewness denotes a deviation or disproportion in a collection of data that differs from the normal distribution or symmetrical bell curve. If the curve is shifted to the right or left, it is said to be skewed. The degree of divergence of a distribution from the normal distribution is measured by skewness. The normal distribution has a skewness of zero, and the lognormal distribution has right skewness [31].

The median of positively biased data is less than the mean. For negatively skewed data, the opposite is true: the median of negatively skewed data is greater than the mean. If data graphs are symmetrical, then they show zero skewness and do not depend on the structure of the tails.

In mathematical statistics, skew is frequently referred to as the third standardized instant:

$$E\left\{\frac{(X-\mu)}{\sigma}\right\}^3 \tag{15.4}$$

where μ = mean and σ = standard deviation.

15.4 Classification

15.4.1 *k*-nearest neighbors

k-NN is an ML technique used for regression and classification applications [16]. It is a form of memory-based or instance-based learning system that compares new problem situations to previously learned ones. Each class is labeled, and the data to be used for training are shown as vectors in a multidimensional feature space. Because the new data and previous instances are presumed to be comparable, the new case is placed in the group that is closest to the current group. Using *k* data points from the training set, the algorithm seeks the label of each data point that is not in the training set.

15.4.2 Support vector machine

This sorts two data sets by drawing lines (hyperplanes) between them based on patterns. It creates a hyperplane that reduces the distance between the separation corners of two classes by increasing the separation between the segregated planes for all feature vectors [16].

SVM is a supervised machine learning method that is linear and non-probabilistic. Mappings are built so that the dot products of input data vector pairs can be computed using kernel functions for the variables in the original space, $k(x_i,\ x_j)$. The application determines which kernel function should be used. We define the Gaussian kernel or radial basis function kernel as $k(x_i,\ x_j) = \exp(-x_i - x_j)$.

15.4.3 Linear discriminant analysis

This is a straightforward approach when the performances have been assessed and intraclass frequencies are unequal for randomly generated test data [32]. It optimizes the ratio of interclass variation to intraclass variation in each data set, providing maximum divisibility. Speech recognition classification issues employ this method for data categorization. The categorization of data is the responsibility of LDA.

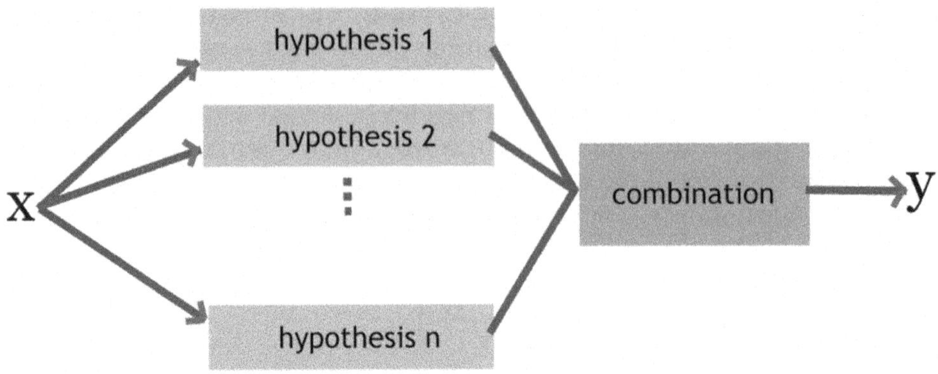

Figure 15.2. General ensemble architecture.

15.4.4 Ensemble techniques

Ensemble techniques are learning algorithms that use the ensemble architecture to generate a collection of many models and then categorize incoming data points according to a subset of their predictions [33].

A set of hypotheses or learners is produced from training data using a simple learning algorithm to construct an ensemble. Figure 15.2 shows the general ensemble architecture.

The most common ensemble approaches are as follows:

(a) **Boosting**

This is an algorithm that may be regarded as a form of model averaging. It is the most widely used ensemble method and one of the most successful learning strategies. This approach was created with classification in mind; however, it may also be used with regression. By merging three weak learners, the original boosting algorithm developed a strong learner.

(b) **Stacking**

Stacking is the process of stacking numerous classifiers created by various learning algorithms using a single data set, including pairs of feature vectors and classifications. This technique is divided into two phases: the first stage is the generation of a collection of base-level classifiers, which are then combined with the outputs of the base-level classifiers to create a metalevel classifier.

15.4.5 Decision tree

A DT is a flowchart with a tree structure, where each internal node denotes a characteristic test, each branch indicates the test results, and every terminal node represents the test results. Leaf nodes contain a class label [33]. This algorithm predicts or categorizes results based on the solution to an earlier set of problems. The model is trained and evaluated on a set of data that contains the classification to be made.

There is the possibility that a decision tree may not always output a clear solution or decision. Instead, it might provide options that a data scientist can use to arrive at their own educated judgment. Data scientists find it very easy to understand and assess the results because decision trees are meant to replicate human cognition. Decision trees work with variables and numeric or categorical data; they are used to model issues involving numerous outputs. Noisy data and huge data sets with uncertainty and multiple related outcomes reduce the effectiveness of data trees.

15.5 Results and discussion

The suggested technique for detecting human attention states is a step-by-step process that includes SSA, feature identification, feature selection, and classification. After SSA is used, the input EEG signal is split into 16 sub-bands (SBs), namely SB1 to SB16. Initially, as many features as possible are retrieved, and then the Kruskal–Wallis (KW) test is applied to the features to see which ones perform best. The skewness feature is selected to distinguish between the 'focused' and 'drowsy' classes derived from these SBs. The probability (p-value) yielded by the KW test is also used to statistically investigate all the channel feature characteristics. The p-values yielded by the KW test for all channels and features are shown in table 15.1.

The individual feature dimensions for each channel, including all SBs, are 480 × 16 for the focused class and 1380 × 16 for the drowsy class. The classification accuracy (ACC) of these features is presented per channel in table 15.2. Classification was performed for each channel (CH) using various classification methods, namely ensemble subspace discriminant, linear discriminant, medium tree, medium Gaussian SVM, ensemble boosted, coarse k-NN, and coarse Gaussian SVM.

From table 15.2, it can be observed that CH 5 provides the best classification ACC with most classifiers compared to the other channels. The reason for this phenomenon is that features based on CH 5 obtained lower p values for most of the SBs compared to the other channels. The CH 5 SB-based features yield the highest classification ACC of 81.1% when used by a medium Gaussian SVM classifier. The ACC is defined as

$$\mathrm{ACC} = \frac{\mathrm{TP} + \mathrm{TN}}{\mathrm{TP} + \mathrm{TN} + \mathrm{FP} + \mathrm{FN}}. \tag{15.5}$$

Here, true positive = TP, true negative = TN, false positive = FP, and false negative = FN.

For the classifiers, the performance characteristic is determined using the tenfold cross validation approach. Figure 15.3 depicts the confusion matrix of the medium Gaussian SVM.

Figure 15.4 presents the receiver operating characteristic (ROC) plot, which contains the whole sensitivity (SEN)/specificity (SPE) report. It is used to analyze and scrutinize the proposed method's classification performance. It is a two-dimensional graph in which the true positive rate (SEN) is displayed against the false positive rate (1-SPE) at various feature thresholds. The true positive rate (TPR)

Table 15.1. *p*-values for different sub-bands (SBs) on different channels (CHs).

SB	CH 1	CH 2	CH 3	CH 4	CH 5	CH 6	CH 7
1	3.86325e−05	0.5771	0.206	0.0049	0.1577	0.8997	0.0016
2	0.9766	0.9964	0.4817	0.1144	0.025	0.2941	0.5527
3	0.0223	0.2094	0.0013	0.1663	2.44367e−05	0.441	0.9768
4	0.8633	0.0482	0.0214	0.3166	2.70934e−07	0.4357	0.4223
5	0.1704	0.3754	0.0015	0.0187	0.5835	0.237	0.2219
6	0.4856	0.092	0.0038	0.0511	0.0011	0.967	0.4083
7	0.9687	0.2269	2.15796e−05	0.0027	5.74723e−18	0.9751	0.0446
8	0.2124	0.2228	0.3039	0.0007	0.2218	0.0075	0.8678
9	0.2635	0.0862	0.036	0.291	0.0195	0.9318	0.0014
10	0.9521	0.2675	0.0041	1.16678e−05	0.0023	0.8718	0.1732
11	0.7912	0.002	0.0344	0.0007	2.41702e−06	0.4518	0.0115
12	0.0264	0.0031	0.2768	0.1325	0.0009	0.3767	0.9336
13	1.90132e−06	0.0158	0.5451	0.0528	6.15772e−05	0.2021	0.2271
14	0.0013	0.1821	0.6669	8.84873e−05	0.6561	0.0006	0.1587
15	2.61317e−05	4.47836e−05	0.3967	0.9436	0.241	7.20589e−06	0.0002
16	0.0155	0.6492	4.97814e−07	0.2492	0.0267	0.0003	2.40054e−05

Table 15.2. Accuracy for different classification methods for different channels.

Methods	CH 1	CH 2	CH 3	CH 4	CH 5	CH 6	CH 7
Ensemble subspace discriminant	74.3%	74.1%	73.5%	73.8%	73.75%	74.1%	74.1%
Linear discriminant	74.2%	74%	73.2%	74.1%	74.5%	74%	73.9%
Medium tree	73%	71.6%	73.1%	75.6%	79%	71.1%	71.7%
Medium Gaussian SVM	74.1%	74.1%	74.8%	78.7%	**81.1%**	74.1%	74.1%
Ensemble boosted	74%	73.8%	76.6%	75.7%	78.3%	73.5%	74.1%
Coarse *k*-NN	74.2%	74.2%	74.5%	75.8%	75.4%	74.2%	74.2%
Cubic SVM	54.6%	27.2%	58%	43.5%	73.9%	58.6%	36.2%
Coarse Gaussian SVM	74.2%	74.2%	74.2%	73.8%	74.15	74.2%	74.2%

denotes the rate at which focused states are detected, whereas the false positive rate (FPR) denotes the rate at which drowsy states are misclassified [4]. Figure 15.4 indicates that the TPR rises swiftly with a smaller change in FPR and a significantly greater area under the curve (AUC) value of 0.84. The acquired ROC curve characteristics indicate that the suggested feature extraction approach is capable of properly distinguishing between focused and drowsy classes.

15.6 Conclusions

Our study aimed to develop a solution for the BCI-based prediction of two states of mind, namely focused and drowsy. We analyzed and compared eight existing prediction techniques for SSA-based features: ensemble subspace discriminant,

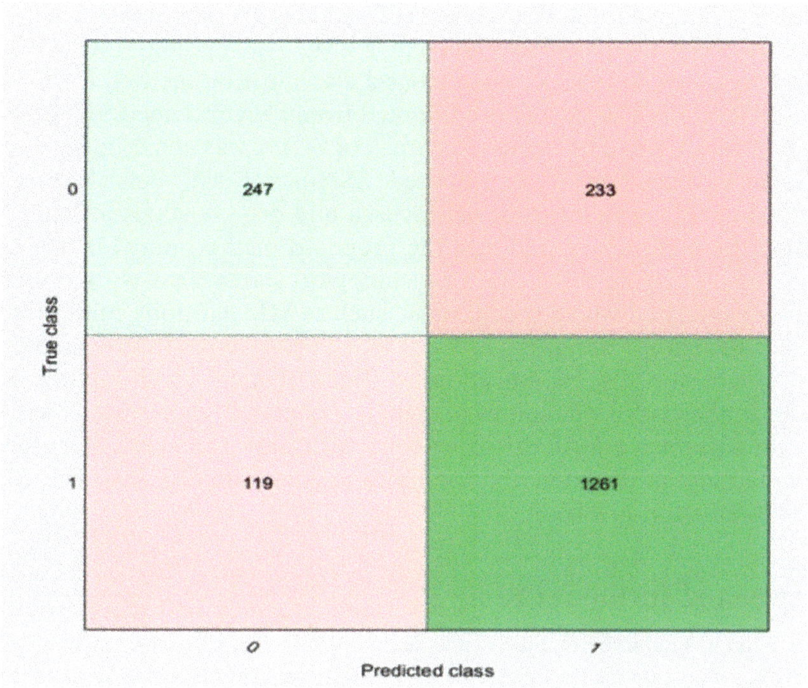

Figure 15.3. Confusion matrix for the medium Gaussian SVM.

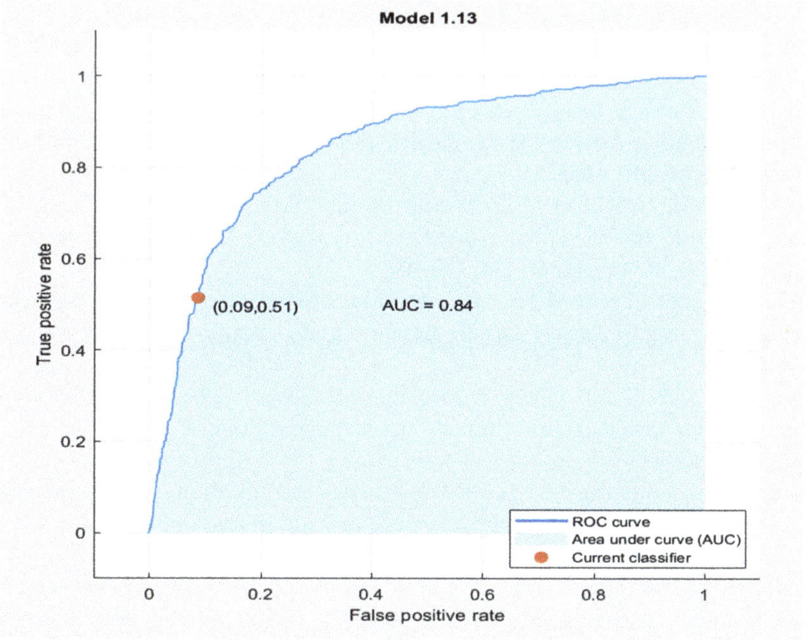

Figure 15.4. ROC curve for the medium Gaussian SVM classifier.

linear discriminant, medium tree, medium Gaussian SVM, ensemble boosted, coarse *k*-NN, cubic SVM, and coarse Gaussian SVM. The findings for our proposed method are as follows: (i) SSA was used as a classification method for focused and drowsiness states. (ii) The skewness computed from SSA-provided SBs gave the best classification result. (iii) The highest accuracy of 81.1% was achieved by the medium Gaussian SVM classifier. The proposed SSA-based skewness feature can be implemented in BCI systems to detect focused and drowsy states in humans.

Based on the preliminary findings, the proposed method may also be useful for analyzing and classifying other brain psychological states. This work only explored EEG signals associated with a specific task, such as MI, emotions, and mental states, which is insufficient for designing modern BCI applications. Improved ML models are thus sought for the classification of EEG signals, event-related potentials (ERPs), and other types of biological signals associated with various and discrete tasks within a framework at the same time with improved precision. Addressing missing values and anticipated abnormalities in contaminated data sets might help to increase prediction precision.

References and further reading

[1] Taran S, Bajaj V, Sharma D, Siuly S and Sengur A 2018 Features based on analytic IMF for classifying motor imagery EEG signals in BCI applications *Measurement* **116** 68–76 ISSN0263–2241

[2] Chaudhary S, Taran S, Bajaj V and Sengur A 2019 Convolutional neural network based approach towards motor imagery tasks EEG signals classification *IEEE Sens. J.* **19** 4494–500

[3] Taran S and Bajaj V 2019 Motor imagery tasks-based EEG signals classification using tunable-Q wavelet transform *Neural Comput. Appl.* **31** 6925–32

[4] Chaudhary S, Taran S, Bajaj V and Siuly S 2020 A flexible analytic wavelet transform based approach for motor-imagery tasks classification in BCI applications *Comput. Methods Programs Biomed.* **187** 105325

[5] Neuper C, Müller G, Kübler A, Birbaumer N and Pfurtscheller G 2003 Clinical application of an EEG-based brain–computer interface: a case study in a patient with severe motor impairment *Clin. Neurophysiol.* **114** 399–409

[6] Hassan A R and Bhuiyan M I H 2017 An automated method for sleep staging from EEG signals using normal inverse Gaussian parameters and adaptive boosting *Neurocomputing* **219** 76–87

[7] Hassan A R, Siuly S and Zhang Y 2016 Epileptic seizure detection in EEG signals using tunable-Q factor wavelet transform and bootstrap aggregating *Comput. Methods Programs Biomed.* **137** 247–59

[8] Hassan A R and Bhuiyan M I H 2017 Automated identification of sleep states from EEG signals by means of ensemble empirical mode decomposition and random under sampling boosting *Comput. Methods Programs Biomed.* **140** 201–10

[9] Hassan A R and Bhuiyan M I H 2016 Automatic sleep scoring using statistical features in the EMD domain and ensemble methods *Biocybernet. Biomed. Eng.* **36** 248–55

[10] Hassan A R and Subasi A 2016 Automatic identification of epileptic seizures from EEG signals using linear programming boosting *Comput. Methods Programs Biomed.* **136** 65–77

Arns M, Gunkelman J, Olbrich S, Sander C and Hegerl U 2010 EEG vigilance and phenotypes in neuropsychiatry: implications for intervention *Neurofeedback and Neuromodulation Techniques and Applications.* (Amsterdam: Elsevier) p 4

[11] Lotte F, Congedo M, Lécuyer A, Lamarche F and Arnaldi B 2007 A review of classification algorithms for EEG-based brain–computer interfaces *J. Neural Eng.* **4** R1

[12] Yong X, Ward R K and Birch G E 2008 Sparse spatial filter optimization for EEG channel reduction in brain-computer interface *Int. Conf. on Acoustics, Speech and Signal Processing. ICASSP 2008IEEE2008* (Piscataway, NJ: IEEE) 417–20

[13] Wu W, Gao X, Hong B and Gao S 2008 Classifying single-trial EEG during motor imagery by iterative spatio-spectral patterns learning (ISSPL) *IEEE Trans. Biomed. Eng.* **55** 1733–43

[14] Suk H-I and Lee S-W 2013 A novel Bayesian framework for discriminative feature extraction in brain-computer interfaces *IEEE Trans. Pattern Anal. Mach. Intell.* **35** 286–99

[15] Li M and Lu C 2012 The recognition of EEG with CSSD and SVM *2012 10th World Congress on Intelligent Control and Automation (WCICA)* (Piscataway, NJ: IEEE) 4741–6

[16] Siuly, Li Y, Wen P P *et al* 2011 Clustering technique-based least square support vector machine for EEG signal classification *Comput. Methods Programs Biomed.* **104** 358–72

[17] Bashar S K, Hassan A R and Bhuiyan M I H 2015 Motor imagery movements classification using multivariate EMD and short time fourier transform *2015 Annual IEEE India Conf. (INDICON)* (Piscataway, NJ: IEEE) 1–6

[18] Taran S, Khare S K, Bajaj V and Sinha G R 2020 Classification of motor-imagery tasks from EEG signals using the rational dilation wavelet transform *Modelling and Analysis of Active Biopotential Signals in Healthcare, Volume 2* (Bristol: IOP Publishing) p 1–1

[19] Taran S, Khare S K, Bajaj V and Sinha G R 2021 Classification of alertness and drowsiness states using the complex wavelet transform-based approach for EEG records *Analysis of Medical Modalities for Improved Diagnosis in Modern Healthcare* (Boca Raton, FL: CRC Press) 1–15

[20] Kardam V S, Taran S and Pandey A 2023 Motor imagery tasks based electroencephalogram signals classification using data-driven features *Neurosci. Inform.* **3** 100128

[21] Taran S and Bajaj V 2018 Drowsiness Detection Using Adaptive Hermite Decomposition and Extreme Learning Machine for Electroencephalogram Signals *IEEE Sens. J.* **18** 8855–62

[22] Taran S, Bajaj V, Sharma D, Siuly S and Sengur A 2018 Features based on analytic IMF for classifying motor imagery EEG signals in BCI applications *Measurement* **116** 68–76

[23] Taran S and Bajaj. V 2019 Motor imagery tasks-based EEG signals classification using tunable-Q wavelet transform *Neural Comput. Appl.* **31** 6925–32

[24] Bajaj V, Taran S, Khare S K and Sengur A 2020 Feature extraction method for classification of alertness and drowsiness states EEG signals *Appl. Acoust.* **163** 107224

[25] Taran S and Bajaj V 2018 Drowsiness detection using instantaneous frequency based rhythms separation for EEG signals *2018 Conf. on Information and Communication Technology (CICT)* (Piscataway, NJ: IEEE) 1–6

[26] Dutta A, Kour S and Taran S 2020 Automatic drowsiness detection using electroencephalogram signal *Electron. Lett.* **56** 1383–6

[27] Aci Ç, Kaya M and Mishchenko Y 2019 EEG data for Mental Attention State Detection. https://www.kaggle.com/datasets/inancigdem/eeg-data-for-mental-attention-state-detection (accessed 10 April 2019)

[28] Çīgdem İ A, Kaya M and Mishchenko Y 2019 Distinguishing mental attention states of humans via an EEG-based passive BCI using machine learning methods *Expert Syst. Appl.* **134** 153–66

[29] Vautard R, Yiou P and Ghil M 1992 Singular-spectrum analysis: A toolkit for short, noisy chaotic signals *Phys. D: Nonlinear Phenom.* **58** 95–126

[30] Golyandina N, Korobeynikov A, Shlemov A and Usevich K 2015 Multivariate and 2D Extensions of Singular Spectrum Analysis with the Rssa Package *J. Stat. Softw.* **67** 1–78

[31] Von Hippel P T 2005 Mean, median, and skew: correcting a textbook rule *J. Stat. Educ.* **13** 1–13

[32] Zhang R, Xu P, Guo L, Zhang Y, Li P and Yao D 2013 Z-score linear discriminant analysis for EEG based brain-computer interfaces *PLoS One* **8** e74433

[33] Pant H, Dhanda H K and Taran S 2022 Sleep apnea detection using electrocardiogram signal input to FAWT and optimize ensemble classifier *Measurement* **189** 110485

[34] Taran S, Bajaj V, Sinha G R and Polat K 2021 Detection of sleep apnea events using electroencephalogram signals *Appl. Acoust.* **181** 108137

www.ingramcontent.com/pod-product-compliance
Ingram Content Group UK Ltd.
Pitfield, Milton Keynes, MK11 3LW, UK
UKHW051904100926
8556IPUK00005B/753

9 780750 359627